PREP

RADIOGRAPHY

Third Edition

D. A. Saia, MA, RT(R) (M)
Director, Radiography Program
The Stamford Hospital
Stamford, Connecticut

Appleton & Lange Reviews/McGraw-Hill
Professional

New York   Chicago   San Francisco   Lisbon   London
Madrid   Mexico City   Milan   New Delhi
San Juan   Seoul   Singapore   Sydney   Toronto

PREP Radiography, Third Edition

1 2 3 4 5 6 7 8 9 0 PBT/PBT 0 9 8 7 6 5 4 3

Notice

Medicine is an ever-changing science. As new research and clinical experience broaden our knowledge, changes in treatment and drug therapy are required. The authors and the publisher of this work have checked with sources believed to be reliable in their efforts to provide information that is complete and generally in accord with the standards accepted at the time of publication. However, in view of the possibility of human error or changes in medical sciences, neither the authors nor the publisher nor any other party who has been involved in the preparation or publication of this work warrants that the information contained herein is in every respect accurate or complete, and they disclaim all responsibility for any errors or omissions or for the results obtained from use of the information contained in this work. Readers are encouraged to confirm the information contained herein with other sources. For example and in particular, readers are advised to check the product information sheet included in the package of each drug they plan to administer to be certain that the information contained in this work is accurate and that changes have not been made in the recommended dose or in the contraindications for administration. This recommendation is of particular importance in connection with new or infrequently used drugs.

This book was set in Garamond Light by Matrix Publishing Services.
The editors were Michael Brown and Karen G. Edmonson.
The production supervisor was Richard Ruzycka.
The Index was prepared by Michael Ferreira.
Phoenix Book Technologies was the printer and binder.

Library of Congress Cataloging-in-Publication Data

Saia, D. A. (Dorothy A.)
    Radiography : PREP : program review & exam preparation / D.A. Saia.—3rd ed.
        p. cm.
    Includes bibliographical references and index.
    ISBN 0-07-138769-2 (alk. paper)
    1. Radiography, Medical—Outlines, syllabi, etc.   I. Title: At head of title: PREP.
II. Title.

RC78.15 .S255 2003
616.07'572'076—dc21

                                                            2002044389

ISBN: 0-07-138769-2 (domestic)

Please tell the author and publisher what you think of this book by sending your comments to radtech@mcgraw-hill.com. Please put the author and title of this book in the subject line.

With all my love, to Tony

Reviewers

Brenda Grant, MPH, BSN, RN, CIC, CHES
Nurse Epidemiologist
The Stamford Hospital
Stamford, Connecticut

Craig T. Shephard, MS, RT(R), RDMS
Program Director
School of Radiologic Technology
Metropolitan Nashville General Hospital
Nashville, Tennessee

Michael L. Walker, BA, RT(R)
Program Director
San Joaquin General Hospital School of Radiologic Technology
Stockton, California

Contents

Preface

Radiography: Program Review and Exam Preparation (PREP), Third Edition, is for use throughout all phases of radiography education. This text is useful for regular coursework, helping the student extract fundamental key concepts from reading assignments and class notes, and for making study and test preparation easier and more productive.

PREP is also useful for students preparing for their American Registry of Radiologic Technologists (ARRT) certification examination. It helps students direct their study efforts toward exam-related material, and includes registry-type multiple choice questions designed to help students practice test taking skills they will need for the ARRT radiography examination.

The ARRT's *Content Specifications for the Examination in Radiography* lists the exam's five content categories and provides a detailed list of the topics addressed in each category. *Radiography: PREP* is divided into five parts reflecting each of the five content categories. Part content reflects changes to the ARRT Content Specifications implemented January 2001. It includes material on Digital/Electronic Imaging and the most recent Centers for Disease Control Isolation Precautions. Thus, study becomes even more directed and focused on exam-related material. Used with its companion book, A&L's *Review for the Radiography Examination*, PREP provides a thorough preparation for the certification examination administered by the ARRT.

KEY FEATURES AND USE

- More than 280 ***illustrations*** appeal to the visual learner as well as the verbal learner. The essence of radiography is visual and *PREP's* graphics and radiographic images visually express the written words.
- The ***summary boxes*** serve to call the student's attention to the most important facts in a particular section. Students can use summary boxes as an overview of key information.
- ***Endpapers*** list a number of formulae, body surface landmarks, and a brief list of processing chemicals and their functions. A "last-minute cheat sheet" is provided for some things that students often forget because they don't use them on a regular basis.
- The ***final review sections*** allow students to assess chapter material in two ways. The first review section, ***Chapter Exercises,*** requires short essay answers; exact page references follow each question, providing answers in chapter material. The second section, ***Chapter Review Questions,***

consists of registry-type multiple choice questions followed by detailed explanations.

- The new Chapter 17 is a practice test; a simulation of the actual certification examination with questions designed to test your problem-solving skills and your ability to integrate facts that fit the situation. The questions are designed to provide focus and direction for your review, thus helping you do your very best on your certification examination.

Following completion of the chapter review questions and the practice test, the student is ready for final self-evaluation by answering more "registry-type" questions in the companion text, *Appleton & Lange's Review for the Radiography Examination, 5/e.*

Acknowledgments

One of my most satisfying tasks is having the opportunity to thank those who have most generously contributed their insights, talents, and concerns to this project. Foremost among those are my teachers and colleagues who have contributed to my knowledge over the years, my students on whom I have the privilege of sharpening my knowledge and skills; I'd like to make special acknowledgement of my *distinctive* class of 2004: Fobert, Christine, Lisa, Stephanie, Mike, and Marina. In particular, I appreciate the friendship, encouragement, and support generously offered by my colleague Olive Peart, M.S., R.T.(R) (M). I am grateful to the professional staff of McGraw-Hill, with special notes of appreciation to Jack Farrell, Michael Brown, Janene Matragrano Oransky, and John Williams for their support and assistance. Everyone at McGraw-Hill has been helpful in the development of this project; it is always a pleasure to work with them.

An outstanding group of reviewers were recruited: Brenda Grant, Craig Shephard, and Michael L. Walker are invaluable resources to health care and the radiologic technology community. They reviewed the manuscript and offered suggestions to improve style and remove ambiguities and inaccuracies. Their participation on this project is deeply appreciated.

I would like to thank the American College of Radiology for the use of many radiographs from their teaching file, and The Stamford Hospital Department of Radiology for permission to use many of their radiographic images.

I wish to acknowledge and thank Bob Wong for permission to use several of his excellent teaching films throughout the text.

Several people were helpful in securing permission and providing photographs for illustration. Special thanks goes to Landauer Inc, especially Judith Mangan for providing and granting permission to use their dosimeter graphics. Mr. Dick Burkhart at Burkhart Roentgen and Mr. Steve Schaaf, Marketing Administration Manager at Landauer, Inc. were very helpful and supportive. A special thank you goes to Mr. Artie Swayhoover, Advertising Manager at Nuclear Associates, for patiently answering questions and returning calls; his help is greatly appreciated.

The preparation of this text would have been a far more difficult task without the help and encouragement of my husband, Tony. His understanding, support, and advice are lovingly appreciated.

MASTER BIBLIOGRAPHY

Adler AM, Carlton RR. *Introduction to Radiography and Patient Care* (2nd ed). Philadelphia: W. B. Sanders, 1999.

Ballinger PW, Frank ED. *Merrill's Atlas of Radiographic Positions and Radiologic Procedures,* Vols 1, 2, and 3 (9th ed). St. Louis, MO: Mosby, 1999.

Bontrager KL. *Textbook of Radiographic Positioning and Related Anatomy* (5th ed). St. Louis, MO: Mosby, 2001.

Bushong SC. *Radiologic Science for Technologists* (7th ed). St. Louis, MO: Mosby, 2001.

Carlton RR, Adler AM. *Principles of Radiographic Imaging* (3rd ed). Albany, NY: Delmar, 2001.

Chusid JG. *Correlative Neuroanatomy & Functional Neurology* (19th ed). East Norwalk, CT: Appleton & Lange, 1985.

Cornuelle AG, Gronefeld DH. *Radiographic Anatomy and Positioning: An Integrated Approach.* Stamford, CT: Appleton & Lange, 1998.

Dowd SB, Tilson ER. *Practical Radiation Protection and Applied Radiobiology* (2nd ed). WB Saunders, 1999.

Ehrlich RA, McCloskey ED. *Patient Care in Radiography* (5th ed). St. Louis, MO: Mosby, 1999.

Fauber TL. *Radiographic Imaging and Exposure* (1st ed). Mosby, 2000.

Fosbinder RA, Kelsey CA. *Essentials of Radiologic Science* (1st ed). McGraw-Hill, 2002.

Gurley LT, Callaway WJ. *Introduction to Radiologic Technology* (5th ed). St. Louis, MO: Mosby, 2002.

Haus, AG, Jaskulski SM. *Film Processing in Medical Imaging.* Madison, WI: Medical Physics Publishing, 1997.

Hendee WR, Ritenour ER. *Medical Imaging Physics* (4th ed). Wiley-Liss, 2002.

Laudicina P. *Applied Pathology for Radiographers.* Philadelphia: W. B. Saunders, 1989.

Linder HH. *Clinical Anatomy* (1st ed). East Norwalk, CT: Appleton & Lange, 1989.

Mill WR. The relation of bodily habitus to visceral form, tonus, and motility. *Am J. Roentgengr* 1917;4:155–169.

McKinney WEJ. *Radiographic Processing and Quality Control.* Philadelphia: Lippincott, 1988.

NCRP Report no 116: *Recommendations on Limits for Exposure to Ionizing Radiation.* NCRP, 1987.

Peart O. *A&L Mammography Review* (1st ed). McGraw-Hill, 2002.

Saia DA. *A&L Review for the Radiography Examination* (3rd ed). East Norwalk, CT: Appleton & Lange, 1997.

Selman J. *The Fundamentals of X-ray and Radium Physics* (9th ed). Springfield, IL: Charles C Thomas, 2000.

Shephard, CT. *Radiographic Image Production and Manipulation* (1st ed). McGraw-Hill, 2003.

Sherer MA, Visconti PJ, Ritenour ER. *Radiation Protection for Student Radiographers* (3rd ed). St. Louis, MO: Mosby, 1998.

Simon RR, Koenigsknecht SJ. *Emergency Orthopedics—The Extremities* (3rd ed). East Norwalk, CT: Appleton & Lange, 1995.

Taber's Cyclopedic Medical Dictionary (19th ed). Thomas CL, ed. Philadelphia: F. A. Davis, 2001.

Thompson, Hattaway, Hall, et al. *Principles of Imaging Science and Protection* (1st ed). Philadelphia: WB Saunders Co, 1994.

Torres, LS. *Basic Medical Techniques and Patient Care for Radiologic Technologists* (5th ed). Philadelphia: Lippincott, 1997.

Tortora GJ, Grabowski SR. *Principles of Anatomy and Physiology* (10th ed). New York: Harper and Row, 2003.

Travis EL. *Primer of Medical Radiobiology* (2nd ed). Chicago: Year Book, 1989.

Way LW. ed *Current Surgical Diagnosis & Treatment* (10th ed). East Norwalk, CT: Appleton & Lange, 1994.

Wolbarst, AB. *Physics of Radiology* (1st ed). Stamford, CT: Appleton & Lange, 1993.

part

I

Patient Care

Legal and Professional Responsibilities

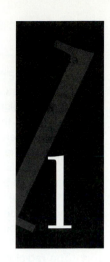

I. LEGAL CONSIDERATIONS IN RADIOLOGY

Practitioners of the profession of radiologic technology, like other health care professionals, have an ethical responsibility to adhere to principles of professional conduct and to provide the best services possible to the patients entrusted to their care. These principles are detailed in the American Registry of Radiologic Technologists (*ARRT*) Code of Ethics (Fig. 1–1) and the American Hospital Association (*AHA*) Patient's Bill of Rights.

A. PATIENT RIGHTS

All health care practitioners must recognize that their patients compose a community of people of all religions, races, and economic backgrounds and that each patient must be afforded their best efforts. Every patient should be treated with consideration of his or her worth and dignity. Patients must be provided *confidentiality* and *privacy*. They have the right to be informed, to make informed consent, and to refuse treatment. The American Hospital Association publishes a *Patient's Bill of Rights* that details 12 specific areas of patients' rights and the health professional's ethical (and often, legal) responsibility to adhere to those rights. The *Patient's Bill of Rights* is summarized as follows:

1. The right to considerate and respectful care;
2. The right to be informed completely and understandably;
3. The right to refuse treatment;
4. The right to have an advance directive (eg, a living will, health care proxy);
5. The right to privacy;
6. The right to confidentiality;
7. The right to review his or her records;
8. The right to request appropriate and medically indicated care and services;
9. The right to know about institutional business relationships that could influence treatment and care;
10. The right to be informed of, consent to, or decline participation in proposed research studies;

The Code of Ethics forms the first part of the Standards of Ethics. The Code of Ethics shall serve as a guide by which Registered Technologists and Candidates may evaluate their professional conduct as it relates to patients, health care consumers, employers, colleagues and other members of the health care team. The Code of Ethics is intended to assist Registered Technologists and Candidates in maintaining a high level of ethical conduct and in providing for the protection, safety and comfort of patients. The Code of Ethics is aspirational.

1. The radiologic technologist conducts herself or himself in a professional manner, responds to patient needs and supports colleagues and associates in providing quality patient care.

2. The radiologic technologist acts to advance the principle objective of the profession to provide services to humanity with full respect for the dignity of mankind.

3. The radiologic technologist delivers patient care and service unrestricted by the concerns of personal attributes or the nature of the disease or illness, and without discrimination on the basis of sex, race, creed, religion or socioeconomic status.

4. The radiologic technologist practices technology founded upon theoretical knowledge and concepts, uses equipment and accessories consistent with the purposes for which they were designed, and employs procedures and techniques appropriately.

5. The radiologic technologist assesses situations; exercises care, discretion and judgment; assumes responsibility for professional decisions; and acts in the best interest of the patient.

6. The radiologic technologist acts as an agent through observation and communication to obtain pertinent information for the physician to aid in the diagnosis and treatment of the patient and recognizes that interpretation and diagnosis are outside the scope of practice for the profession.

7. The radiologic technologist uses equipment and accessories, employs techniques and procedures, performs services in accordance with an accepted standard of practice, and demonstrates expertise in minimizing radiation exposure to the patient, self and other members of the health care team.

8. The radiologic technologist practices ethical conduct appropriate to the profession and protects the patient's right to quality radiologic technology care.

9. The radiologic technologist respects confidences entrusted in the course of professional practice, respects the patient's right to privacy, and reveals confidential information only as required by law or to protect the welfare of the individual or the community.

10. The radiologic technologist continually strives to improve knowledge and skills by participating in continuing education and professional activities, sharing knowledge with colleagues and investigating new aspects of professional practice.

Figure 1–1. The American Registry of Radiologic Technologists code of ethics. (Copyright The American Registry of Radiologic Technologists; effective July 2002.)

11. The right to continuity of care; and
12. The right to be informed of hospital policies and procedures relating to patient care, treatment, and responsibilities.

The above *Patient's Rights* can be exercised on the patient's behalf by a *designated surrogate or proxy* decision maker if the patient lacks decision-making capacity, is legally incompetent, or is a minor.

Patient *consent* can be verbal, written, or implied. For example, if a patient arrived for emergency treatment alone and unconscious, implied consent is assumed. A patient's previously granted or presumed consent can be withdrawn at any time. Written patient consent is required before any examination that involves greater than usual risk—for example, invasive vascular examinations requiring the use of injected iodinated contrast agents. For lower-risk procedures, the consent given on admission to the hospital is generally sufficient.

Conditions for Valid Patient Consent

- The patient must be of legal age.
- The patient must be of sound mind.
- The patient must give consent freely.
- The patient must be adequately informed of the procedure about to take place.

It is imperative that the radiographer take adequate time to thoroughly explain the procedure or examination to the patient. An informed patient is a more cooperative patient, and a better examination is more likely to result. Patients should be clear about what will be expected of them and what they may expect from the radiographer. This must be considered the *standard of care* for each patient, not only to fulfill legal mandates, but to also fulfill professional and humanistic obligations.

B. PROFESSIONAL LIABILITY

It is essential that radiographers, like other health care professionals, be familiar with their *Practice Standards* (formerly Scope of Practice) publsihed by the ASRT. The Standards provide role definition and identify Clinical, Quality, and Professional Standards of practice—each Standard has its own rationale and identifies general and specific criteria related to that Standard. Figure 1–2 is the *Introduction to Radiography Practice Standards*. The student radiographer can access the individual standards, their rationale, and criteria on the ASRT website.

The four primary *sources of law* are the Constitution of the United States, statutory law, regulations and judgments of administrative bureaus, and court decisions.

The *Constitution* expresses the categorical laws of the country. Its impact with respect to health care and health care professionals lies, in part, in its insurance of the *right to privacy*. The right to privacy indicates that the patient's modesty and dignity will be respected. It also refers to the health care professional's obligation to respect the confidentiality of privileged information. Inappropriate communication of privileged information to anyone but the appropriate health care professionals is inexcusable.

Statutory law refers to laws enacted by congressional, state, or local legislative bodies. The enforcement of statutory laws is frequently delegated to administrative bureaus such as the Board of Health, the Food and Drug Administration, or the Internal Revenue Service. It is the responsibility of these agencies to enact *rules and regulations* that will serve to implement the statutory law.

Court decisions involve the interpretation of *statutes* and various regulations in decisions involving individuals. For example, the decision of an administrative bureau can be appealed and the court would decide if the agency acted appropriately and correctly. Court decisions are referred to as common law.

There are two basic kinds of law: *public law* and *private (civil) law*. *Public* laws are any that regulate the relationship between individuals and government. *Private,* or civil, law includes laws that regulate the relationships among people. *Litigation* involving a radiographer's professional practice is most likely to involve the latter.

A private (civil) injustice or injury is a *tort,* and the injured party may seek reparation for damage incurred. Torts are described as either *intentional* or *negligent*.

Examples of *intentional* torts include false imprisonment, *assault* and *battery,* defamation, and invasion of privacy. *False imprisonment* is the illegal restriction of an individual's freedom. Holding a person against his or her will or using unauthorized restraints can constitute false imprisonment.

Introduction to Radiography Practice Standards

The complex nature of disease processes involves multiple imaging modalities. Although an inter-disciplinary team of radiologists, radiographers and support staff plays a critical role in the delivery of health services, it is the radiographer who performs the radiographic examination that creates the images needed for diagnosis. Radiographay integrates scientific knowledge and technical skills with effective patient interaction to provide quality patient care and useful diagnostic information.

Radiographer

Radiographers must demonstrate an understanding of human anatomy, physiology, pathology and medical terminology.

Radiographers must maintain a high degree of accuracy in radiographic positioning and exposure technique. He or she must maintain knowledge about radiation protection and safety. Radiographers prepare for and assist the radiologist in the completion of intricate radiographic examinations. They prepare and administer contrast media and medications in accordance with state and federal regulations.

Radiographers are the primary liaison between patients and radiologists and other members of the support team. They must remain sensitive to the physical and emotional needs of the patient through good communication, patient assessment, patient monitoring and patient care skills.

Radiographers use professional and ethical judgment and critical thinking when performing their duties. Quality improvement and customer service allow the radiographer to be a responsible member of the health care team by continually assessing professional performance. Radiographers embrace continuing education for optimal patient care, public education and enhanced knowledge and technical competence.

Education and Certification

Radiographers prepare for their role on the interdisciplinary team by satisfactorily completing an accredited educational program in radiologic technology. Two-year certificate, associate degree and four-year baccalaureate degree programs exist throughout the United States.

Accredited programs must meet specific curricular and educational standards. The Joint Review Committee on Education in Radiologic Technology (JRCERT) is the accrediting agency for radiologic technology programs recognized by the U.S. Department of Education.

Upon completion of a course of study in radiologic technology, individuals may apply to take the national certification examination. The American Registry of Radiologic Technologists (ARRT) is the recognized certifying agency for radiographers. Those who successfully complete the certification examination in radiography may use the credential R.T.(R) following their name; the R.T. signifies registered technologist and the (R) indicates radiography.

To maintain ARRT certification, a level of expertise and awareness of changes and advances in practice, radiographers must complete 24 hours of appropriate continuing education every two years.

Practice Standards

The practice standards define the practice and establish general criteria to determine compliance. Practice standards are authoritative statements enunciated and promulgated by the profession for judging the quality of practice, service and education. They include desired and achievable levels of performance against which actual performance can be measured.

Professional practice constantly changes and actual practice varies from state to state as determined by

Figure 1–2. Introduction to Radiography Practice Standards. *(Continued)*

local law and community custom. Recognizing this, the profession has adopted standards that are general in nature. The general format was favored over a "cookbook" style or "step-by-step" approach that would be difficult to maintain in a changing environment and confining for those practitioners with an expanded practice.

The standards focus on the dynamic nature of the health care delivery system. The standards are adaptable not only to the area of practice but also the locality of practice and institutional needs. While a minimum standard of acceptable performance is appropriate and should be followed by all practitioners in a specific area, it is unrealistic and highly inappropriate to assume that professional practice is the same in all regions of the United States.[1] State statue or regulation may dictate practice parameters. To conduct an appropriate review of the standards, one must look to the professional standard as well as local or state law that may impact the nature and scope of practice.

Format

The cohesive nature and inherent differences of medical imaging and radiation therapy are recognized in the general format of the standards. The standards are divided into three sections: clinical performance, quality performance and professional performance.

Clinical Performance Standards. The clinical performace standards define the activities of the practitioner in the care of patients and delivery of diagnostic or therapeutic procedures and treatment. The section incorporates patient assessment and management with procedural analysis, performance and evaluation.

---

[1] The term "practitioner" is used in all areas of the standards in place of the various names used in medical imaging and radiation therapy, such as radiologic technologist, sonographer or radiation therapist. Practitioner is defined as any individual practicing in a specific area or discipline. The profession believes that any individual practicing in one of the defined disciplines or specialties should be held to a minimum standard of performance to protect the patients who receive professional services.

Quality Performance Standards. The quality performance standards define the activities of the practitioner in the technical areas of performance including equipment and material assessment, safety standards and total quality management.

Professional Performance Standards. The professional performance standards define the activities of the practitioner in the areas of education, interpersonal relationships, personal and professional self-assessment and ethical behavior.

Each section of the standards is subdivided into individual standards. The standards are numbered and followed by a term or set of terms that identify the standards, such as "assessment" or "analysis/ determination." The next statement is the expected performance of the practitioner when performing the procedure or treatment. A rationale statement follows and explains why a practitioner should adhere to the particular standard of performance.

Criteria. Criteria are used in evaluating a practitioner's performance. Each set of criteria is divided into two parts, the general criteria and the specific criteria. Both the measurement and specific criteria should be used when evaluating performance.

General Criteria. General criteria are written in a general style that applies to either medical imaging or radiation therapy practitioners. These criteria are the same in all sections of the standards and should be used for the appropriate area of practice. For example, a radiographer should use good professional judgment to make decisions concerning the adaptation of eqipment and technical variables for a diagnostic procedure. Under these circumstances, the evaluation of the decision-making process concerning radiation therapy procedures would not be appropriate and should not be applied unless the procedure is diagnositc in nature, such as simulation.

Specific Criteria. Specific criteria meet the needs of the practitioners in the various areas of professional performance. While many areas of

Figure 1–2 *(Continued).*

performance within medical imaging and radiation therapy are similar, others are not. The specific criteria are drafted with these differences in mind. For example, a criterion that calls for daily review of patient treatment records and doses to ensure that treatment does not exceed prescribed dose or normal tissue tolerance is imperative for those who practice in radiation therapy yet is not applicable to those who practice in the imaging professions.

A profession's practice standards serve as a guide for appropriate practice. Standards provide role definition for practitioners that can be used by individual facilities to develop job descriptions and practice parameters. Those outside the medical imaging and radiation therapy community can use the standards as an overview of the role and responsibilities of the practitioner as defined by the profession.

Figure 1–2. Introduction to Radiography Practice Standards. (Reprinted with the permission of the American Society of Radiologic Technologists. All right reserved, Copyright 2000.)

Assault is to threaten harm; *battery* is the carrying out of the threat. A patient may feel sufficiently intimidated to claim assault by a radiographer who threatens to repeat a difficult examination if the patient does not try to cooperate better. A radiographer who performs an examination on a patient without his or her consent, or after the patient has refused the examination, can be guilty of *battery*. A charge of battery may also be made against a radiographer who treats a patient roughly or who performs an examination on the *wrong* patient.

A radiographer who discloses confidential information to unauthorized individuals may be found guilty of *invasion of privacy*. A radiographer whose disclosure of confidential information is in some way detrimental to the patient (causing ridicule or loss of job, for example) may be accused of *defamation. Spoken defamation* is *slander; written defamation* is *libel*.

The assessment of *duty* (what *should* have been done) is determined by the professional *standard of care* (that level of expertise generally possessed by reputable members of the profession). The determination of whether or not the standard of care was met is usually made by determining what another reputable practitioner would have done in the same situation. Examples of negligent torts may include patient injury as a result of a fall while unattended on an x-ray table, in a radiographic room, or on a stretcher without side rails or safety belt. Radiographing the wrong patient or opposite limb are other examples of *negligence*.

The term *malpractice* is usually used with reference to negligence. Three areas of frequent litigation in radiology involve patient falls and positioning injuries, pregnancy, and errors or delays in *diagnosis*.

Patient falls and positioning injuries. Examples: A sedated patient left unattended in the radiographic room falls from the x-ray table; a patient with a spinal injury is moved from the stretcher to the x-ray table, resulting in irreversible damage to the spinal cord.

Pregnancy. Example: The radiographer fails to inquire about a possible pregnancy before performing a radiologic examination. Some time later, the patient contacts the health care facility expressing concern about the fetus.

For Liability for a Negligent Tort, Four Elements Must be Present:

- Duty (what *should* have been done)
- Breach (deviation from duty)
- Injury sustained
- Cause (as a result of breach)

Errors or delays in diagnosis. Example: The patient has an x-ray examination in the emergency department (ED) and is sent home. The radiologist reads the films and fails to notify the ED physician of findings. The physician gets a written report 2 days later. Meanwhile, the patient suffers permanent damage from an untreated condition.

If patient injury results from misperformance of a duty in the routine scope of practice of the radiographer, most courts will apply *res ipsa loquitur,* that is, "the thing speaks for itself." If the patient is obviously injured as a result of the radiographer's actions, it becomes the radiographer's burden to *disprove* negligence. In many instances, the hospital and/or radiologist will also be held responsible according to *respondeat superior,* or, "the master speaks for the servant."

Summary

- The ARRT Code of Ethics details guidelines for the radiographer's professional conduct.
- The AHA Patient's Bill of Rights details 12 specific areas of patient rights that the health care professional is obligated to respect.
- The American Society of Radiologic Technologists (ASRT) Practice Standards identifies the level of knowledge and skill required of a professional radiographer.
- The two kinds of law are public law and private (civil) law. Litigation involving health care practitioners usually involves private (civil) law.
- A civil injustice is a tort; a tort can be intentional or negligent.
- Negligence litigation in radiology most frequently involves injuries from falls and positioning injuries, pregnancy, and errors or delay in diagnosis.

II. REQUISITION AND CONSULTATION CONSIDERATIONS

A. AUTHORIZATION

Request forms for radiologic examinations should be carefully reviewed by the radiographer prior to commencement of the examination. Many hospitals and radiology departments have specific rules about exactly what kind(s) of information must appear on the requisition.

The requisition is usually stamped with the patient's personal information (name, address, age, admitting physician's name, and the patient's hospital identification number). The requisition should also include the patient's mode of travel to the radiology department (eg, wheelchair versus stretcher), the type of examination to be performed, pertinent diagnostic information, and any *infection control* or *isolation* information. Many institutions now have computerized, paperless systems that accomplish the same information transmittal. The healthcare professional generally has access to the computerized system via personal password, thus ensuring confidentiality of patient information. X-ray examinations can be requested only by a physician.

The radiographer should carefully review the patient information before bringing the patient into the radiographic room. This will enable the radiographer to have the x-ray room prepared, having all equipment and accessories readily available.

B. ACCURATE TERMINOLOGY AND APPROPRIATE REQUEST

The radiographer must be certain to understand and, if necessary, clarify the information provided, for example, any abbreviations used, any vague terms such as "leg" or "arm" (versus femur or humerus). The radiographer must also be alert to note and clarify conflicting information, for example, a request for a left ankle examination when the patient complains of, or has obvious injury to, the right ankle. Computerized systems or department policy may require that there be appropriate and accurate diagnosis information accompanying every request for diagnostic procedure.

C. ADEQUATE PATIENT HISTORY

It is important that the radiographer obtain a short, pertinent patient history of why the examination has been requested. Because patients are rarely examined or interviewed by the radiologist, observations and information obtained by the radiographer can be a significant help in making an accurate diagnosis.

D. VERIFICATION OF PATIENT IDENTITY

Care must be taken when making the initial patient identification. If the radiographer calls out a name at the door of a rather full waiting room, or asks a patient if he or she is Mr. or Ms. So-and-so, an anxious patient may readily respond in the affirmative without actually having heard his or her name called. It is always advisable to ask a patient to tell you his or her name or, if an inpatient, for you to check his or her wristband.

E. MODIFIED AND ADDITIONAL PROJECTIONS

If a patient is unable to assume or maintain the routine position used for a particular examination, the radiographer should be able to modify the projection to provide the required information. It is not within the radiographer's scope of practice to supply additional, unrequested positions, but the radiographer should advise the physician of other projections or modifications that might enable him or her to better visualize the affected area.

F. SCHEDULING AND PREPARATION CONSIDERATIONS

When the patient must be scheduled for multiple x-ray examinations, each requiring the use of a *contrast medium*, the examinations must be scheduled in the correct sequence. For example, if a particular patient must be scheduled for an upper gastrointestinal (UGI) series, barium enema (BE), and intravenous urogram (IVU), what sequence will permit optimal visualization of the required structures? Remember that it is important that residual barium not overlie structures of interest. Radiographic examinations of the gallbladder (GB) are rarely requested today, but should that exam be requested, the accompanying chart indicates when that exam would be scheduled among the others.

Generally speaking, those examinations with a contrast medium that is excreted quickly and completely should be scheduled first. Therefore, the IVU should be scheduled first, then the GB, if requested. If the UGI series were scheduled next, residual barium would be in the large bowel the next day, thus preventing adequate investigation. So the BE should be scheduled third; any residual barium should not interfere with an UGI examination, although a preliminary scout film should first be taken in each case.

If it is desired to expedite the studies, perhaps to reduce the length of hospital stay, some examinations can be performed on the same day; for example, GB and IVU. If the patient's GB is studied first and a *fatty meal* is used to evaluate its emptying function, there should be little contrast medium left to obscure the right urinary collecting system. Another example of paired examinations is the IVU and BE. IVU contrast medium is excreted rapidly by the kidneys and should not interfere with visualization of the barium and air-filled large bowel.

Patient preparation is somewhat different for each of these examinations. An iodinated contrast agent, usually in the form of several pills, is taken by the patient the evening before a scheduled *GB* examination and only water is allowed the morning of the examination. The patient scheduled for an *UGI* series must receive npo (nothing by mouth) after midnight. A barium enema (*lower GI*) requires that the large bowel be very clean prior to the administration of barium; this requires the administration of *cathartics* (laxatives) and cleansing enemas. Preparation for an *IVU* requires that the patient be npo after midnight; some institutions also require that the large bowel be cleansed of gas and fecal material. Aftercare for barium examinations is very important. Patients are typically instructed to take milk of magnesia, increase their intake of fiber, drink plenty of water, to expect change in stool color until all barium is evacuated, and to call their physician if they do not have a bowel movement within 24 hours. Because water is removed from the barium sulfate suspension in the large bowel, it is essential to make patients understand the importance of these instructions to avoid barium impaction in the large bowel.

The use of barium sulfate suspensions is contraindicated when ruling out *visceral perforation*. Barium could enter the peritoneal cavity and cause the serious condition, *peritonitis*. When performing examinations on patients suspected or known to have stomach or intestinal perforation, *water-soluble iodinated contrast media* should be used instead of barium sulfate. If this water-soluble medium leaks through a perforation into the peritoneal cavity, it will simply be absorbed and excreted by the kidneys.

Diabetic patients who are scheduled for an UGI series are generally instructed to withhold their morning insulin until the meal following the examination. Should the patient take insulin before the examination and remain npo, a reaction might occur, especially if the examination was delayed for any reason. Upper GI examinations on diabetic patients should be among the first examinations scheduled each day and priority should be given these patients.

Summary
- **Radiologic examinations can be requested only by a physician.**
- **The radiographer should examine the requisition carefully prior to bringing the patient to the radiographic room.**

Sequence and Combining of Contrast Exams

Sequence
IVU
GB
BE
GI

Exams that can be performed together
GB and IVU
IVU and BE
GB and GI

Patient Preparation

GB
Iodinated contrast evening before exam; water only in AM
UGI
NPO after midnight
BE
Cathartics, cleansing enemas
IVU
NPO after midnight, cleansing enemas, empty bladder before scout film

- Most health care facilities require that examination requests include pertinent diagnostic information and any infection control or isolation information.
- The patient should be identified by asking his or her name and/or by checking the wristband.
- It is the radiographer's responsibility to clarify any vague or conflicting information found on the requisition.
- Multiple radiologic examinations must be scheduled in a sequence that will allow prompt and adequate visualization of structures of interest.
- Patients must be appropriately prepared for the contrast examination(s) for which they are scheduled.

Chapter Exercises

⭐ *Congratulations!* *You have completed this chapter. If you are able to answer the following group of comprehensive questions, you can feel confident that you have mastered this section. You are then ready to go on to the "Registry-type" questions that follow.* ***For greatest success, do not go to the multiple choice questions without first completing the short answer questions below****.*

1. Discuss the ARRT Code of Ethics with respect to legal considerations pertinent to radiology *(p. 4)*.

2. Discuss the AHA Patient's Bill of Rights with respect to legal considerations pertinent to radiology *(pp. 3–5, 11)*.

3. Discuss the ASRT Practice Standards for the Radiographer with respect to legal considerations pertinent to radiology *(p. 5)*.

4. List the conditions necessary for valid consent *(p. 4)*.

5. Explain the importance of explaining the procedure to the patient *(p. 5)*.

6. Discuss public versus private (civil) law *(p. 5)*.

7. Differentiate between assault and battery; slander and libel *(pp. 5, 8)*.

8. Give examples of intentional and unintentional torts *(pp. 8, 9)*.

9. List the four elements of a negligent tort *(p. 8)*.

10. Identify the three areas of litigation that most frequently involve radiology *(pp. 8, 9)*.

11. Explain the importance of reviewing the examination request and other patient information prior to bringing the patient to the radiographic room *(pp. 9, 10)*.

12. List the patient information usually found on examination request forms *(p. 9)*.

13. Identify the kinds of clarification that may be required prior to starting the examination *(p. 10)*.

14. Explain the importance of obtaining a patient history *(p. 10)*.

15. Discuss the best way(s) to ensure correct identification of a patient *(p. 10)*.

16. Explain how best to correctly schedule multiple contrast examinations on the same patient; identify which examinations can be performed together *(p. 10).*

17. Explain the appropriate patient preparation for GB, UGI, BE, and IVU/IVP *(p. 11).*

18. Explain why diabetic patients who are required to receive nothing by mouth beginning the preceding midnight should be scheduled as the first AM appointment *(p. 11).*

A&U Chapter Review Questions
REVIEW SERIES

1. A cathartic is almost always required before performing which of the following examinations?
   (A) upper GI
   (B) lower GI
   (C) sialogram
   (D) IVU

2. In what order should the following examinations be performed?
   1. UGI
   2. IVU
   3. barium enema
   (A) 3, 1, 2
   (B) 1, 3, 2
   (C) 2, 1, 3
   (D) 2, 3, 1

3. The usual patient preparation for an upper GI examination is:
   (A) npo 8 hours before the exam
   (B) light breakfast only the morning of the exam
   (C) clear fluids only the morning of the exam
   (D) 2 ounces of castor oil and enemas until clear

4. When a GI series has been requested on a patient with a suspected perforated ulcer, the type contrast medium that should be used is:
   (A) thin barium sulfate suspension
   (B) thick barium sulfate suspension
   (C) water-soluble iodinated medium
   (D) oil-base iodinated medium

5. A radiographer who discloses confidential information to unauthorized individuals may be found liable for:
   (A) assault
   (B) battery
   (C) intimidation
   (D) defamation

6. Patients' rights include which of the following?
    1. the right to refuse treatment
    2. the right to confidentiality
    3. the right to possess one's radiographs
   (A) 1 only
   (B) 1 and 2 only
   (C) 1 and 3 only
   (D) 1, 2, and 3

7. Which of the following examinations require(s) restriction of the patient's diet?
    1. GI series
    2. abdominal survey
    3. urogram
   (A) 1 only
   (B) 1 and 2 only
   (C) 1 and 3 only
   (D) 2 and 3 only

8. Which of the following instructions should the patient be given following a barium enema examination?
    1. increase fluid and fiber intake for a few days
    2. changes in stool color will occur until all barium is evacuated
    3. contact your physician if you do not have a bowel movement within 24 hours
   (A) 1 only
   (B) 2 only
   (C) 1 and 3 only
   (D) 1, 2, and 3

9. Which of the following refer(s) to the patient's right to privacy?
    1. patient modesty must be preserved
    2. patient dignity must be respected
    3. patient confidentiality must be respected
   (A) 1 only
   (B) 2 only
   (C) 1 and 3 only
   (D) 1, 2, and 3

10. The threat to do harm is referred to as:
   (A) assault
   (B) battery
   (C) slander
   (D) libel

Answers and Explanations

1. (B) Patient preparation varies among contrast examinations. A patient scheduled for an UGI series must be npo (receive nothing by mouth) after midnight. A barium enema (lower GI) *requires* that the large bowel be very clean prior to the administration of barium; this requires the administration of *cathartics* (laxatives) and *cleansing enemas.* Preparation for an IVU/IVP requires that the patient be npo after midnight; *some* institutions also require that the large bowel be cleansed of gas and fecal material.

2. (D) When scheduling patient examinations, it is important to avoid the possibility of residual contrast medium overlying areas of interest of later examinations. The IVU should be scheduled first because the contrast medium used is excreted very rapidly. The barium enema should be scheduled next. The UGI is scheduled last. Any barium remaining from the previous BE is unlikely to interfere with the stomach or duodenum, although a preliminary scout film should be taken in each case.

3. (A) Patient preparation differs for various contrast examinations. To obtain a diagnostic examination of the stomach, it must first be empty. The usual *UGI* preparation is npo (nothing by mouth) after midnight (approximately 8 hours before the exam). Any material in the stomach can simulate the appearance of disease. An iodinated contrast agent, usually in the form of several pills, is taken by the patient the evening before a scheduled *GB* examination and only water is allowed the morning of the examination. The patient scheduled for a *barium enema* (lower GI) requires a large bowel that is very clean prior to the administration of barium; this requires the administration of cathartics (laxatives) and cleansing enemas. Preparation for an *IVU* requires that the patient be npo after midnight; some institutions may require that the large bowel be cleansed of gas and fecal material. *Aftercare* for barium examinations is also very important. Patients are typically instructed to take milk of magnesia and to drink plenty of water. Because water is removed from the barium sulfate suspension in the large bowel, it is essential to make patients understand the importance of these instructions to avoid barium impaction in the large bowel.

4. (C) The use of barium sulfate suspensions is contraindicated when ruling out visceral perforation. Barium could enter the peritoneal cavity and cause the very serious condition, *peritonitis.* When performing examinations on patients suspected or known to have stomach or intestinal perforation, *water-soluble iodinated contrast media* (such as Gastrografin or Oral Hypaque) should be used instead of barium sulfate. If this water-soluble medium leaks through a perforation into the peritoneal cavity, it will simply be absorbed and excreted by the kidneys. Water-soluble contrast agents may also be used in place of barium sulfate when the possibility of barium impaction exists.

5. (D) A radiographer who discloses confidential information to unauthorized individuals may be found guilty of *invasion of privacy or defamation.* A radiographer whose disclosure of confidential information is in some way detrimental to the patient may be accused of defamation. Spoken defamation is *slander;* written defamation is *libel. Assault* is to threaten harm; *battery* is to carry out the threat.

6. (B) The American Hospital Association identifies 12 important areas in their "Patient's Bill of Rights." These include the right to refuse treatment (to the extent allowed by law), the right to confidentiality of records and communication, and the right to continuing care. Other patient rights identified are the right to informed consent, privacy, respectful care, *access* to personal records, refusal to participate in research projects, and an explanation of one's hospital bill.

7. (C) A patient having a GI series is required to receive npo for at least 8 hours prior to the exam; food or drink in the stomach can simulate disease. A patient scheduled for a urogram must have the preceding meal withheld to avoid the possibility of aspirating vomitus in case of an allergic reaction. An abdominal survey does not require the use of contrast media, and no patient preparation is necessary.

8. (D) A mild laxative is often recommended to aid in the elimination of barium sulfate. The patient may also be instructed to increase dietary fiber and fluid and monitor bowel movement (should have at least one within 24 hours, or physician should be notified). Patients should also be aware of the white-colored appearance of the stool. It will be present until all barium is expelled.

9. (D) The *Constitution of the United States* expresses the categorical laws of the country. Its impact with respect to health care and health care professionals lies, in part, in its insurance of the *right to privacy*. The right to privacy indicates that the patient's modesty and dignity will be respected. It also refers to the health care professional's obligation to respect the confidentiality of privileged information. Inappropriate communication of privileged information to anyone but the appropriate health care professionals is inexcusable.

10. (A) *Assault* is to threaten harm; *battery* is to carry out the threat. A patient may feel sufficiently intimidated to claim assault by a radiographer who threatens to repeat a difficult examination if the patient doesn't try to cooperate better. A radiographer who performs an examination on a patient without the patient's consent or after the patient has refused the examination, may be liable for battery. A charge of battery may also be made against a radiographer who treats a patient roughly or who performs an examination on the wrong patient. A radiographer who discloses confidential information to unauthorized individuals may be found liable for *invasion of privacy* or *defamation*. A radiographer whose disclosure of confidential information is in some way detrimental to the patient may be accused of defamation. Spoken defamation is *slander;* written defamation is *libel*.

Patient Education, Safety, and Comfort

2

I. COMMUNICATION WITH PATIENTS

Effective communication with patients often begins with a review of relevant patient history. The acquisition of pertinent clinical history is one of the most valuable contributions to the diagnostic process. Because the diagnostic radiologist rarely has the opportunity to speak with the patient, this is a crucial responsibility of the radiographer. For instance, to report that your patient indicates most pain at his medial malleolus is far more valuable than simply saying that his ankle hurts.

The importance of effective patient and professional *communication* skills cannot be overstressed; the interaction between patient and radiographer generally leaves a lasting impression of the patient's health care experience. Of course, communication refers not only to the spoken word but also to unspoken communication. Facial expression can convey caring and reassurance or impatience and disapproval. Similarly, a radiographer's touch can convey his or her commitment to considerate care, or it can convey a rough, uncaring, hurried attitude.

A. Verbal and Nonverbal Communication

Consider the nonverbal messages communicated to a patient brought into a disorderly radiographic room, or by a radiographer presenting a sloppy, poorly groomed appearance. What about the grim-faced professional who hurries the patient along to the radiographic room, gives rapid-fire instructions on what to do while searching about for missing markers and cassettes, tosses the patient about on the x-ray table, and finally dismisses the patient with a curt "you can go now"?

Another patient is greeted by a smiling professional who introduces himself or herself and brings the patient to a neat and orderly radiographic room, where everything is in readiness for the procedure. The radiographer explains the procedure and answers the patient's questions. At the end of the examination, the patient is escorted back to the waiting area and clear instructions are given for appropriate postprocedural care.

Which patient has a more comfortable, anxiety-free examination? Which leaves the hospital or clinic environment with a more favorable impression of his or her health care experience? Which experience would *you* prefer for yourself or a loved one?

The volume of the radiographer's voice and his or her rate of speech are also important factors to consider in effective communication. Loud, rapid speech is particularly uncomfortable for the sick patient. A conscious effort should be made to use a well-modulated tone. The radiographer should face the patient and make eye contact during communication.

Gaining the patient's confidence and trust through effective communication is an essential part of the radiographic examination. Some patients will require a greater use of the radiographer's communication skills—patients who are seriously ill or injured; traumatized patients; patients who have impaired vision, hearing, or speech; pediatric patients; non–English-speaking patients; the elderly and infirm; the physically or mentally impaired; alcohol and drug abusers—the radiographer must adapt his or her communication skills to meet the needs of many types of individuals.

Elderly patients, for example, dislike being pushed or hurried about. They appreciate the radiographer who is compassionate enough to take the extra few minutes necessary for comfort. Some elderly patients are easily confused; it is best to address them by their full name and to keep instructions simple and direct. The elderly deserve the same courteous, dignified care as all other patients.

B. EXPLANATION OF PROCEDURE

It is imperative that the radiographer take adequate time to thoroughly explain the procedure or examination to the patient. The radiographer requires the cooperation of the patient throughout the course of the examination. A thorough explanation will alleviate the patient's anxieties and permit fuller cooperation. Patients should be clear about what will be expected of them and what they may expect from the radiographer. Effective communication skills help to ensure this cooperation.

Patients often have questions about other scheduled diagnostic imaging procedures such as mammography, computed tomography (CT), magnetic resonance imaging (MRI), sonography, or nuclear medicine studies. The diagnostic radiographer must be able to respond knowledgeably to questions regarding diet restrictions or other preparation that might be needed for CT or sonography, concerns or contraindications for some exams such as MRI, and positioning techniques such as compression used in mammography.

C. EXPLANATION OF AFTERCARE

Radiographers must be certain to provide patients with appropriate aftercare instructions (eg, plenty of fluids following barium examinations). Patients sometimes need to repeat explanations or instructions (to the radiographer) to be certain they understand; some have an additional question or two they must ask to clarify their thoughts. The radiographer's patience and understanding at these times is greatly appreciated by the anxious patient or relative.

Summary

- **Communication may be verbal or nonverbal. Verbal communication involves the tone and rate of speech as well as what is being said. It involves personalization and respect. Nonverbal communication involves facial expression, professional appearance, orderliness of the radiographic room, and the preparation and efficiency of the radiographer.**
- **A thorough explanation of procedures reduces the patient's anxiety, increases cooperation, and results in a better examination.**

II. EVALUATING PATIENT CONDITION

The radiographer must *assess* a patient's condition prior to bringing the patient to the radiographic room, and as the examination progresses. A good place to begin is with a review of the patient's chart. Other useful information includes the admitting diagnosis and recent nurses' notes including information regarding the patient's degree of ambulation, any preparation for the x-ray procedure and how it was tolerated, notes regarding laboratory tests, and saving the patient's urine.

As the radiographer obtains a brief pertinent clinical history, he or she also assesses the patient's condition by observing and listening. To provide safe and effective care, the radiographer must be able to assess the severity of a trauma patient's injury, the patient's degree of motor control, and the need for support equipment or radiographic accessories. Can the patient move or be moved from the stretcher? Can the part be imaged adequately and with less pain on the stretcher or in the wheel chair? Will the use of sponges and/or sandbags result in a more comfortable, safer, and better imaged examination?

A. PHYSICAL SIGNS

When the patient is first approached, and as the examination progresses, the radiographer should be alert to the patient's appearance and condition, and any subsequent changes in them. Notice the color, temperature, and moistness of the patient's skin. Paleness frequently indicates weakness; the *diaphoretic* patient has pale, cool skin. Fever is frequently accompanied by hot, dry skin. "Sweaty" palms may indicate *anxiety*. A patient who becomes *cyanotic* (bluish lips, mucous membranes, or nail beds) needs oxygen and requires immediate medical attention.

B. VITAL SIGNS

If a medical emergency arises, the radiographer may be required to assist by obtaining the patient's vital signs. Although checking vital signs is not a routine function, the radiographer should be proficient and confident if and when the need arises. Practicing vital signs during "slow" periods will benefit the patient who needs those skills during an emergency; also, those on whom you practice will learn their vital signs—valuable information for all.

Normal Body Temperatures

Adult	
Oral	98.6°F
Rectal	99.1°–99.6°F
Axillary	97.6°–98.1°F
Infant to 3 years	99°–99.7°F
Children 5–13 years	97.8°–98.6°F

Common Pulse Points

Artery	Location
Radial	wrist; at base of thumb
Carotid	neck; just lateral to midline
Temporal	in front of upper ear
Femoral	inguinal region; groin
Popliteal	posterior knee

Normal Pulse Rates (beats/min)

Men	70–72
Women	78–82
Children	90–100
Infants	120

Obtaining *vital signs* involves the measurement of *body temperature, pulse* rate, *respiratory rate,* and arterial *blood pressure.* Increased body temperature, or *fever,* usually signifies infection. Symptoms of fever include general *malaise,* increased pulse and respiratory rates, flushed skin that is hot and dry to the touch, and occasional chills. Very high, prolonged fevers can cause irreparable brain damage.

Normal body temperature varies from person to person depending on several factors, including age. A normal *adult* body temperature taken orally is 98.6°F (37°C). Rectal temperature is generally 0.5° to 1.0° higher, whereas axillary temperature is usually 0.5° to 1.0° lower. A variation of 0.5° to 1.0° is generally considered within normal limits. Body temperature is usually lowest in the early morning and highest at night. Infants up to 3 years of age have normal body temperatures of between 99°F and 99.7°F. *Children* ages 5 to 13 years have a normal range of 97.8°F to 98.6°F.

Body areas having superficial arteries are best suited for determination of a patient's pulse rate. The *five most readily palpated pulse points* are the radial, carotid, temporal, femoral, and popliteal pulse. Of these, the radial pulse is the most frequently used. The apical pulse, at the apex of the heart, may be readily evaluated with the use of a stethoscope.

Pulse rate depends on the person's age, sex, body exertion and position, and general state of health. The very young and the very old have higher pulse rates. The pulse rate increases in the standing position and after exertion. The pulse rate also increases with certain conditions, such as fever, organic heart disease, *shock,* and alcohol and drug use. Certain variations in the regularity and strength of the pulse are characteristic of various maladies. Pulse rates vary between men and women and among adults, children, and infants; athletes often have lower pulse rates.

The act of *respiration* serves to deliver oxygen to all the body's cells and rid the body of carbon dioxide. The radiographer must be able to recognize abnormalities or changes in patient respiration. The general term used to describe difficult breathing is *dyspnea.* More specific terms used to describe abnormal respirations include *uneven, spasmodic, strident* (shrill, grating sound), *stertorous* (labored, eg, snoring), *tachypnea* (abnormally rapid breathing), *orthopnea* (difficulty breathing while recumbent), *oligopnea* (abnormally shallow, slow).

A patient's respirations should be counted after counting the pulse rate, while still holding the patient's wrist. Respiratory action may become more deliberate and less natural in the patient who is aware that his or her respirations are being counted. The normal *adult* respiratory rate is 12 to 18 breaths per minute. The respiratory rate of young *children* is somewhat higher, up to 30 breaths per minute. While the radiographer is counting respirations, he or she should also be assessing the respiratory pattern (even, uneven) and depth (normal, shallow, deep).

Blood encounters a degree of resistance as it travels through the peripheral vascular system; thus, a certain amount of pressure exists within the walls of the vessels. *Blood pressure* among individuals varies with age, sex, fatigue, mental or physical stress, disease, and trauma. The blood pressure within vessels is greatest during ventricular *systole* (contraction) and lowest during *diastole* (relaxation). Blood pressure measurements are recorded with the systolic pressure on top and the diastolic pressure on the bottom, as in 100/80 (read: "one hundred over eighty"). Normal *adult* systolic pressure ranges between 100 and 140 mm Hg; the normal diastolic range is between 60 and 90 mm Hg. Blood pressure consistently above 140/90 is considered *hypertension*. Left undiagnosed and untreated, hypertension can lead to renal, cardiac, or brain damage. Hypotension is characterized by a systolic pressure of less than 90 mm Hg. Hypotension is seen in individuals with a decreased blood volume as a result of hemorrhage, infection, fever, and anemia. *Orthostatic* hypotension occurs in some individuals when they rise quickly from a recumbent position.

Blood pressure is measured using a *sphygmomanometer* and stethoscope. The patient may be recumbent or seated with the arm supported. The cuff of the sphygmomanometer is wrapped snugly around the arm, with its lower edge just above the *antecubital fossa*. With the stethoscope earpieces in place, the brachial artery pulse is palpated in the antecubital fossa and the bell (diaphragm) of the stethoscope is placed over the brachial artery. The valve on the bulb pump is closed and the cuff inflated enough to collapse the brachial artery (about 180 mm Hg). The valve is then opened very slowly. The first sound heard is the systolic pressure; as the valve pressure is slowly released, the sound becomes louder, then suddenly gets softer—this is the diastolic pressure. After the blood pressure measurements are recorded, the stethoscope earpieces and bell should be cleaned.

Summary

- Patient condition may be assessed through chart information, observation, questioning, and vital signs.
- A patient's vital signs are temperature, pulse and respiration rate, and blood pressure.
- A normal adult oral body temperature is 98.6°F, axillary temperatures are 0.5° to 1° lower, and rectal temperatures are 0.5° to 1° higher.
- The arterial pulse points include radial, carotid, temporal, femoral, and popliteal.
- The normal adult pulse rate is 70 to 80 beats per minute; infant and children pulse rates are higher.
- The normal adult respiratory rate is 12 to 18 breaths per minute, with children's respirations being higher (up to 30 per minute).
- Dyspnea refers to difficulty breathing; other terms are used to describe specific respiratory abnormalities.
- Blood pressure is measured using a sphygmomanometer and stethoscope.
- The average normal adult blood pressure is 120/80; blood pressure varies with a person's age, sex, fatigue and stress level, and disease, and with trauma.
- Systolic pressure (contraction) is the top number, diastolic pressure (relaxation) is the bottom number.

III. BODY MECHANICS AND PATIENT TRANSFER

Radiographers work with many patients whose capacities for *ambulation* vary greatly. Outpatients are usually *ambulatory*, that is, able

Other Rules of Good Body Mechanics

1. When carrying a heavy object, hold it close to the body.
2. The back should be kept straight; avoid twisting.
3. When lifting an object, bend the knees and use leg and abdominal muscles to lift (rather than back muscles).
4. Whenever possible, push or roll heavy objects (rather than lifting or pulling).

to walk and not confined to bed. Ambulatory inpatients generally travel by wheelchair, while patients confined to bed must travel by stretcher. It is essential for the radiographer to use proper technique and body mechanics when transferring patients, for the safety of the patient and the radiographer.

To transfer the patient with maximum safety for the patient and himself or herself, the radiographer must correctly use certain concepts of body mechanics. First, a broad base of support lends greater stability; therefore, the radiographer should stand with his or her feet about 12 inches apart and with one foot slightly forward. Secondly, stability is achieved when the body's center of gravity (center of the pelvis) is positioned over its base of support. For example, leaning away from the central axis of the body makes the body more vulnerable to losing balance; if the feet are close together, balance is even more difficult to keep.

Even the ambulatory outpatient may be somewhat unsteady, so a ready, supporting hand at the elbow can be very helpful. The radiographer should keep a watchful eye on the patient and assist him or her as needed. Not all patients need, or want, well-intentioned assistance. Many prefer to manage on their own. The radiographer should recognize this, but be ever alert and watchful should the patient need assistance. Other patients find it reassuring and feel an added sense of security with an attentive radiographer. The professional radiographer develops a sense of awareness of each patient's needs and concerns.

Before helping a patient into or out of a wheelchair, it must first be locked. Then, the footrests must be moved aside to avoid tripping over them or tilting the wheelchair forward. Once the patient is seated, the footrests should be lowered into place for the patient's comfort.

When transferring a patient between the x-ray table and a stretcher, the stretcher is first securely locked. Often a smooth piece of plastic, placed partially under the patient and used in conjunction with the drawsheet, is used to facilitate patient transfer. Patient transfer should involve pulling, not pushing; pushing increases friction and makes the transfer more difficult. Use the biceps muscles for pulling; do not bend at the waist and pull, as this motion increases back strain.

It is essential that someone be responsible for keeping any IV tubing, *catheters,* oxygen lines, or other equipment free from entanglement during wheelchair and/or stretcher transfers.

The patient may be adjusted into the Fowler's position (head higher than feet) for comfort or ease of breathing. The radiographer must be certain that safety belts and/or side rails are appropriately used for any patient on a stretcher.

IV. PATIENT SAFETY AND COMFORT

It is the health care practitioner's responsibility to ensure patient safety and comfort while the patient is in his or her care. The radiographer should make mental notes of what the patient has when he or she enters the department, such as glasses or a purse. Patient belongings should be properly secured according to institution or department policy. The radiographer must be certain that the radiographic room is hazard free, that all equipment and accessories are used properly and safely, and that the patient is as comfortable as possible.

When moving to or from the wheelchair or stretcher, patients should always be assisted or, at least, given careful attention. It is exceedingly unwise to finish a radiographic examination and say "OK, you can get off the x-ray table now," or something to that effect. The x-ray tube must be moved away from the x-ray table, a footstool must be in place to assist the patient from the table, and the radiographer must be there to guide or assist the patient safely to the correct dressing room.

Should an injured patient require assistance with dressing and undressing, it is important to remember that clothing should be *removed* from the *un*injured side first and *placed* on the *injured* side first.

Special consideration must be given to each patient according to his or her condition. Elderly and very thin patients, and those who will be required to lie on the x-ray table for a lengthy period of time, benefit greatly from a foam pad between them and the x-ray table. Lumbar strain is relieved by a pillow or positioning sponge placed under the knees. An extra pillow for the head or cushioning under the heels or ischial tuberosities can make a big difference in patient care. Special care and attention should be given to the skin of the elderly, as it bruises and bleeds easily.

Patients that are sedated, senile, in shock, or under the influence of alcohol or drugs must never be left unattended. Patients who arrive in the radiology department with restraints in place must never be left alone on the x-ray table, since they are usually active, disoriented, and occasionally, combative. Indeed, many radiology departments have rules stating that *no* patient may *ever* be left unattended in the radiographic room.

Just as health care practitioners provide for patient safety and comfort, they must ensure their own safety by practicing good body mechanics, infection control, and standard precautions.

Should an accident ever occur and a patient or health care practitioner be injured, no matter how small or insignificant the injury seems, it must be reported to the supervisor and an incident report completed. The risk management team, or similar group, requires all such information for legal documentation and as a means of identifying and resolving potential hazards.

Summary

- **Modes of patient transportation include ambulation, wheelchair, and stretcher.**
- **Patient and radiographer safety require the use of proper and safe body mechanics.**
- **Wheelchairs and stretchers must be locked and wheelchair footrests positioned out of the way prior to patient transfer.**
- **One person should be responsible for the safe transport of IV lines, catheters, and other tubes.**
- **Patient transfer between the radiographic table and stretcher should involve pulling, not pushing; a smooth plastic board often helps.**
- **The knees should be bent when lifting heavy objects; leg and abdominal muscles are used instead of back muscles.**
- **Heavy objects should be carried close to the body.**

- The back should be kept straight and twisting motions should be avoided.
- Heavy objects should be pushed or rolled (instead of pulled or lifted) whenever possible.
- Patient belongings should be properly secured according to policy while the patient is in the radiographer's care.
- The radiographer must be alert for patient safety and comfort at all times; patients should not be left unattended in the radiographic room.
- Should an accident occur involving the patient and/or radiographer, an incident report should be completed regardless how minor the incident.

Chapter Exercises

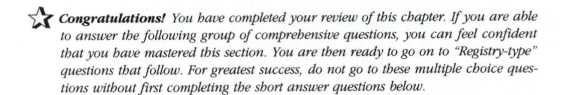

Congratulations! You have completed your review of this chapter. If you are able to answer the following group of comprehensive questions, you can feel confident that you have mastered this section. You are then ready to go on to "Registry-type" questions that follow. For greatest success, do not go to these multiple choice questions without first completing the short answer questions below.

1. Discuss five ways in which the radiographer can send verbal messages to the patient *(pp. 19, 20)*.

2. Discuss five ways in which the radiographer can send nonverbal messages to the patient *(pp. 19, 20)*.

3. Discuss some qualities of verbal communication likely to evoke a positive response from the patient; a negative response *(p. 20)*.

4. Explain the value of making as many preparations as possible prior to bringing the patient into the radiographic room *(pp. 19, 20, 24–25)*.

5. Discuss five types of patients who might require special communication efforts on the part of the radiographer *(p. 20)*.

6. List five benefits of effective communication skills *(pp. 19, 20)*.

7. Discuss the importance of being alert to initial patient condition and any subsequent changes in condition *(p. 21)*.

8. Identify the following with respect to body temperature: *(p. 22)*

   A. normal adult, infant, and child temperature

   B. the significance of fever, that is, what it usually indicates

   C. symptoms usually associated with fever

   D. difference among oral, rectal, and axillary temperatures

9. Identify the following with respect to pulse rate: *(p. 22)*

   A. the normal, average adult pulse rate for men and women

   B. normal and abnormal conditions under which pulse rate will vary/change

   C. the usual site of pulse determination; other possible sites

10. Identify the following with respect to respiration: *(p. 22)*

    A. its function

    B. the ideal time to determine patient respiration rate; why

    C. the normal, average adult respiratory rate

11. Identify the following with respect to blood pressure: *(pp. 22, 23)*

    A. equipment necessary

    B. position of patient

    C. position of cuff and bell

    D. first and second sounds heard

12. Discuss three modes of patient transport *(pp. 23, 24)*.

13. Identify, with respect to body mechanics and patient transfer: *(p. 24)*

    A. position of radiographer's feet (as base of support)

    B. the body's center of gravity (versus stability) and when moving heavy objects: push versus pull; use of knees, legs, and back; proximity of object to body

    C. position of footrests and locks during wheelchair transfers

    D. position of locks, use of drawsheet and plastic mover, push versus pull in stretcher transfer

    E. care of IV lines, catheters, O2, safety belts, and side rails

14. Identify the manner in which patients should be directed onto, and removed from, the x-ray table *(p. 25)*.

15. Explain how clothing should be removed from a patient with unilateral injury *(p. 25)*.

16. Identify techniques used to reduce patient discomfort of elderly and/or thin patients recumbent on the radiographic table *(p. 25)*.

17. Discuss the types of patients likely to be at greater risk left unattended on the radiographic table *(p. 25)*.

A&U Chapter Review Questions

1. Which of the following communicate messages to the patient?
   1. tone of voice
   2. eye contact
   3. appearance of radiographer
   (A) 1 only
   (B) 1 and 2 only
   (C) 3 only
   (D) 1, 2, and 3

2. When an injured patient requires assistance dressing or undressing, the radiographer must remember to:
   1. *remove* clothing *from* the uninjured side first
   2. *place* clothing *on* the injured side first
   3. always start with the injured side
   (A) 1 only
   (B) 1 and 2 only
   (C) 3 only
   (D) 1, 2, and 3

3. What number of breaths per minute represents the average rate of respiration for a normal adult?
   (A) 8 to 15
   (B) 10 to 20
   (C) 30 to 60
   (D) 60 to 90

4. The normal adult rectal temperature is:
   (A) higher than oral temperature
   (B) lower than oral temperature
   (C) the same as oral temperature
   (D) the same as axillary temperature

5. The period of relaxation of the heart is termed:
   (A) systole
   (B) diastole
   (C) hypertension
   (D) dyspnea

6. A patient who is diaphoretic has:
   (A) pale, cool, clammy skin
   (B) hot, dry skin
   (C) dilated pupils
   (D) warm, moist skin

7. Which pulse can be detected only by the use of a stethoscope in which of the following locations?
    (A) wrist
    (B) neck
    (C) groin
    (D) apex of the heart

8. Rules for good body mechanics when transferring patients include:
    1. the radiographer's feet should be about 12 inches apart
    2. the radiographer's trunk should lean toward the patient
    3. the radiographer's pelvis should be positioned over his or her feet
    (A) 1 only
    (B) 1 and 2 only
    (C) 1 and 3 only
    (D) 2 and 3 only

9. To reduce the back strain associated with transferring patients from stretcher to x-ray table, you should:
    (A) pull the patient
    (B) push the patient
    (C) hold the patient away from your body and lift
    (D) bend at the waist and pull

10. Instruments needed to assess vital signs include:
    1. tongue blade
    2. watch with second hand
    3. thermometer
    (A) 1 only
    (B) 1 and 2 only
    (C) 2 and 3 only
    (D) 1, 2, and 3

Answers and Explanations

1. (D) The interaction between patient and radiographer generally leaves a lasting impression of the patient's health care experience. Communication may be verbal or nonverbal. *Verbal communication* involves tone and rate of speech as well as what is being said. It involves personalization and respect. *Nonverbal communication* involves facial expression, professional appearance, orderliness of radiographic room, and preparation and efficiency of the radiographer.

2. (B) Special consideration must be given to each patient according to his or her condition. Elderly and very thin patients, and those who will be required to lie on the x-ray table for a lengthy period of time benefit greatly from a foam pad between them and the x-ray table. Should an injured patient require assistance with dressing and undressing, it is important to remember that clothing should be *removed from* the *un*injured side first and *placed on* the *injured* side first.

3. (B) A patient's respirations should be counted after counting the pulse rate, while still holding the patient's wrist. Respiratory action may become more deliberate, or less natural, in the patient who is aware that his or her respirations are being counted. *The normal respiratory rate is 12 to 18 breaths per minute.* The respiratory rate of young *children* is somewhat *higher,* up to 30 breaths per minute. While the radiographer is counting respirations, he or she should be assessing the respiratory pattern (even, uneven) and depth (normal, shallow, deep) as well.

4. (A) Obtaining *vital signs* involves the measurement of *body temperature, pulse rate, respiratory rate, and arterial blood pressure.* Increased body temperature, or fever, usually signifies infection. Symptoms of fever include general malaise, increased pulse and respiratory rates, flushed skin that is hot and dry to the touch, and occasional chills. Very high, prolonged fevers can cause irreparable brain damage.

Normal body temperature varies from person to person depending on several factors, including age. Normal adult body temperature taken orally is 98.6°F (37°C). *Rectal* temperature is generally 0.5° to 1.0° *higher,* whereas *axillary* temperature is usually 0.5° to 1.0° *lower.* Variation of 0.5° to 1.0° is generally considered within normal limits. Body temperature is usually lowest in the early morning and highest at night. Infants up to 3 years of age have normal body temperatures of between 99° and 99.7°F. Children ages 5 to 13 years have a normal range of 97.8° to 98.6°F.

5. (B) Blood pressure within vessels is greatest during ventricular *systole* (contraction) and lowest during *diastole* (relaxation). Blood pressure measurements are recorded with the systolic pressure on top and the diastolic pressure on the bottom, as in 100/80 (read: "one hundred over eighty"). Normal adult systolic pressure ranges between 100 and 140 mm Hg; the normal diastolic range is between 60 and 90 mm Hg. Blood pressure consistently above 140/90 is considered *hypertension. Dyspnea* is the medical term used to describe difficulty in breathing.

6. (A) The radiographer should be alert to the patient's appearance and condition, and any subsequent changes in them. Notice the color, temperature, and moistness of the patient's skin: paleness frequently indicates weakness; the *diaphoretic* patient has pale, cool skin; *fever* is frequently accompanied by hot, dry skin; "sweaty" palms may indicate *anxiety,* a patient who becomes *cyanotic* (bluish lips, mucous membranes, nail beds) needs oxygen and requires immediate medical attention.

7. (D) Body areas having superficial arteries are best suited for determination of a patient's pulse rate. The five most readily palpated pulse points are the radial, carotid, temporal, femoral, and popliteal pulse. Of these, the radial pulse is the most frequently used. *The apical pulse, at the apex of the heart, may be readily evaluated with the use of a stethoscope.*

8. (C) It is essential for the radiographer to use proper technique and body mechanics when transferring patients, for the safety of the patient and the radiographer. To transfer the patient with maximum safety to the patient and himself or herself, the radiographer must correctly use certain concepts of body mechanics. First, a good base of support lends greater stability; therefore, the radiographer should stand with *his or her feet approximately 12 inches apart,* with one foot slightly forward. Second, stability is achieved when the body's *center of gravity* (center of the *pelvis) is positioned over its base of support.* For example, leaning away from the central axis of the body makes the body more vulnerable to losing balance; if the feet are close together, balance is even more difficult to keep.

9. (A) When transferring a patient from stretcher to x-ray table, several rules apply that will help reduce back strain. *Pull*, do not push the patient; pushing increases friction and makes the transfer more difficult. *Use the biceps* muscles for pulling; do not bend at the waist and pull, as this motion increases back strain.

10. (C) Obtaining vital signs involves the measurement of *body temperature,* pulse rate, *respiratory rate,* and *arterial blood pressure.* A *thermometer* is used to take the patient's temperature. A *watch* with a second hand is required to time the patient's pulse rate and respirations. To measure blood pressure, a *sphygmomanometer* and *stethoscope* are required. A tongue blade is used to depress the tongue for inspection of the throat and is not part of vital sign assessment.

Infection Control and Prevention

3

I. MEDICAL AND SURGICAL ASEPSIS

Antisepsis is a practice that retards the growth of pathogenic bacteria. *Medical asepsis* refers to the destruction of pathogenic microorganisms through the process of *disinfection*. Examples of disinfectants are hydrogen peroxide, chlorine, and boric acid. *Surgical asepsis (sterilization)* refers to the removal of all microorganisms *and* their spores (reproductive cells) and is practiced in the surgical suite. Health care practitioners must practice medical asepsis at all times.

The most important precaution in the practice of aseptic technique is proper hand washing. The radiographer's hands should be thoroughly washed with soap and warm, running water for at least 10 seconds after each patient examination. If the faucet cannot be operated with the knee, it should be opened and closed using paper towels (to avoid contamination of or by the faucet). The radiographer's uniform should not touch the sink. The hands and forearms should always be kept lower than the elbows; care should be taken to wash all surfaces and between fingers. Hand lotions should be used to prevent hands from chapping; broken skin permits the entry of microorganisms. *Disinfectants, antiseptics, and germicides, are substances used to kill pathogenic bacteria*; they are frequently used in hand-washing substances. Alcohol-based hand sanitizers were recently recommended as an alternative to hand washing with soap and water (according to the HICPAC 2001 Draft Guideline for Hand Hygiene in Healthcare Settings).

Uniforms are recommended because clothing that is worn in patient areas should not be worn elsewhere. Because clothing becomes contaminated in the patient area, a clean uniform should be worn daily. Microorganisms can find safe harbor in jewelry, especially rings with stones and other crevices, and in cracked nail polish. It is recommended that the only jewelry a health care practitioner wear is a wristwatch and unadorned wedding band. *Remember that many microorganisms can remain infectious while awaiting transmission to another host.*

Sterile technique is employed during invasive procedures, such as biopsies, and for the administration of contrast media via the intravenous and *intrathecal* routes (eg, IV urography and myelography). When radiography is required in the surgical suite, every precaution must be made to maintain the surgical asepsis required in surgical procedures. This requires proper dress, cleanliness of equipment, and restricted access to certain areas. One example of a restricted area is the *"sterile corridor,"* the area between the draped patient and the instrument table. This area is occupied only by the surgeon and the instrument nurse.

II. MODES OF TRANSMISSION

The control and prevention of infection must be a hospital-wide effort; each department is required to have its own infection-control protocol, designed according to the risks unique to the services provided. Because radiography often involves exposure to sickness and disease, the radiographer must be aware of, and conscientiously practice, infection control and effective preventative measures.

Infectious microorganisms can be transmitted from patients to other patients or to health care workers, and from healthcare workers to patients. They are transmitted by means of either direct or indirect contact. *Direct contact* involves *touch*. The courteous act of handshaking is a simple way of transmitting infection from one individual to another. Diseases transmitted by direct contact include skin infections such as boils, and sexually transmitted diseases such as syphilis and acquired immunodeficiency syndrome (AIDS). Direct contact with droplets of nasal or oral secretions from a sneeze or cough is referred to as *droplet* contact.

Indirect contact involves transmission of microorganisms via *airborne* contamination, *fomites,* and *vectors. Pathogenic microorganisms* expelled from the respiratory tract through the mouth or nose can be carried as evaporated droplets through the air or on dust and settle on clothing, utensils, or food. Patients with respiratory infections or disease transported to the radiology department, therefore, should wear a mask to prevent such transmission during a cough or sneeze; it is not necessary for the health care worker to wear a mask (as long as the patient does). Many microorganisms can remain infectious while awaiting transmission to another host. A contaminated inanimate object such as a food utensil, doorknob, or IV pole is referred to as a *fomite*. A *vector* is an insect or animal carrier of infectious organisms, such as a rabid animal, a mosquito that carries malaria, or a tick that carries Lyme disease. They can transmit disease through either direct or indirect contact.

It is somewhat surprising, yet understandable, that many infections can be *acquired in the hospital*; surprising because hospitals are places where people go to regain their health, yet understandable because individuals weakened by illness or disease are more susceptible to infection than are healthy individuals. Infections acquired in hospitals, especially by patients whose resistance to infection has been diminished by their illness, are termed *nosocomial*. The most common nosocomial infection is the *urinary tract infection* (UTI), often related to the use of urinary catheters which can allow passage of pathogens into the patient's body. Other types of nosocomial infections include sepsis, wound infection and respiratory infection.

Health care practitioners must exercise strict infection-control precautions so that their equipment and/or technique will not be the source of nosocomial infection. *Contaminated* waste products, soiled linen, and improperly sterilized equipment are all means by which microorganisms can travel. Not every patient will come in contact with these items; however, the health care professional is in constant contact with patients and is therefore a constant threat to spread infection. Microorganisms are most commonly spread by way of the hands; spread of infection can be effectively reduced by proper disposal of contaminated objects and proper hand washing before and after each patient. *Disinfectants, antiseptics,* and *germicides,* are used in many hand-washing liquids to kill microorganisms.

Summary

- **Antiseptics retard the growth of bacteria.**
- **Medical asepsis refers to the destruction of bacteria through the use of disinfectants/antiseptics.**
- **Surgical asepsis refers to the destruction of all microorganisms and their spores through sterilization.**
- **The practice of medical asepsis is required at all times, while surgical asepsis is required for invasive procedures.**
- **The single most important component of medical asepsis is proper and timely hand washing.**
- **A clean uniform must be worn daily; uniforms become contaminated and should not be worn elsewhere; pathogenic microorganisms thrive in jewelry crevices and cracked nail polish.**
- **Infectious microorganisms are transmitted by either direct or indirect contact. Direct contact involves touch. Indirect contact includes airborne contamination, fomites, and vectors.**
- **Infections acquired in hospitals are called nosocomial infections; the most common nosocomial infection is the UTI.**
- **Disinfectants (germicides) are used in hand-washing liquids to kill microorganisms.**

III. STANDARD PRECAUTIONS

The Centers for Disease Control and Prevention (*CDC*) and the Hospital Infection Control Practices Advisory Committee (*HICPAC*) have revised and simplified infection control guidelines for hospitals and other health care facilities. The various types of isolation techniques, disease-specific precautions, and varied terminology have been reviewed, revised and updated. All these considerations are now incorporated in *standard precautions* and *transmission-based precautions.*

Exposure to infectious microorganisms is a daily concern for health care professionals, especially with the rapid spread of human immunodeficiency virus (*HIV*), *AIDS,* and the hepatitis B virus (*HBV*) infection. HIV-infected individuals may be symptomless and go undiagnosed for 10 years or more, yet they are carriers of the infection and have the potential to spread the disease. *Epidemiologic* studies indicate that HIV infection can be transmitted only by intimate contact with blood or body fluids of an infected individual. This can occur through the sharing of contaminated needles, through sexual contact, from mother to baby at childbirth, and from transfusion of contaminated blood. HIV *cannot* be transmitted by inanimate objects such as water fountains, telephone surfaces, or toilet seats. Hepatitis B is another bloodborne infection; it affects the liver. It is thought that more than one million people in the United States have chronic hepatitis B and, as such, can transmit the disease to others.

Because no symptoms may be evident in patients infected with particular diseases, such as HIV, AIDS, and HBV, all patients must be treated as potential sources of infection from blood and other body fluids. The practices associated with this concept are called *standard precautions.* This rationale treats *all* body fluids and substances as infectious and serves to prevent the spread of microorganisms to other patients by the radiographer, as well as to protect the radiographer from contamination. Body fluids and substances that may be considered infectious include blood, breast milk, vaginal secretions, amniotic fluid, semen, peritoneal fluid, synovial fluid, cerebrospinal fluid, feces, urine, secretions from the nasal and oral cavities, and secretions from the lacrimal and sweat glands.

It is essential, then, that the radiographer make the practice of blood and body fluid precautions *standard,* that is, they must be practiced on all patients without exception. This involves the use of barriers, such as gloves, to provide a separation between a patient's blood and body fluids and the radiographer or other health care worker. *Special precautions must also be taken with the disposal of biomedical waste,* such as laboratory and pathology waste, all sharp objects, and liquid waste from suction, bladder catheters, chest tubes, and IV tubes, as well as drainage containers.

Biomedical waste is generally packaged in easily identifiable impermeable bags and removed from the premises by an approved biomedical waste hauler.

IV. TRANSMISSION-BASED PRECAUTIONS

Adherence to standard blood, body fluids, and substances precautions in the care of all patients will minimize the risk of transmission of HIV and other blood and body substance-borne pathogens from the patient to the radiographer and from the radiographer to patient. The use of standard precautions also minimizes the need for category specific isolation. These have been replaced by *transmission-based precautions: airborne, droplet,* and *contact.* Under these guidelines, some conditions/diseases can fall into more than one category.

Medical asepsis and blood and body fluids precautions are used when performing radiographic examinations on *all* patients, but additional precautions may be required when a patient is suspected or known to have a *particular communicable disease.* For example, *airborne precaution* is employed with patients suspected or known to be infected with the *tubercle bacillus (TB), chickenpox (varicella),* and *measles (rubeola).* Airborne precaution *requires the patient to wear a mask* to avoid the spread of acid-fast bacilli (in bronchial secretions) or other pathogens during coughing. If the patient is unable or unwilling to wear a mask, the radiographer must wear one. An N95 Particulate Respirator mask, which requires fit-testing, is the mask to be worn by health care workers. The radiographer should wear gloves, but a gown is required only if flagrant contamination is

---

Guidelines for Standard Precautions

The radiographer is now legally, as well as ethically, responsible for strict adherence to standard precaution principles identified in the following guidelines:

- Shielding for the face and eyes must be in place whenever the possibility of blood or body fluid splashes may occur near the face.
- Plastic aprons must be worn whenever the possibility of blood or body fluid splashes may occur on the clothing.
- Gloves must be worn whenever touching blood or body fluids is possible, and whenever handling equipment or touching surfaces contaminated with blood or body fluids is possible.
- Gloves must be changed and the hands washed after every patient contact.
- Blood and body fluid spills should be carefully cleaned and disinfected using a solution of 1 part bleach to 10 parts water.
- Used needles must not be separated from the syringe and must be placed in designed puncture-proof containers.
- Prescribed procedures must be followed and sufficient care and attention given risky tasks to avoid needle sticks and other skin penetrations from cutting instruments ("sharps").
- Emergency cardiopulmonary resuscitation (CPR) equipment must include resuscitation bags and mouthpieces.

likely. Patients infected with *airborne diseases* require a *private, specially ventilated (negative pressure) room* (Table 3–1).

A private room is indicated for all patients on *droplet precaution*, that is, diseases transmitted via large droplets expelled from the patient while speaking, sneezing, or coughing. The pathogenic droplets can infect others when they come in contact with mouth or nasal mucosa or conjunctiva. *Rubella* ("German measles"), *mumps*, and *influenza* are among the diseases spread by droplet contact; *a private room is required* for the patient, and health care practitioners must wear a regular (string) *mask* to enter a droplet-precautions isolation room.

Any diseases spread by direct or close *contact*, such as *MRSA* (methicillin-resistant *Staphylococcus aureus*), *Clostridium difficile (C-diff)*, and *some wounds*, require *contact precautions. Contact precaution* procedures require a *private patient room*, and the use of *gloves and gown* for anyone coming in direct contact with the infected individual or the infected person's environment. Some facilities require health care workers to wear a mask when caring for a patient with MRSA.

Patients in *contact isolation* occasionally have to be transported to the radiology department for examination. When this is the case, the department should be notified first in order to prepare properly. The patient should wear a mask and gown. The wheelchair or stretcher should first be covered with a clean sheet, followed by a second sheet or thin blanket. After transferring the patient to the wheelchair or stretcher, the inner sheet is wrapped around the patient, and the outer sheet over it (thus, the inner sheet is the contaminated one). The radiographic room should be available and ready for the patient to be taken in directly. The x-ray table should be covered with a clean sheet before the patient is transferred to it. One radiographer (wearing gloves) must be responsible for patient positioning and the other for equipment controls and operation (to avoid contamination of equipment and possible transmission of disease to others via indirect contact or fomites).

After the examination is completed, the patient is transferred to the wheelchair or stretcher and wrapped in the same way. Any con-

TABLE 3–1. TRANSMISSION-BASED PRECAUTIONS

EXAMPLES	PROTECTION
Airborne	
TB	Patient: wears mask, private, negative-pressure room
Varicella	Radiographer: wears gloves; gown for blatant
Rubeola	contamination
Droplet	
Rubella	Patient: wears mask, private room
Mumps	Radiographer: gown and gloves as indicated
Influenza	
Contact	
MRSA	Patient: private room, wears mask if required by
C-diff	your facility
Some wounds	Radiographer: gloves and gown, mask for MRSA
	if required by facility

C-diff, *clostridium difficile;* MRSA, methicillin-resistant *Staphylococcus aureus.*

taminated linens should be placed in a plastic bag and contaminated disposables such as tissues are placed in a separate bag; both are returned with the patient to his private room.

The radiographic table and other equipment should be cleaned with a disinfectant and hands should be washed carefully when the task is completed.

Mobile radiography performed on patients on *contact isolation* generally requires special precautions and the teamwork of *two* radiographers. The first (or "dirty") radiographer dons gown, gloves (gloves must cover gown cuffs), and mask, usually available just outside the patient's room. The necessary cassette(s) must be placed in a plastic bag or pillowcase to protect them from contamination. This radiographer must remember to bring an extra pair of gloves into the patient room. The mobile x-ray unit is brought into the room, and all possible adjustments must be made before the radiographer touches anything else.

The equipment and cassette are positioned, and patient adjusted properly. *At this point, the mobile x-ray unit must not be touched* until the radiographer disposes of the gloves he or she has on and replaces them with the clean extra pair.

The exposure is then made; the covered cassette is removed from behind/under the patient and brought to the door. The "dirty" radiographer slides the pillowcase or plastic cover away from the cassette and the second member of the team (the "clean" radiographer) grasps the uncovered cassette. Just inside the patient room door, the contaminated gloves should be removed properly and the hands washed thoroughly. The mask and gown ties are then untied with clean hands; the gown is removed by placing a clean hand under the cuff and pulling the arm down from underneath. The other sleeve is also removed *by touching only the inside of the gown.* The gown is slipped off and folded forward with the contaminated surfaces touching.

The discarded garments must be placed in the container provided. The radiographer should then carefully rewash his or her hands, dry them with paper towels, and take care not to touch the faucets. After leaving the room, *the mobile unit must be thoroughly cleaned* with a disinfectant and the hands carefully washed once again.

It should be noted that these patients may feel ostracized and relegated to a kind of solitary confinement. The radiographer must remember that these patients have the same needs as other patients (indeed, perhaps greater needs) and be certain to treat them with dignity and care.

Protective, or reverse, isolation is used to keep the susceptible patient from becoming infected. Burn patients who have lost their means of protection, their skin, have increased susceptibility to bacterial invasion. Patients whose immune systems are compromised (eg, transplant recipients, leukemia) are unable to combat infection and are more susceptible to infection. These patients are treated with strict isolation technique, taking care to protect the *patient* from contamination.

Summary

■ **Because no symptoms may be evident in patients afflicted with certain diseases such as HIV, AIDS, and hepatitis B, *all* patients must be treated as potential sources of infection** from blood and other body fluids; this is the *standard precautions* concept.

■ The practice of standard precautions helps prevent transmission of infection to the health care professional and to other patients.

■ The health care professional is legally and ethically responsible for adhering to standard precautions principles; *they must be practiced on all patients at all times without exception.*

■ Biomedical waste (body substances and their containers) must be disposed of in carefully controlled circumstances.

■ Transmission-based precautions include airborne, droplet, and contact.

■ Airborne precaution requires that the patient wear a mask and be admitted to a private, specially ventilated room.

■ Droplet precaution and a private room are required for measles, mumps, and influenza; the radiographer requires a mask (if the patient is not wearing one), and may also need to wear gown and gloves.

■ Contact precaution (C-diff, MRSA, some wounds) require that the radiographer use mask, gown, and gloves when in direct contact with the patient, and for MRSA may be needed.

■ Mobile radiography on a patient with contact precaution requires the teamwork of two radiographers.

■ Protective, or reverse, isolation is used to keep the susceptible patient from being infected.

Chapter Exercises

 Congratulations! You have completed your review of this chapter. If you are able to answer the following group of comprehensive questions, you can feel confident that you have mastered this section. You are then ready to go on to "Registry-type" questions that follow. For greatest success, do not go to these multiple choice questions without first completing the short answer questions below.

1. Identify and differentiate between the two basic means of transmitting infectious microorganisms *(p. 34)*.

2. List three means of indirect transmission of pathogenic microorganisms *(p. 34)*.

3. Identify the most common type of hospital-acquired infection *(p. 34)*.

4. List five possible sources of nosocomial infection in the radiology department *(p. 35)*.

5. Describe the type protection required for patients with respiratory infections *(p. 36)*.

6. Identify the means by which microorganisms are spread *(p. 34)*.

7. What substances are added to hand-washing liquids to kill microorganisms *(p. 33)?*

8. Discuss the rationale of body fluid and substance (standard) precautions *(pp. 35, 36)*.

9. Discuss each of the following with respect to standard precautions *(p. 36)*:

    A. when a face shield should be used

    B. when a plastic apron should be used

    C. when hands should be washed

    D. when gloves should be used

    E. how body fluid and substance spills should be cleaned

    F. care of used needles

    G. special devices available for CPR

    H. on whom standard precautions should be practiced

10. Differentiate between medical and surgical asepsis *(p. 33)*.

11. Identify and explain the most important practice in good aseptic technique *(p. 33)*.

12. Discuss the function of uniforms worn by health care practitioners; the hazards of jewelry and nail polish *(p. 33)*.

13. List the three types of transmission-based precautions *(p. 36)*.

14. Explain the precautionary measures taken in airborne precaution; ie, apparel (and for whom), patient room *(pp. 36, 37)*.

15. List three communicable diseases spread by droplet contact that require droplet precaution *(p. 37)*.

16. Describe the method of performing mobile chest radiography on patients with contact precaution, to include: *(p. 38)*

    A. number of persons needed

    B. radiographer's apparel

    C. how to protect cassettes from contamination

    D. why an extra pair of gloves is needed in the patient room

    E. role played by the second individual

    F. how protective clothing should be removed

    G. care of x-ray machine at completion of exam

17. Describe the proper method of transporting a contact precaution patient to the radiology department *(p. 37)*.

18. Describe the purpose of reverse isolation *(p. 38)*.

19. Discuss any special needs the isolation patient may have *(p. 38)*.

A&I Chapter Review Questions

1. Diseases that can be transmitted by direct contact include:
   1. skin infections
   2. syphilis
   3. malaria
   (A) 1 only
   (B) 1 and 2 only
   (C) 2 and 3 only
   (D) 1, 2, and 3

2. Which of the following can be transmitted via infected blood?
   1. TB
   2. AIDS
   3. HBV
   (A) 1 only
   (B) 1 and 2 only
   (C) 2 and 3 only
   (D) 1, 2, and 3

3. Which of the following are means of indirect transmission of microorganisms?
   1. vector
   2. fomite
   3. airborne
   (A) 1 only
   (B) 1 and 2 only
   (C) 3 only
   (D) 1, 2, and 3

4. What is the single most-effective means of controlling the spread of infectious microorganisms?
   (A) [wearing gloves
   (B) wearing masks
   (C) hand washing
   (D) sterilization

5. What technique is practiced when all patients are treated as potential sources of infection from blood and other body fluids?
   (A) standard precautions
   (B) sterilization
   (C) disinfection
   (D) contamination precautions

6. What is the name of the practice that serves to retard the growth of pathogenic bacteria?
   (A) antisepsis
   (B) bacteriogenesis
   (C) sterilization
   (D) disinfection

7. Which of the following diseases require(s) airborne precaution?
   1. TB
   2. varicella
   3. rubella
   (A) 1 only
   (B) 1 and 2 only
   (C) 3 only
   (D) 1, 2, and 3

8. The radiographer must perform the following procedure(s) prior to entering an isolation room with a mobile x-ray unit:
   1. wear gown and gloves
   2. wear gown, mask, and gloves
   3. clean the mobile x-ray unit
   (A) 1 only
   (B) 2 only
   (C) 1 and 3 only
   (D) 2 and 3 only

9. Lyme disease is a condition caused by bacteria carried by deer ticks. The tick bite may cause fever, fatigue, and other associated symptoms. This is an example of transmission of an infection by:
   (A) droplet contact
   (B) the airborne route
   (C) a vector
   (D) a vehicle

10. In which of the following conditions is protective or reverse isolation indicated?
    1. transplant recipient
    2. burns
    3. leukemia
    (A) 1 only
    (B) 1 and 2 only
    (C) 2 and 3 only
    (D) 1, 2, and 3

Answers and Explanations

1. (B) Infectious microorganisms can be transmitted from one patient to other patients or to health care workers, and from health care workers to patients. They are transmitted by means of either direct or indirect contact. *Direct contact* involves touch. Diseases transmitted by direct contact include skin infections such as boils and sexually transmitted diseases such as syphilis.

    Indirect contact involves transmission of microorganisms via airborne contamination, fomites, and vectors. Pathogenic microorganisms expelled from the respiratory tract through the mouth or nose can be carried as evaporated droplets through the air or on dust and settle on clothing, utensils, or food. Patients with respiratory infections and disease transported to the radiology department, therefore, should wear a mask to prevent such transmission during a cough or sneeze; it is not necessary for the health care professional or transporter to wear a mask (as long as the patient does). Many such microorganisms can remain infectious while awaiting transmission to another host. A contaminated inanimate object such as a food utensil, doorknob, or IV pole is referred to as a fomite. A vector is an insect or animal carrier of infectious organisms, such as a rabid animal (eg, rabies; and although the rabid animal is the vector, rabies is contracted by contact), a mosquito that carries malaria, or a tick that carries Lyme disease.

2. (C) Epidemiologic studies indicate that HIV and AIDS can be transmitted only by intimate contact with blood or body fluids of an infected individual. This can occur through the sharing of contaminated needles, through sexual contact, from mother to baby at childbirth, and from transfusion of contaminated blood. HIV and AIDS cannot be transmitted by inanimate objects. HBV is another bloodborne infection and affects the liver. It is thought that more than one million people in the United States have chronic hepatitis B and, as such, can transmit the disease to others. Acid-fast bacillus (AFB) isolation is employed with patients suspected or known to be infected with the TB. AFB isolation requires that the patient wear a mask to avoid the spread of acid-fast bacilli (in bronchial secretions) during *coughing.*

3. (D) *Indirect* contact involves transmission of microorganisms via *airborne* contamination, *fomites,* and *vectors.* Pathogenic microorganisms expelled from the respiratory tract through the mouth or nose can be carried as evaporated droplets through the air or on dust and settle on clothing, utensils, or food. A contaminated inanimate object such as a pillowcase, x-ray table, or IV pole is referred to as a *fomite.* A *vector* is an insect or animal carrier of infectious organisms, such as a rabid animal (rabies), a mosquito that carries malaria, or a tick that carries Lyme disease.

4. (C) Health care practitioners must exercise strict infection-control precautions so that they or their equipment will not be the source of nosocomial infection. Contaminated waste products, soiled linen, and improperly sterilized equipment are all means by which microorganisms can travel. Not every patient will come in contact with these items; however, the health care professional is in constant contact with patients and is therefore a constant threat to spread infection. *Microorganisms are most commonly spread by way of the hands; therefore hand washing before and after each patient is the most effective means of controlling the spread of microorganisms.* Disinfectants, antiseptics, and germicides are used in many hand-washing liquids to kill microorganisms.

5. (A) Standard precautions treats *all* body fluids and substances as infectious. Its use prevents the spread of microorganisms to other patients and protects the radiographer from contamination. Body fluids and substances that may be considered infectious include blood, breast milk, vaginal secretions, amniotic fluid, semen, peritoneal fluid, synovial fluid, cerebrospinal fluid, feces, urine, secretions from the nasal and oral cavities, and secretions from the lacrimal and sweat glands.

 Sterilization (surgical asepsis) refers to the removal of all microorganisms and their spores (reproductive cells) and is practiced in the surgical suite. The destruction of pathogenic microorganisms is the process of *disinfection* (medical asepsis). Examples of disinfectants are hydrogen peroxide, chlorine, and boric acid.

6. (A) *Antisepsis* retards the growth of pathogenic bacteria. Alcohol is an example of an antiseptic. *Medical asepsis* refers to the destruction of pathogenic microorganisms through the process of *disinfection.* Examples of disinfectants are hydrogen peroxide, chlorine, and boric acid. *Surgical asepsis (sterilization)* refers to the removal of all microorganisms *and* their spores (reproductive cells) and is practiced in the surgical suite. *Bacteriogenesis* refers to the formation of bacteria.

7. (B) A*irborne precaution* is employed with patients suspected or known to be infected with the tubercle bacillus (TB), chickenpox (varicella) and measles (rubeola). Airborne precaution requires the patient to wear a mask to avoid the spread of acid-fast bacilli (in bronchial secretions) and other pathogens during coughing. If the patient is unable or unwilling to wear a mask, the radiographer must wear one. An N95 Particulate Respirator is the mask required for health care workers. The radiographer should wear gloves, but a gown is required only if flagrant contamination is likely. Patients with airborne precautions require a private, specially ventilated (negative pressure) room (see Table 3–1).

A private room is indicated for all patients on *droplet precaution,* that is, diseases transmitted via large droplets expelled from the patient while speaking, sneezing, or coughing. The pathogenic droplets can infect others when they come in contact with mouth or nasal mucosa or conjunctiva. Rubella ("German measles"), mumps, and influenza are among the diseases spread by droplet contact; a private room is required for the patient, and health care practitioners must wear a mask.

8. (B) When performing bedside radiography in an isolation room, the radiographer should wear a gown, gloves, and mask. The cassettes are prepared for the examination by placing a pillowcase over them to protect them from contamination. Whenever possible, one person should manipulate the mobile unit and remain "clean," while the other handles the patient. The mobile unit should be cleaned with a disinfectant before exiting the patient's room.

9. (C) Lyme disease is a condition that results from transmission of an infection by a vector (deer tick). *Vectors* are insects and animals carrying disease. *Droplet contact* involves contact with secretions (from the nose, mouth) that travel via a sneeze or cough. *Airborne* route involves evaporated droplets in the air that transfer disease.

10. (D) *Protective, or reverse, isolation is used to keep the susceptible patient from becoming infected.* Burn patients who have lost their means of protection (their skin) have increased susceptibility to bacterial invasion. Patients whose immune systems are compromised (eg: transplant recipients, leukemia) are unable to combat infection and are more susceptible to infection. These patients are treated with strict isolation technique, taking care to protect the *patient* from contamination.

Patient Monitoring

I. ROUTINE MONITORING

Routine monitoring of patient condition, physical signs, and *vital signs* were discussed in Chapter 2.

In review, obtaining *vital signs* involves the measurement of *body temperature, pulse rate, respiratory rate, and arterial blood pressure.* Elevated body temperature, or *fever*, often signifies infection. Symptoms malaise, increased pulse and respiratory rates, flushed, hot and dry skin, and occasional chills.

Normal body temperature varies from person to person depending on several factors, including age. Normal adult body temperature taken orally is 98.6°F (37°C). *Rectal* temperature is generally 0.5° to 1.0° *higher*, whereas *axillary* temperature is usually 0.5° to 1.0° *lower*. Slight variation of 0.5° to 1.0° is generally considered within normal limits. Body temperature is usually lowest in the early morning and highest at night. Infants up to 3 years of age have normal body temperatures of between 99° and 99.7°F. Children ages 5 to 13 years have a normal range of 97.8° to 98.6°F.

Superficial arteries are best suited for determination of *pulse rate*. The five most easily palpated pulse points are the radial, carotid, temporal, femoral, and popliteal pulse. The radial pulse is the most frequently used. The apical pulse, at the apex of the heart, can be evaluated with the use of a stethoscope.

Respirations should be counted after counting the pulse rate, while still holding the patient's wrist. *The normal respiratory rate is 12 to 18 breaths per minute.* The respiratory rate of young children is higher, up to 30 breaths per minute. While the radiographer is counting respirations, he or she should be assessing the respiratory pattern (even, uneven) and depth (normal, shallow, deep) as well.

Blood pressure within vessels is greatest during ventricular *systole* (contraction) and lowest during *diastole* (relaxation). Blood pressure is recorded with the systolic pressure on top and the diastolic pressure on the bottom, as in 100/80 (read: "one hundred over eighty"). Normal adult systolic pressure ranges between 100 and 140 mm Hg; the normal diastolic range is between 60 and 90 mm Hg. Blood pressure consistently above 140/90 is considered *hypertension*.

47

The radiographer should be alert to the patient's appearance and condition, and any subsequent changes in them, such as changes in the color, temperature, and moistness of the patient's skin. Paleness can indicate weakness; the *diaphoretic* patient has pale, cool skin; *fever* is frequently accompanied by hot, dry skin; "sweaty" palms may indicate *anxiety,* a patient who is *cyanotic* (bluish lips, mucous membranes, nail beds) needs oxygen and requires immediate attention.

II. PATIENT SUPPORT EQUIPMENT

One of a human being's most basic physiologic needs is an adequate supply of oxygen. Diminished oxygen supply *(hypoxia)* can result from an airway obstructed by *aspirated* material, laryngeal edema as a result of *anaphylaxis*, or a pathologic process such as *emphysema*. The radiographer must be knowledgeable enough to recognize symptoms and respond appropriately. The proper response to respiratory distress might be to perform the *Heimlich maneuver,* to summon the code team, or to check the flow of oxygen already in place.

Oxygen is taken into the body and supplied to the blood to be delivered to all body tissues. Any tissue(s) lacking in, or devoid of, an adequate blood supply can suffer permanent damage or die. Oxygen may be required in cases of severe anemia, pneumonia, pulmonary edema, and shock.

Symptoms of inadequate oxygen supply include *dyspnea, cyanosis, diaphoresis,* and distention of the veins of the neck. The patient who experiences any of these symptoms will be very anxious and must not be left unattended. The radiographer must *call* for help, assist the patient to a sitting or semi-*Fowler's position* (the recumbent position makes breathing more difficult), and have oxygen and emergency drugs available.

In areas that patients will occupy for extended periods (eg, patient rooms, operating room, emergency room, and radiology department), oxygen is available through wall outlets at a pressure of 60 to 80 psi (pounds per square inch) equipped with an easily adjustable flowmeter to regulate the administration of oxygen. It is important to administer *humidified* oxygen to avoid drying and irritation of the respiratory mucosa. In other areas, oxygen will be available in tanks having one valve to regulate its flow and another to indicate the amount of oxygen remaining in the tank.

There are various devices available to deliver oxygen to the patient. Their use is determined by the amount of oxygen required by the patient. They are frequently classified as *low* or *high flow*.

The *nasal cannula* is the most frequently used device and is used to supplement the oxygen in room air. The nasal cannula is a low-flow oxygen device. It is convenient and fairly comfortable for the patient, although it can be somewhat easily moved out of position, during sleep for example.

There are various types of oxygen *masks* available for delivery of oxygen. The *simple face mask* (low-flow) is best suited for short-term oxygen therapy. With extended use, the plastic becomes warm and sticky. Communication is difficult, the mask is easily displaced, and it must be removed at mealtime. The *partial rebreathing mask* (low-flow) and *nonrebreathing mask* (low-flow) deliver more precise concentrations of oxygen to the patient.

Mechanical ventilators (high-flow) are most frequently encountered in a hospital critical care unit. Patients on ventilators have an artificial airway in place, while the ventilator controls the respiratory rate and volume.

Although oxygen is not a flammable substance, it does support combustion, so care must be taken to avoid spark or flame where oxygen is in use.

The use of a *suction* device is occasionally required to maintain a patient's airway by *aspirating* secretions, blood, or other fluids when the patient is unconscious or otherwise unable to do so. Suction is available from a wall outlet, similar to oxygen, or as a mobile apparatus. It is unlikely that the radiographer would be required to suction a patient, but he or she might be needed to assist with the procedure. Suction tubing must have a disposable catheter attached to its end for collection of airway secretions. The radiographer should be familiar with the location of suction equipment and replacement disposable catheters.

Intravenous equipment includes needles, syringes, fluids such as normal saline or D5W (a solution of 5% dextrose in water), IV catheters, heparin locks, IV poles, and infusion sets.

The diameter of a needle is identified as its *gauge*. As the diameter of its *bore* increases, the gauge decreases. Hence, an 18-gauge needle has a larger diameter bore than a 23-gauge needle. Hypodermic needles are generally used for phlebotomy, while butterflies and IV catheters are used more frequently for injections such as contrast media. If an *infusion* injection is required, an IV catheter is generally preferred. The *hub* of the hypodermic needle is attached to a syringe, while the hub of the butterfly tubing or IV catheter may be attached to a syringe or an IV bottle or bag via an IV infusion set.

Medication or contrast material is often mixed with normal saline or D5W. Some intravenous medications are given at intervals through an established heparin lock. A *heparin lock* consists of a venous catheter established for a certain length of time to make a vein available for medications that have to be administered at frequent intervals. This helps prevent the formation of scarred, sclerotic veins as a result of frequent injections at the same site.

The IV bottle or bag should be hung 18 to 24 inches *above the level of the vein*. If placed lower than the vein, the solution will stop flowing and blood will return into the tubing. If hung too high, the solution can run too fast. Occasionally, the position of the needle or catheter in the vein will affect the flow rate. If the bevel is adjacent to the vessel wall, flow may decrease or stop altogether. Often, just changing the position of the patient's arm will remedy the situation.

Extravasation occurs when medication or contrast medium is introduced into the tissues surrounding a vein rather than into the vein itself. It can occur when the patient's veins are particularly deep or small. The needle should be removed, pressure applied to prevent formation of a *hematoma,* and *warm moist heat* applied to relieve pain.

The *antecubital* vein is the most commonly used injection site for contrast medium administration. It is not used for infusions that take longer than 1 hour due to its location at the bend of the elbow. The *basilic* vein, located on the dorsal surface of the hand, is used when the antecubital vein is inaccessible. The *cephalic* vein may also be used. Strict aseptic technique must be used for all intravenous injections.

Following thoracic surgery, *chest tubes* may be put in place for the purpose of removing air and/or fluid from the pleural space. The chest drainage system usually has three compartments; one is the suction control chamber, another is the collection chamber, and the third is the water seal chamber, which prevents atmospheric air from entering the chest cavity. The drainage system must always be kept below the level of the patient's chest. Radiographers might encounter chest drainage systems when performing mobile radiographic examinations on postsurgical patients. The radiographer must be careful not to disturb the chest tubes during patient or equipment manipulation.

Nasogastric (NG) and *nasointestinal* (NI) *tubes* are frequently employed following digestive tract surgery to remove gastric fluids and air. NG and NI tubes may be single or double *lumen* and can sometimes be temporarily disconnected for radiographic exams. The single-lumen NG or NI tube can be clamped, but the double-lumen tube must never be clamped. If clamped, the walls of the double-lumen tube could adhere permanently. Instead, the tip of a syringe is inserted into the lumen and the syringe and tube then pinned (open side up) to the patient's gown. Care must be taken not to disturb the placement of the NG or NI tube.

Urinary catheterization may be employed postsurgically to assist in the healing of tissues or to assist the incontinent patient in the elimination of urine. It is essential that equipment used for the catheterization procedure is sterile, and that subsequent care is given to the catheterized patient to prevent infection, as *urinary tract infections (UTIs) account for the greatest number of nosocomial infections.* Urinary catheters are made of plastic, rubber, PVC (polyvinylchloride), and silicone. The type selected is dependent on how long it is expected to remain in the bladder. Plastic and rubber are generally employed for short-term use, while PVC or silicone catheters can be in place for up to 3 months. The urine collection bag must be kept below the level of the bladder; backflow of urine into the bladder can lead to infection. When transporting or transferring the catheterized patient, care must be taken that the catheter does not become entangled or dislodged.

II. MEDICAL AND LIFE-THREATENING EMERGENCIES

The importance of the radiographer's careful evaluation of his or her patient is never more obvious than when an emergency arises. An emergency is defined as *a sudden change in a patient's condition requiring immediate medical intervention.* Most patients arrive in the radiology department in a stable condition; a few arrive for diagnostic evaluation of a medical crisis. The radiographer must note the patient's condition on arrival and be alert to any subsequent sudden change in that condition. The value of continual review of the knowledge and skills required for emergency situations cannot be overemphasized. Many of these emergencies can occur with little or no warning. Many can be life-threatening if not dealt with immediately and correctly.

A. VOMITING

Vomiting patients who are seated or standing should be provided with a basin, tissues, and water for rinsing their mouth. It is essential that the recumbent patient have his or her head turned to the side to prevent choking from aspiration of vomitus. A patient who reports feeling nauseous is often apprehensive and may get some relief by breathing slowly and deeply through his or her mouth.

B. FRACTURES

An *unsplinted* fracture must be moved with great care, with *areas proximal and distal to the fracture site adequately supported.* Any motion is very painful and can result in further injury to tissues surrounding the fracture. Muscle spasm can cause additional pain and can interfere with proper reduction of the fracture. A *splint* should never be removed from an extremity except by or under the direct supervision of the physician. Some splinting devices are not radiolucent and removal may be required before the radiographic examination.

Rib fractures may be associated with lung trauma, and sternum fractures with heart lacerations. Rib fractures can be very painful— the patient experiences pain just from breathing. *Pelvic* fractures are often associated with injuries to pelvic and abdominal viscera, and extreme care must be taken to avoid *hemorrhage.*

C. SPINAL INJURIES

Patients arriving for radiographic evaluation with possible spinal injuries must not be moved. The position of any sandbags or other supportive mechanisms must not be changed. A *horizontal (cross-table) lateral projection* should be evaluated by the physician first to determine the extent of injury and necessity for further radiographs. If the patient must be placed in a lateral position, the logrolling method is usually advised. *A physician must be present whenever the patient's position is changed.*

D. EPISTAXIS

A nosebleed *(epistaxis)* may be a result of any one of many causes, including *hypertension,* dry nasal mucous membranes, sinusitis, or trauma. The patient should be seated or in a Fowler's position. The radiographer should place cold cloths over the patient's nose and back of the neck. Compressing the sides of the nose against the nasal septum for 6 to 8 minutes is also helpful. Continued hemorrhage should be brought to the attention of the physician, because cautery or nasal packs might be required.

E. POSTURAL HYPOTENSION

Orthostatic, or postural, *hypotension* is a decrease in blood pressure that occurs on rising to the erect position. It can be severe enough to cause fainting in individuals who have been confined to bed for several days. The radiographer should assist patients slowly and be watchful for signs of weakness.

F. VERTIGO

Objective vertigo is the sensation of having *objects* (or "the room") spinning about the person; *subjective* vertigo is the sensation of the *person* spinning about. It is usually associated with an inner-ear disturbance. Patients experiencing true vertigo (as opposed to dizziness or lightheadedness) are often very nauseous and must be protected from falls by the use of side rails and/or safety belts.

G. Syncope

A patient who reports feeling dizzy or faint should be immediately assisted to a chair. Bending forward and placing the head between the knees will often help relieve the lightheadedness as blood flow to the brain increases. In more severe cases, a patient who cannot be assisted to a chair should be *lowered to a recumbent position*. Elevation of the lower legs or use of the Trendelenburg position is helpful. If the patient loses consciousness, the radiographer should make certain that the airway is open and that clothing, especially at the collar, is loose. Once the patient is recumbent, recovery is usually swift; however, a physician should be notified and the cause of *syncope* identified.

H. Convulsion

Involuntary muscular contractions and relaxations, often associated with epilepsy, characterize a *convulsion*. *Febrile* convulsions are associated with fever, especially in children. During convulsion, no attempt must be made to restrain the patient's movements. The radiographer's responsibility is to keep the patient from injuring himself or herself. Tight clothing can be loosened and objects that could harm the patient should be moved out of the way. A padded tongue blade or other suitable object should be placed between the patient's teeth to prevent biting the tongue.

I. Unconsciousness

The unconscious patient is unaware of and unresponsive to his or her surroundings. Unconsciousness can be caused by a wide variety of conditions including insulin overdose, uremia, concussion, heat *stroke,* and intoxication.

There are various levels of consciousness and the condition of an acutely ill patient can rapidly deteriorate from being fully aware and responsive, to diminished or inappropriate responsiveness, to complete unresponsiveness. The unconscious patient must never be left unattended. The radiographer must be alert to changes in the patient's level of consciousness and notify the physician immediately of any deterioration.

J. Acute Abdomen

Patients arriving for radiographic evaluation having a diagnosis of "acute abdomen" are usually suffering severe abdominal pain, are nauseous and vomiting, and are frequently close to being in shock. These are indeed very sick patients. The radiographer must perform the examination swiftly and efficiently and remain alert for any sudden changes in patient condition.

K. Shock

Shock is a general term and is characterized by diminished peripheral blood flow and insufficient oxygen supply to body tissues. Shock can be caused by a number of conditions including allergic reaction, trauma, hemorrhage, myocardial infarction, and infection. The patient is pale and may become cyanotic; the pulse is rapid and weak, breathing is shallow and rapid, and blood pressure drops sharply. The radiographer should keep the patient warm and flat, or in the Trendelenburg position, and be prepared to assist with emergency procedures.

L. Seizure

The type of *seizure* known as *petit mal* is so subtle as to go unnoticed by the patient and observer. It is characterized by brief loss of consciousness (10 to 30 seconds) and accompanied by eye or muscle fluttering. A *grand mal* seizure is characterized by loss of consciousness and falling, followed by generalized muscle spasms. The radiographer should remove any objects in the area that could harm the patient and loosen any tight clothing. The patient's head should be turned to the side to allow any secretions to flow from the mouth. A padded tongue blade should be placed between the patient's teeth to help avoid biting the tongue.

M. Respiratory Failure

The inability of the lungs to perform ventilating functions is respiratory distress and may be described as *acute* or *chronic*. Acute respiratory distress can be due to impaired gas exchange processes (requiring positive-pressure ventilation) or airway obstruction (requiring the Heimlich maneuver). Chronic respiratory failure is a result of a disease process that impairs breathing, such as emphysema, bronchitis, *asthma,* or cystic fibrosis.

   The radiographer should be able to distinguish between respiratory arrest (absence of chest movement and breathing sounds) and cardiopulmonary arrest (absence of pulse and respiration with loss of consciousness) and be able to initiate life-saving actions.

N. Cardiopulmonary Arrest

The *sudden cessation of productive ventilation and circulation* is called cardiopulmonary arrest. The radiographer should be trained in the ABCs (airway, breathing, and circulation) of cardiopulmonary resuscitation (CPR) and be able to initiate the appropriate care until the arrival of the emergency team.

   Many health care facilities require their employees to be certified in basic life saving (BLS) skills. It is wise for radiographers to be familiar with skills such as the Heimlich maneuver (abdominal thrust) and CPR should the need arise.

O. Stroke

A *stroke,* or cerebrovascular accident *(CVA),* is an interference with blood supplied to the brain as a result of occlusion or rupture of a cerebral vessel. If the condition results from a partial vessel occlusion, the interference is usually mild and temporary and is referred to as a *transient ischemic attack (TIA).* The patient may experience temporary blindness in one eye, *dysphasia* or *aphasia, hemiparesis* or hemiplegia, or anesthesia.

   If the cerebral vessel is totally occluded or ruptures into the brain or subarachnoid space, a much more serious event has occurred. The patient frequently experiences sudden loss of consciousness and one-sided paralysis (*hemiparesis*), although the onset can be slower if the *occlusion* is caused by *thrombus* formation. Other symptoms include speech disturbances and cool, sweaty skin. The patient should have his or her head and shoulders elevated or be in the lateral recumbent position; an open airway must be maintained. Because a stroke can occur without warning at any time, the radiographer should be familiar with the signs of an impending stroke and be able to provide appropriate immediate care.

Summary

- Symptoms of inadequate oxygen supply include dyspnea, cyanosis, diaphoresis, and neck vein distention.
- Seated or semi-Fowler's positions are most helpful for the dyspneic patient.
- Oxygen is usually available through wall outlets with adjustable flowmeters, or in tanks having a flow-regulation valve and an indicator showing the quantity of oxygen left in the tank.
- Oxygen can be administered via nasal cannula, masks, or mechanical ventilators.
- Oxygen supports combustion so it must be used away from flame.
- Suction devices are used for aspiration of secretions; suction is available from wall outlets or portable suction mechanisms.
- Needle size is indicated by gauge; larger gauge = smaller needle bore.
- Butterfly sets or IV catheters are generally used for IV injection of a contrast medium.
- A heparin lock makes a vein accessible for medications administered at frequent intervals.
- IV solutions should be elevated 18 to 24 inches above the injection site.
- The antecubital vein is generally used for injection of contrast material.
- Chest tubes function to remove fluids or air from the thoracic cavity.
- NG and NI tubes assist in the removal of gastric secretions or air following GI surgery and/or for the administration of water-soluble contrast material.
- Urinary collection bags must be kept below the level of the bladder; to prevent UTIs, catheterization procedures must be sterile.
- It is essential that the radiographer be alert for any sudden changes in patient condition; how well the radiographer recognizes and is prepared to meet the challenges of emergency situations can largely determine the outcome of the emergency.

Chapter Exercises

 Congratulations! *You have completed your review of this chapter. If you are able to answer the following group of comprehensive questions, you can feel confident that you have mastered this section. You are then ready to go on to "Registry-type" questions that follow. For greatest success, do not go to these multiple choice questions without first completing the short answer questions below.*

1. Identify illnesses and conditions that might require supplemental oxygen *(p. 48)*.

2. List the subjective symptoms of inadequate oxygen; identify the body position frequently helpful for the dyspneic patient *(p. 48)*.

3. Describe four methods of oxygen therapy and identify when each might be indicated *(pp. 48, 49)*.

4. Identify any hazards involved in the use of oxygen *(p. 49)*.

5. Describe the circumstance(s) in which suction might be required; identify types of suction devices available *(p. 49)*.

6. Identify how needle bore changes with increasing gauge *(p. 49)*.

7. Describe the function and uses of a heparin lock *(p. 49)*.

8. Identify the height at which IV bottles and bags should be hung *(p. 49)*.

9. Explain how contrast medium extravasation should be treated *(p. 49)*.

10. Identify the vein(s) frequently used for introduction of contrast medium *(p. 49)*.

11. Explain the function of chest tubes and precautions that should be taken by the radiographer *(p. 50)*.

12. Describe the function of NG and NI tubes and any precautions that should be taken by the radiographer *(p. 50)*.

13. Describe the function of urinary catheters and any precautions that should be taken by the radiographer *(p. 50)*.

14. Identify the level at which urinary collection bags should be kept *(p. 50)*.

15. Discuss the importance of observing initial patient condition and any subsequent changes *(p. 50)*.

16. Describe care provided to the nauseous or vomiting patient; identify the body position required for the recumbent patient *(pp. 50, 51)*.

17. Describe precautions the radiographer should take when examining a patient with a fracture *(p. 51)*.

18. Discuss precautions that should be taken with patients having suspected spinal injuries *(p. 51)*.

19. Describe first aid for epistaxis *(p. 51)*.

20. Distinguish between postural hypotension, vertigo, and syncope; discuss precautions taken and care given by the radiographer *(pp. 51, 52)*.

21. Describe any precautions that should be taken with the unconscious patient *(p. 52)*.

22. Describe symptoms of acute abdomen and shock; indicate any precautions that should be taken by the radiographer *(pp. 52, 53)*.

23. Distinguish between grand mal and petit mal seizures; discuss the care appropriate for a patient experiencing a grand mal seizure *(p. 53)*.

24. Distinguish between respiratory arrest and cardiopulmonary arrest; discuss the responses appropriate to the radiographer *(p. 53)*.

25. Describe "stroke," to include some symptoms and responses appropriate for the radiographer *(pp. 53, 54)*.

Chapter Review Questions

1. Which of the following is/are symptoms of inadequate oxygen supply?
    1. diaphoresis
    2. cyanosis
    3. dyspnea
   (A) 1 only
   (B) 1 and 2 only
   (C) 2 and 3 only
   (D) 1, 2, and 3

2. A patient's IV bottle or bag should be hung:
   (A) 8 to 24 inches above the vein
   (B) 8 to 24 inches below the vein
   (C) 8 to 24 inches above the heart
   (D) 8 to 24 inches below the heart

3. Which of the following gauge needles has the largest bore?
   (A) 12
   (B) 18
   (C) 20
   (D) 23

4. Proper treatment for contrast media extravasation into tissues around a vein includes:
      1. application of cold wet towel to affected area
      2. application of moist heat to affected area
      3. application of pressure to injection site
   (A) 1 only
   (B) 2 only
   (C) 1 and 2 only
   (D) 2 and 3 only

5. What is the most frequently used site for intravenous injection of contrast agents?
   (A) basilic vein
   (B) cephalic vein
   (C) antecubital vein
   (D) femoral vein

6. What precaution should be taken with a vomiting patient?
   (A) place the patient in the Trendelenburg position
   (B) place the patient in Fowler's position
   (C) turn the patient's head to the side
   (D) turn the patient prone

7. A decrease in blood pressure which occurs on suddenly arising from the recumbent position is called:
   (A) orthostatic hypotension
   (B) epistaxis
   (C) vertigo
   (D) syncope

8. What is the correct response by the radiographer when a patient suffers a convulsion?
      1. gently restrain the patient
      2. keep the patient from injuring himself
      3. loosen tight clothing
   (A) 1 only
   (B) 1 and 2 only
   (C) 2 and 3 only
   (D) 1, 2, and 3

9. A patient's feeling of spinning, or the room spinning about him, is called:
   (A) orthostatic hypotension
   (B) epistaxis
   (C) vertigo
   (D) syncope

10. All of the following statements are true, *except:*
    (A) A heparin lock makes a vein accessible for medications administered at frequent intervals.
    (B) Aseptic technique is employed for catheterization of the urinary bladder.
    (C) Oxygen may be administered via nasal cannula, masks, and mechanical ventilators.
    (D) Oxygen supports combustion so it must be used away from flame.

Answers and Explanations

1. (D) Symptoms of inadequate oxygen supply include dyspnea, *cyanosis, diaphoresis,* and distention of the veins of the neck. The patient who experiences some or all of these symptoms will be very anxious and must not be left unattended. The radiographer must *call* for help, assist the patient to a sitting or semi-Fowler's position (the recumbent position makes breathing more difficult), and have oxygen and emergency drugs available.

2. (A) The IV bottle or bag should be hung 18 to 24 inches *above the level of the vein.* If placed lower than the vein, solution will stop flowing and blood will return into the tubing. If hung too high, solution can run too fast. Occasionally, the position of the needle or catheter in the vein will affect the flow rate. If the bevel is adjacent to the vessel wall, flow may decrease or stop altogether. Usually just changing the position of the patient's arm will remedy the situation.

3. (D) The diameter of a needle is identified as its *gauge.* As the diameter of its *bore* decreases the *gauge* increases. Hence, a 23-gauge needle has a smaller diameter bore than an 18-gauge needle. Hypodermic needles are generally used for phlebotomy (ie, blood samples), while butterflies and IV catheters are used more frequently for injections such as contrast media. If an infusion injection is required, an IV catheter is generally preferred. The hub of the hypodermic needle is attached to a syringe, while the hub of the butterfly tubing or IV catheter may be attached to a syringe or an IV bottle or bag via an IV infusion set.

4. (D) *Extravasation* occurs when medication or contrast medium is introduced into the tissues surrounding a vein rather than into the vein itself. It can occur when the patient's veins are particularly deep or small. The needle should be removed, pressure applied to prevent formation of a hematoma, and warm moist heat applied to relieve pain.

5. (C) The *antecubital* vein is the most commonly used injection site for contrast medium administration. It is not used for infusions that take longer than 1 hour because of its location at the bend of the elbow. The basilic vein, located on the dorsal surface of the hand, is used when the antecubital vein is inaccessible. The cephalic vein may also be used. Strict aseptic technique must be used for all intravenous injections.

6. (C) Patients who are seated or standing should be provided with a basin, tissues, and water for rinsing their mouth. It is essential that the recumbent patient have his or her head turned to the side to prevent choking from aspiration of vomitus. A patient who reports feeling nauseous is often apprehensive, as well, and may get some relief by breathing slowly and deeply through his or her mouth.

7. (A) *Orthostatic, or postural, hypotension* is a decrease in blood pressure that occurs on rising to the erect position. It can be severe enough to cause fainting in individuals who have been confined to bed for several days. A nosebleed (*epistaxis*) may be a result of any one of many causes, including hypertension, dry nasal mucous membranes, sinusitis, or trauma. The patient should be seated or placed in a Fowler's position. The radiographer should place cold cloths over the patient's nose and back of the neck. *Vertigo* is an individual's sensation of spinning, or the room spinning about. It is often associated with an inner-ear disturbance. Patients experiencing true vertigo are often very nauseous. A patient who reports feeling dizzy or faint should be immediately assisted to a chair; bending forward and placing the head between the knees will often. In more severe cases, *a patient who cannot be assisted to a chair should be lowered to a recumbent position.* Elevation of the lower legs, or use of the Trendelenburg position, is helpful.

8. (C) Involuntary muscular contractions and relaxations, often associated with epilepsy, characterize a *convulsion*. No attempt must be made to restrain the patient's movements. The radiographer's responsibility here is to keep the patient from injury. Tight clothing may be loosened and objects that could harm the patient should be moved out of the way. A padded tongue blade or other suitable object should be placed between the patient's teeth to prevent biting the tongue.

9. (C) *Objective vertigo* is the sensation of having *objects* (or "the room") spinning about the person; *subjective vertigo* is the sensation of the *person* spinning about. It is often associated with an inner-ear disturbance. Patients experiencing true vertigo (as opposed to dizziness or lightheadedness) are often very nauseous and must be protected from falls. A patient who reports feeling dizzy or faint (*syncope*) should be immediately assisted to a chair. Bending forward and placing the head between the knees will often help relieve the lightheadedness as blood flow to the brain increases. In more severe cases, *a patient who cannot be assisted to a chair should be lowered to a recumbent position.* Elevation of the lower legs, or use of the Trendelenburg position, is helpful. *Orthostatic, or postural, hypotension* is a decrease in blood pressure that occurs on rising to the erect position. It can be severe enough to cause fainting in individuals who have been confined to bed for several days. A nosebleed (epistaxis) may be a result of any one of many causes, including hypertension, dry nasal mucous membranes, sinusitis, or trauma. The patient should be seated or placed in a Fowler's position. The radiographer should place cold cloths over the patient's nose and back of the neck.

10. (B) Some intravenous medications are given at intervals through an established heparin lock. A *heparin lock* consists of a venous catheter established for a certain length of time to make a vein available for medications having to be administered at frequent intervals. This helps prevent the formation of scarred, sclerotic veins as a result of frequent injections at the same site.

It is essential that equipment used for urinary catheterization procedures be *sterile,* and that subsequent care of the catheterized patient prevent infection, as UTIs account for the greatest number of nosocomial infections.

Although oxygen is not a flammable substance, it does support combustion, so care must be taken to avoid spark or flame where oxygen is in use. There are various devices available to deliver oxygen to the patient; their use is determined by the amount of oxygen required by the patient. They are frequently classified as *low* or *high flow.*

Contrast Media

5

I. CHARACTERISTICS AND NOMENCLATURE

Although radiographic contrast media are usually administered orally or intravenously, there are a number of *routes* and methods of drug administration (see Table 5–1). Drugs and medications may be administered either *orally* or *parenterally*. *Parenteral* refers to any route other than via the digestive tract and includes *topical, subcutaneous, intradermal, intramuscular, intravenous,* and *intrathecal*.

The purpose of a *contrast medium* is to artificially increase subject contrast in body tissues and areas where there is little natural subject contrast. The abdominal viscera, for example, have very little subject contrast; that is, it is very difficult to identify specific organs or distinguish one organ from another. However, if a contrast agent is introduced into a particular organ such as the kidney or stomach, or into a vessel such as the aorta or one of its branches, we may more readily visualize these anatomic structures and/or evaluate physiologic activity.

Contrast media or *contrast agents* can be described as either positive (radiopaque) or negative (radiolucent). *Positive,* or *radiopaque,* contrast agents have a higher atomic number than the surrounding soft tissue, resulting in a greater attenuation or absorption of x-ray photons. They therefore produce higher radiographic contrast. Examples of positive contrast media are *iodinated agents* (both water and oil-based) and *barium sulfate* suspensions. The inert characteristics of barium sulfate render it the least *toxic* contrast medium. On the other hand, iodinated contrast media have characteristics that increase their likelihood of producing *side effects* and reactions.

Negative, or *radiolucent, contrast agents* used are *air* and various *gases*. Because the atomic number of air is also quite different from that of soft tissue, high subject contrast is produced. Carbon dioxide is absorbed more rapidly by the body than air.

Negative contrast is often used *with* positive contrast in examinations termed *double-contrast studies*. The function of the positive agent is usually to *coat* the various parts under study, while the air *fills* the space and permits visualization through the gaseous medium.

Methods of Administration

<u>Oral</u>
PO (by mouth), through digestive system
<u>Parenteral</u>
topical
subcutaneous
intradermal
intramuscular
intravenous
intrathecal

Qualities of Iodinated Contrast Agents that Contribute to Discomfort, Side Effects, and Reactions

Viscosity More viscid (thick, sticky) agents are more difficult to inject and produce more heat and vessel irritation; the higher the concentration, the greater the viscosity.

Toxicity Potential toxicity is greater with higher-concentration agents and ionic agents; viscosity also increases as room temperature decreases.

Miscibility Contrast agents should be readily miscible (able to mix) with blood.

Osmolality Low-osmolality agents have a fewer number of particles in a given amount of solution and are less likely to provoke an allergic reaction.

TABLE 5–1. COMMON MEDICATIONS AND THEIR APPLICATION

TYPE	EFFECT	EXAMPLE
Adrenergic	Vasopressor, stimulates sympathetic nervous system: increases BP, relaxes smooth muscle of respiratory system	Epinephrine (Adrenalin)
Analgesic	Relieves pain	Aspirin, acetaminophen (Tylenol), codeine, meperidine (Demerol)
Antiarrhythmic	Relieves cardiac arrythmia	Quinidine sulfate, lidocaine (Xylocaine)
Antibacterial	Stops growth of bacteria	Penicillin, tetracycline, erythromycin
Anticholinergic	Depresses parasympathetic system	Atropine, scopolamine, belladonna
Anticoagulant	Inhibits blood clotting; keeps IV lines and catheters free of clots	Heparin, warfarin
Antihistamine	Relieves allergic symptoms	Diphenhydramine hydrochloride (Benadryl)
Antipyretic	Reduces fever	Aspirin, acetaminophen
Barbiturate	Depresses CNS, decreases BP and respiration, induces sleep	Phenobarbital, secobarbital sodium (Seconal)
Cardiac stimulant	Increases cardiac output	Digitalis
Cathartic	Laxative, relieves constipation, prepares colon for diagnostic tests	Bisacodyl (Dulcolax), castor oil
Diuretic	Stimulates urine	Furosemide (Lasix)
Emetic	Stimulates vomiting	Ipecac
Hypoglycemic	Lowers blood sugar	Insulin, chlorpropamide (Diabinese)
Narcotic	Sedative/analgesic; potentially addictive	Morphine, codeine, meperidine (Demerol)
Vasodilator	Relaxes and dilates blood vessels, decreases BP	Nitroglycerine, verapamil

BP, blood pressure; CNS, central nervous system.

Examinations that frequently use double-contrast technique are barium enema (BE), upper gastrointestinal (GI) series, and arthrography.

II. USES AND CONTRAINDICATIONS

Radiopaque contrast media are most frequently employed for radiographic procedures. *Barium sulfate* is one type of radiopaque contrast agent that is used to visualize the GI tract. Mixed with water, it forms a suspension that is usually administered orally for demonstration of the upper GI tract (esophagus, stomach, and progression through the small intestine), and rectally for demonstration of the lower GI tract (large intestine).

Barium sulfate is *contraindicated* if a *perforation* is suspected somewhere along the course of the GI tract (eg, a perforated diverticulum or gastric ulcer). Barium could escape into the peritoneal cavity and result in peritonitis. A water-soluble (absorbable) iodinated contrast medium is generally used instead of barium in these cases. The water-soluble preparations are available as ready-mixed liquid or as powder requiring appropriate dilution with water. A patient with a nasogastric (NG) tube can have the contrast medium administered through it for the purpose of locating and studying any site of obstruction. This procedure is called *enteroclysis.*

Patients can experience constipation following a GI or BE examination unless proper *aftercare instructions* are given to the patient upon completion of the examination. Barium preparations in the large bowel become thickened as a result of absorption of its fluid content, a process called *inspissation,* causing symptoms from mild constipation to bowel obstruction. Constipation can be a serious problem, particularly in the elderly, and fecal impaction or obstruction can result. It is essential that the radiographer provide clear instructions for follow-up care, especially to outpatients. Patients are usually advised to expect light-colored stools for the next few days, to drink plenty of fluids, to increase their intake of fiber, and to take a mild laxative such as milk of magnesia following a barium study.

Iodinated contrast agents are another type of radiopaque contrast media. They may be *oil base or water base.* Oil-base contrast media are infrequently used today. They are not water soluble, not readily absorbed by the body, and remain in body tissues for lengthy periods of time. Examinations that can employ the use of oil-base contrast agents, though infrequently performed, are lymphangiograms, sialograms, and bronchograms. Water-base contrast media may be *ionic* or *nonionic.* These agents are principally used to delineate the urinary and vascular systems, the gallbladder (GB), and the GI tract when barium sulfate is contraindicated.

Ionic contrast media have a *higher osmolality,* that is, a greater number of particles in a given amount of solution. *Nonionic,* or *low-osmolality,* contrast agents are used especially with children, the elderly, patients with renal disease, patients having a history of *allergic* reaction to contrast media, or patients having multiple allergies. Side effects and allergic reactions are less likely and less severe with these media. Nonionic contrast agents are associated with less injection discomfort, and a lower incidence of *nausea,* vomiting, and cardiovascular complications. Their only disadvantage is their cost, which is far greater than that of ionic contrast agents.

Iodinated contrast agents can become more *viscous* at normal room temperatures, making injection more difficult. Warming the contrast to body temperature, in a special warming oven, reduces *viscosity,* permitting an easier and more comfortable injection.

III. REACTIONS AND EMERGENCY SITUATIONS

Anaphylaxis can result from the body's sensitivity and allergic reaction to certain foods, insect bites, drugs, and anesthetics. The reaction can be the result of *ingestion, injection,* or *absorption* of the sensitizing agent.

Because iodinated contrast media are potentially toxic, the radiographer must be knowledgeable and alert to the possible adverse effects of their use (although the risk of a life-threatening reaction is relatively rare). Reactions to contrast media generally occur within 2 to 10 minutes following injection and can affect all body systems.

The body's response to the introduction of contrast material is the production of histamines, which brings about various symptoms. Symptoms of a *mild* reaction include a flushed appearance, nausea, a metallic taste in the mouth, nasal congestion, a few hives *(urticaria),* and, occasionally, vomiting. Treatment of these minor symptoms generally consists of administration of either an *antihistamine* such as diphenhydramine (Benadryl), which blocks the action of the histamine and reduces the body's inflammatory response, or epinephrine to raise the blood pressure and relax the bronchioles (see Table 5–1).

Potentially life-threatening responses include respiratory failure, shock, and death within minutes. A very serious and life-threatening response is an anaphylactic reaction. *Early* symptoms of an anaphylactic reaction include itching of the palms and soles, wheezing, constriction of the throat (possibly caused by laryngeal edema) *dyspnea, dysphagia, hypotension,* and *cardiopulmonary arrest.* The radiographer must maintain the patient's airway, summon the radiologist, and call a "code." The radiographer should then be prepared to stay with the patient and assist until the arrival of the code team.

The diabetic patient requires different and special attention. Metformin (Glucophage) is an antidiabetic agent indicated for the treatment of type II diabetes mellitus. Radiologic examinations requiring the use of intravascular iodinated contrast agents can lead to acute alteration of renal function and have been associated with lactic acidosis in patients taking metformin. The manufacturer recommends that patients taking metformin discontinue it at the time of or prior to the x-ray exam and withhold it for 48 more hours following the examination. The medication should be continued only after adequate renal function has been indicated by blood test (blood urea nitrogen [BUN], creatinine).

Summary

- **Drugs and medications may be administered orally or parenterally.**
- **Parenteral administration includes topical, oral, subcutaneous, intradermal, IM, IV, and intrathecal.**
- **Artificial contrast media function to increase insufficient subject contrast.**
- **Artificial contrast media can be positive (radiopaque) or negative (radiolucent).**
- **Positive contrast media include barium sulfate and iodinated (oil- or water-based) agents.**
- **Qualities of iodinated contrast media that contribute to its risk include viscosity, toxicity, and miscibility.**
- **Negative and positive contrast agents are often used together in "double-contrast" studies.**
- **Water-soluble (absorbable) contrast agents are used in place of barium sulfate when visceral perforation is suspected.**

- Patients require clear and complete postprocedural instructions, particularly following barium examinations.
- Nonionic iodinated contrast agents produce far fewer side effects than do their ionic counterparts; ionic contrast agents are far more expensive.
- Reactions to ionic agents usually occur within 2 to 10 minutes following injection.
- Symptoms of a mild reaction include mild urticaria, flushing, nausea, nasal congestion, metallic taste; an antihistamine is usually given to the patient.
- To avoid renal dysfunction, diabetic patients taking Metformin must discontinue its use for 48 hrs after administration of an intravascular contrast agent.

Chapter Exercises

 Congratulations! You have completed your review of this chapter. If you are able to answer the following group of comprehensive questions, you can feel confident that you have mastered this section. You are then ready to go on to "Registry-type" questions that follow. For greatest success, do not go to these multiple choice questions without first completing the short answer questions below.

1. Describe the difference between oral and parenteral drug administration; list five types of parenteral administration *(p. 61).*

2. Explain the purpose of contrast medium *(p. 61).*

3. Identify the two types of contrast media, describe their characteristics, and give examples of each *(pp. 61, 62).*

4. Describe the risks associated with iodinated contrast media and identify the type of iodinated media associated with less risk *(pp. 62, 63).*

5. Describe three qualities of iodinated contrast media that contribute to the production of side effects *(pp. 62, 63).*

6. Explain how double-contrast examinations can serve to better demonstrate certain anatomic parts *(p. 61).*

7. Describe contraindications to the use of barium sulfate; identify the alternative contrast medium *(p. 63).*

8. Explain the importance of aftercare explanations, especially following barium examinations *(p. 63).*

9. Distinguish between oil- and water-based iodinated contrast media, their uses, and their characteristics *(p. 63).*

10. Identify the basic difference between ionic and nonionic contrast media and identify when use of nonionic agents is indicated *(p. 63).*

11. Identify the major disadvantage of nonionic contrast media *(p. 63).*

12. Describe symptoms a patient having a mild reaction to iodinated contrast media might experience and their usual treatment *(p. 64).*

13. Describe the symptoms of a possible impending anaphylactic reaction and the radiographer's responsibilities *(p. 64).*

A&U Chapter Review Questions

1. Rapid onset of severe respiratory or cardiovascular symptoms after ingestion or injection of a drug, vaccine, contrast agent; or food; or after an insect bite, best describes:
   (A) rhinitis
   (B) myocardial infarct
   (C) anaphylaxis
   (D) asthma

2. Which of the following is used to relax the bronchioles and to treat anaphylactic reaction or cardiac arrest?
   (A) warfarin
   (B) hydrocortisone
   (C) epinephrine
   (D) nitroglycerin

3. Which of the following drugs is considered an anticoagulant?
   (A) warfarin
   (B) hydrocortisone
   (C) epinephrine
   (D) nitroglycerin

4. Parenteral administration of drugs may be performed:
   1. intrathecally
   2. intravenously
   3. orally
   (A) 1 only
   (B) 1 and 2 only
   (C) 3 only
   (D) 1, 2, and 3

5. That quality of a substance that renders it poisonous is referred to as its:
   (A) toxicity
   (B) miscibility
   (C) viscosity
   (D) osmolality

6. Symptoms of a mild reaction to contrast media include:
   1. few hives
   2. nausea
   3. flushed appearance
   (A) 1 only
   (B) 1 and 2 only
   (C) 1 and 3 only
   (D) 1, 2, and 3

7. Early symptoms of anaphylactic reaction include:
     1. sneezing
     2. dyspnea
     3. hypotension
   (A) 1 only
   (B) 1 and 2 only
   (C) 2 and 3 only
   (D) 1, 2, and 3

8. Which of the following is appropriate to administer for treatment of minor symptoms following intravenous injection of contrast media?
   (A) histamine
   (B) antihistamine
   (C) emetic
   (D) cathartic

9. Types of positive contrast agents include:
     1. barium sulfate suspension
     2. water-based iodinated media
     3. carbon dioxide
   (A) 1 only
   (B) 2 only
   (C) 1 and 2 only
   (D) 1 and 3 only

10. The advantages of using nonionic, water-soluble contrast media include:
     1. less patient discomfort
     2. low toxicity
     3. cost-containment benefits
   (A) 1 only
   (B) 1 and 2 only
   (C) 2 and 3 only
   (C) 1, 2, and 3

Answers and Explanations

1. (C) *Anaphylaxis* is an acute reaction characterized by sudden onset of urticaria, respiratory arrest, vascular collapse, or systemic shock, and sometimes leads to death. It is caused by ingestion or injection of a sensitizing agent such as a drug, vaccine, contrast agent, or food, or after an insect bite. *Asthma* and *rhinitis* are examples of allergic reactions. Myocardial infarct (heart attack) describes failure of the myocardium to receive adequate blood supply, usually as a result of an occluded vessel.

2. (C) *and* **3. (A)** *Epinephrine* (trade name Adrenalin) is a vasopressor (*vasoconstrictor*) used to treat cardiac dysrhythmia or arrest, anaphylactic reaction, or to relax the bronchioles. *Nitroglycerin* is a *vasodilator* used especially in angina pectoris. *Hydrocortisone* is a steroid that may be used to treat bronchial asthma, allergic reactions, and inflammatory reactions. *Warfarin* is an anticoagulant used to prevent diseases caused by venous thrombosis, for example myocardial infarction, and to help prevent systemic embolism in patients with atrial fibrillation.

4. (B) Although radiographic contrast media are usually administered orally or intravenously, there are a number of routes or methods of drug administration. Drugs and medications may be administered either *orally* or *parenterally*. *Parenteral* refers to any route other than via the digestive tract (orally) and includes: *topical, subcutaneous, intradermal, intramuscular, intravenous,* and *intrathecal.*

5. (A) A *toxic* substance is a poisonous substance. Contrast agents must have low toxicity. *Viscosity* refers to the degree of thickness or stickiness of a substance. More viscid contrast agents are more difficult to inject, and produce more heat and vessel irritation; the higher the agent's concentration, the greater its viscosity. *Miscibility* refers to the contrast agent's ability to mix with the blood. Contrast agents should be readily miscible. *Osmolality* refers to the number of particles in a given amount of solution. Low osmolality agents are less likely to provoke an allergic reaction.

6. (D) The body's response to the introduction of contrast material is the production of histamines, which brings about various symptoms. Symptoms of a mild reaction include a flushed appearance, nausea, a metallic taste in the mouth, nasal congestion, a few hives *(urticaria),* and occasionally vomiting. Treatment of these minor symptoms generally consists of administration of either an *antihistamine* such as diphenhydramine (Benadryl), which blocks the action of the histamine and reduces the body's inflammatory response, or epinephrine to raise the blood pressure and relax the bronchioles.

7. (A) Potentially life-threatening responses to contrast agents include respiratory failure, shock, and death within minutes. A very serious and life-threatening response is an *anaphylactic reaction* whose early symptoms include itching of the palms and soles, sneezing, and nausea. Constriction of the throat (possibly as a consequence of laryngeal edema), dyspnea, dysphagia, hypotension, and cardiopulmonary arrest may follow. The radiographer's responsibilities include maintaining the patient's airway, summoning the radiologist, and calling a "code." The radiographer should be prepared to stay with the patient and assist in any way possible until the arrival of the code team.

8. (B) Symptoms of a mild reaction include a flushed appearance, nausea, a metallic taste in the mouth, nasal congestion, a few hives *(urticaria),* and occasionally vomiting. Treatment of these minor symptoms generally consists of administration of either an *antihistamine* such as diphenhydramine (Benadryl), which blocks the action of *histamine* and reduces the body's inflammatory response, or epinephrine to raise the blood pressure and relax the bronchioles. An *emetic* is used to induce vomiting; a *cathartic* is a laxative.

9. (C) Contrast media may be described as either positive (radiopaque) or negative (radiolucent). *Positive,* or *radiopaque, contrast agents* have a higher atomic number than the surrounding soft tissue, resulting in a greater attenuation or absorption of x-ray photons, thereby producing a higher radiographic contrast. Examples of positive contrast media are iodinated agents (both water and oil based) and barium sulfate suspensions. *Negative,* or *radiolucent, contrast agents* used are air and various gases. Because the atomic number of air is also quite different from that of soft tissue, an artificially high subject contrast can be produced. The advantage of carbon dioxide over air is that it is absorbed more rapidly by the body.

10. (B) The low-osmolality and nonionic, water-soluble contrast agents available to radiology departments have outstanding advantages, particularly for patients with a history of allergic reaction. They were originally used for intrathecal injections (myelography), but were quickly accepted for intravascular injections. Side effects and allergic reactions are less likely and less severe with these media. Their one significant disadvantage is their increased cost as compared to ionic media.

part

II

Radiographic Procedures

General Procedural Considerations

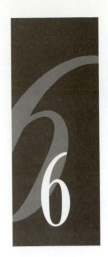

The development of positioning skills requires a thorough knowledge of normal *anatomy* and an awareness of *pathologic conditions* and their impact on positioning limitations and selection of *technical factors*.

A review of basic positioning principles and terminology is essential to an overview of radiographic procedures. Several tables and figures in this chapter summarize body *planes* (Fig. 6–2), body *habitus*, (Fig. 6–3), the *four quadrants* and *nine regions* of the abdomen (Fig. 6–4), *body surface landmarks* and localization points (Fig. 6–5), and *ARRT standard terminology* (Fig. 6–6). The student should be thoroughly acquainted with these before approaching the study of specific positioning skills.

It must be emphasized that a patient's condition very often impacts his or her ability to cooperate. The descriptions of *"Position of Part"* in this section are most easily used on patients who are not severely injured or afflicted with debilitating pathology. One measure of a good radiographer is his or her ability to be cautious and resourceful when examining injured or debilitated patients having pathologic or traumatic conditions such as *metastatic* bone disease, *arthritis,* or bone *fractures.*

The use of *body surface landmarks* and localization points (see Fig. 6–5) as external indicators of anatomic structures can increase the ease and accuracy of positioning.

Thoughtful placement of a cushioning sponge, the use of a horizontal beam for *lateral* projections instead of moving the patient (see Fig. 6–1), performing the examination *erect* if the *recumbent* position is uncomfortable, are examples of modifications that the considerate radiographer can make that will result in an appreciative patient, as well as a diagnostic exam. The radiographer must also be alert to the changes in technical factors that may be necessitated by various pathologic processes.

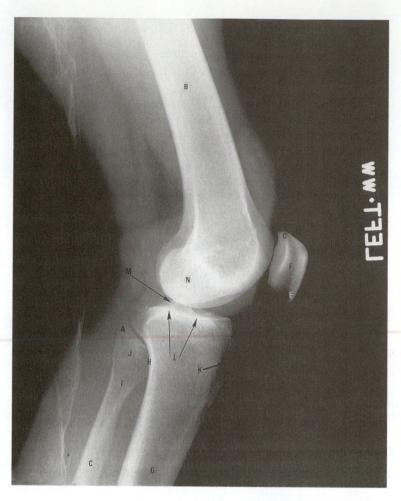

Figure 6–1. Lateral projection of knee performed in supine position on a patient with multiple injuries. A horizontal (cross-table) x-ray beam was used to reduce discomfort and the risk of further injury. Observe the bed sheet artifact from the mattress pad beneath the patient. Use this radiograph to *review the skeletal anatomy* of the knee and correctly identify the lettered parts. (Courtesy of The Stamford Hospital.)

I. BODY PLANES (Fig. 6–2)

- **Midsagittal** or *Median Sagittal Plane* (MSP): divides body into left and right halves.
- **Sagittal Plane:** any plane parallel to the MSP.
- **Midcoronal Plane** (MCP): divides body into anterior and posterior halves.
- **Coronal Plane:** any plane parallel to the MCP.
- **Transverse**/*Horizontal* **Plane:** perpendicular to MSP and MCP, divides body axially into superior and inferior portions.

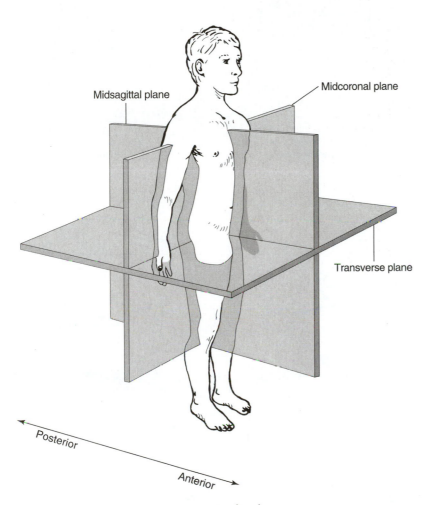

Figure 6–2. Body planes.

Body Types and Habitus

Hypersthenic and asthenic characterize the extremes in body types:

Hypersthenic
- Body is large and heavy
- Bony framework is thick, short and wide
- Lungs and heart are high
- Transverse stomach
- Gallbladder high and lateral
- Peripheral colon

Asthenic
- Body is slender and light
- Bony framework is delicate
- Long, narrow thorax
- Very low, long ("fish hook") stomach
- Gallbladder low and medial
- Low, medial, and redundant colon

Sthenic and hyposthenic types characterize the more average body types:

Sthenic
- Average, athletic build
- Similar to hypersthenic, but modified by elongation of abdomen and thorax

Hyposthenic
- Somewhat slighter, less robust
- Similar to asthenic, but stomach, intestines, and gallbladder situated higher in abdomen

II. BODY TYPES AND HABITUS (Fig. 6–3)

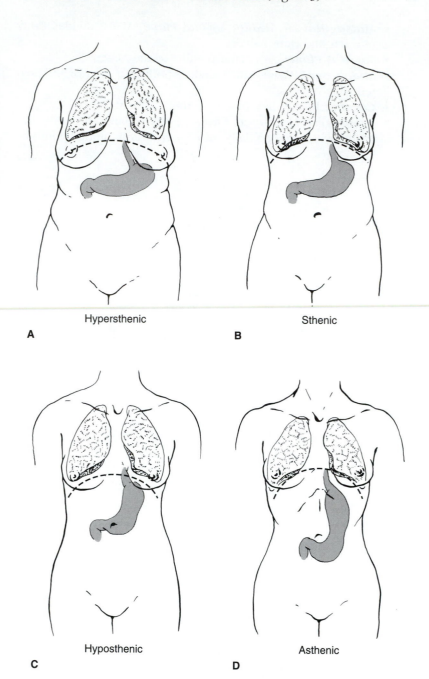

A   Hypersthenic

B   Sthenic

C   Hyposthenic

D   Asthenic

Figure 6–3. The position, shape, and motility of various organs can differ greatly from one *body habitus* to another. Each of the body habitus types is shown and the characteristic variations in shape and position of the diaphragm, lungs, and stomach are illustrated. The radiographer must take these characteristic differences into consideration while performing radiographic examinations on individuals of various body habitus.

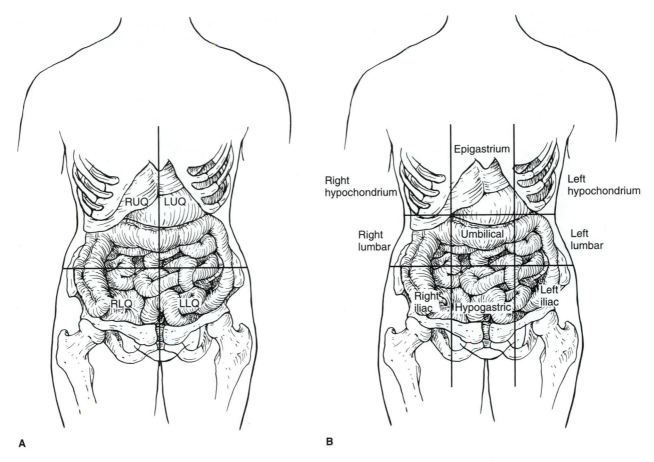

Figure 6–4. **A.** Four quadrants of the abdomen, illustrating position of major organs. **B.** Nine regions of the abdomen, illustrating position of major organs.

III. SURFACE LANDMARKS AND LOCALIZATION POINTS (Fig. 6–5)

	VERTEBRA(E)	LOCALIZATION POINT
Cervical region	C1	mastoid process
	C5	thyroid cartilage (Adam's Apple)
	C7	vertebra prominens
Thoracic region	T2–3	suprasternal (jugular) notch
	T4–5	sternal angle
	T7–8	inferior angle of scapula
	T10	xiphoid (ensiform) process
Lumbar region	T12–L3	kidneys
	L1	transpyloric plane
	L3	inferior costal margin
	L4	iliac crest
Sacral and coccygeal regions	S1–2	anterior superior iliac spine (ASIS)
	Coccyx	symphysis pubis and greater trochanter

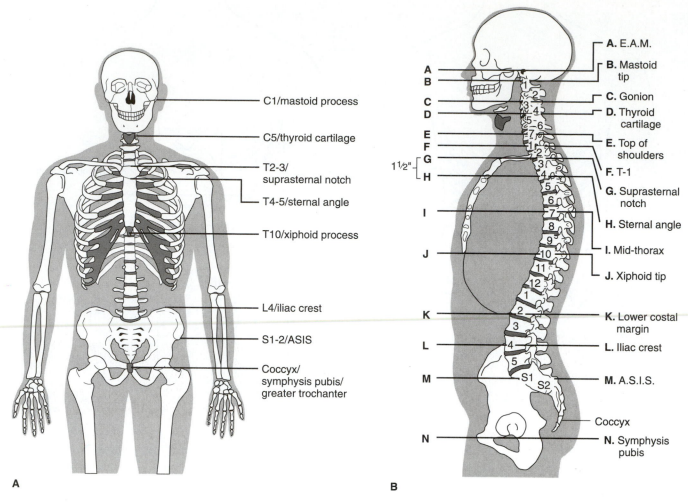

Figure 6–5. Body surface landmarks and localization points.

STANDARD TERMINOLOGY FOR POSITIONING AND PROJECTION

Radiographic view
Describes the body part as seen by an x-ray film or other recording medium, such as a fluoroscopic screen. Restricted to the discussion of a *radiograph* or *image*.

Radiographic position
Refers to a specific body position, such as supine, prone, recumbent, erect, or Trendelenburg. Restricted to the discussion of the *patient's physical position*.

Radiographic projection
Restricted to the discussion of the *path of the central ray*.

Positioning terminology
　　A. *Lying down*
　1. Supine: lying on the back
　2. Prone: lying face downward
　3. Decubitus: lying down with a horizontal x-ray beam
　4. Recumbent: lying down in any position

B. *Erect or Upright*
1. Anterior position: facing the film
2. Posterior position: facing the radiographic tube
3. Oblique positions: erect or lying down

a. Anterior: facing the film
(1) *Left anterior oblique:* body rotated with left anterior portion closest to the film

(2) *Right anterior oblique:* body rotated with right anterior portion closest to the film

b. Posterior facing the radiographic tube
(1) *Left posterior oblique:* body rotated with left posterior portion closest to the film

(2) *Right posterior oblique:* body rotated with right posterior portion closest to the film

Figure 6–6. Standard terminology provides descriptions and interpretation of accepted radiologic positioning language. (*Standard Terminology.* © 2001 The American Registry of Radiologic Technologists. Reproduced with permission.)

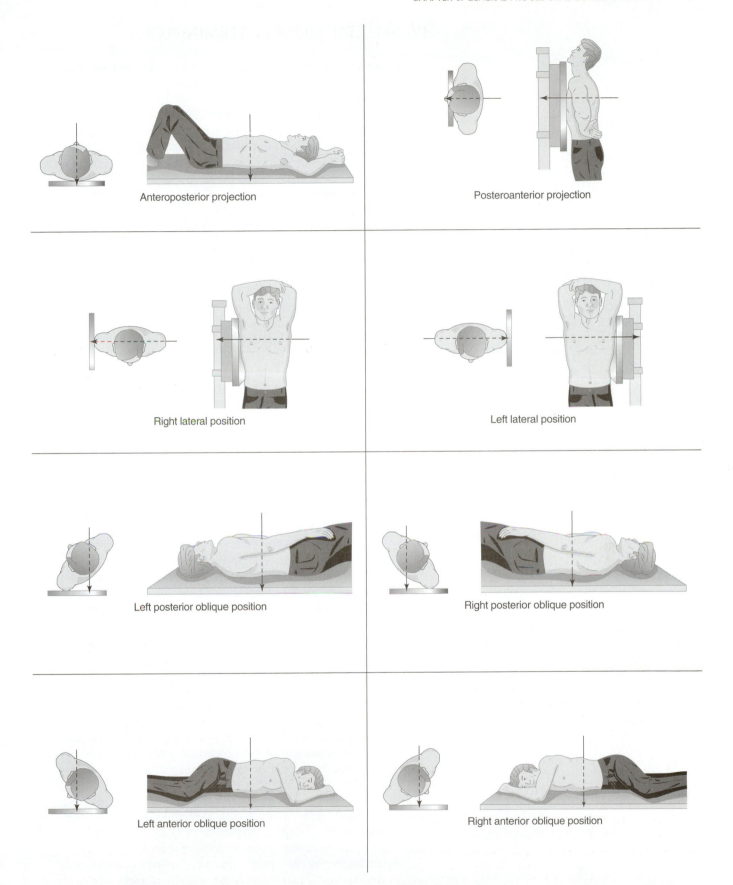

Anteroposterior projection

Posteroanterior projection

Right lateral position

Left lateral position

Left posterior oblique position

Right posterior oblique position

Left anterior oblique position

Right anterior oblique position

Figure 6–6 *(Continued)*.

IV. SKELETAL MOTION TERMINOLOGY

- **Supination:** turns the body or arm so that the palm faces forward, with thumb away from midline of body.
- **Pronation:** turns the body or arm so that the palm faces backward, with thumb toward midline of body.
- **Abduction:** movement of a part away from the body's MSP.
- **Adduction:** movement of a part toward the body's MSP.
- **Flexion:** bending motion of an articulation, decreasing the angle between associated bones.
- **Extension:** bending motion of an articulation, increasing the angle between associated bones.
- **Eversion:** a turning outward or lateral motion of an articulation, sometimes with external tension or stress applied.
- **Inversion:** a turning inward or medial motion of an articulation, sometimes with external tension or stress applied.
- **Rotation:** movement of a part about its central or long axis.
- **Circumduction:** movement of a limb that produces circular motion; circumscribes a small area at its proximal end and a wide area at the distal end.

V. PRELIMINARY STEPS AND PROCEDURAL GUIDELINES

The following are steps and procedures that help ensure high quality patient care and diagnostic radiographs:

1. *Read the request carefully,* noting the type of examination, patient condition, and mode of travel (make mental notes of any modifications or accessory equipment that may be required).
2. *Prepare the radiographic room.* Be certain the x-ray room is neat and orderly with a clean x-ray table and a fresh pillowcase. All accessories needed for the exam should be in the room before bringing in the patient.
3. *Identify the correct patient,* quickly evaluating any special needs; *introduce yourself* and establish rapport en route to the radiographic room, being careful not to discuss confidential issues within earshot of others.
4. *Instruct the patient* to change into a dressing gown (if necessary), removing appropriate clothing and objects (eg, jewelry, dentures, braided hair) that may cast *artifacts* within the area of interest (see Figs. 6–7 and 6–8).
5. Speak in a well-modulated voice, give a clear and succinct *explanation* of the procedure and address any patient questions or concerns. Obtain a short pertinent *patient history* of why the exam has been requested. The radiographer should explain that a number of different positions may be needed to evaluate the area of interest and may require *palpation* of bony landmarks and instructions to turn into various positions.
6. Radiography of most structures *usually requires a minimum of two projections,* usually at right angles to each other. Side-to-side (left/right) relationships are

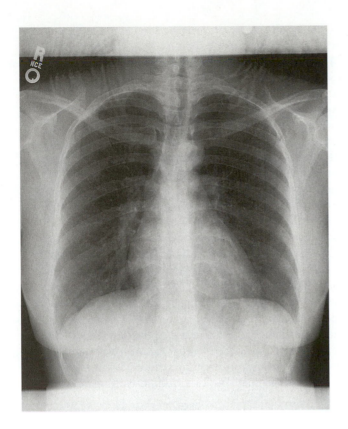

Figure 6–7. The posteroanterior (PA) chest film is well positioned and exposed, but observe the braids of hair that extend past the neck and superimpose on the pulmonary apices. Braided hair should be pinned up or otherwise removed from superimposition on thoracic structures. (Courtesy of The Stamford Hospital.)

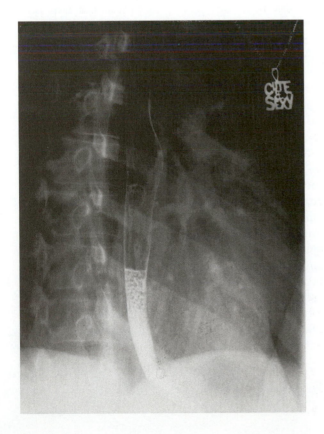

Figure 6–8. Left posterior oblique (LPO) image of the esophagus with a jewelry artifact near the area of interest. The patient must remove clothing and other objects, such as jewelry, from the area to be examined before donning the dressing gown. (Courtesy of The Stamford Hospital.)

demonstrated in the *frontal* projection, while anterior/posterior relationships are seen in the *lateral* projection. This is especially important in localizing foreign bodies and tumors, and demonstrating fracture displacement or alignment.

7. It is customary and economical to use the smallest size film or image recorder that will include all necessary information. Therefore, the smallest possible anatomic area (consistent with a diagnostic examination) will be irradiated to keep patient dose to a minimum.

8. In radiography of the extremities, every effort should be made to *include both articulations* associated with the injured bone, but it is essential to include at least the articulation nearest the injury.

9. So that an accurate diagnosis can be made, supplemental radiographs of any anatomic part may be required; eg, *oblique, axial, tangential, erect,* or *decubitus.* Exposure factors must be correctly adjusted for each change of position.

10. Each radiograph must be accurately *labeled* with patient information such as *name or identification number, institution name, date of examination, and side marker.* Other information may be included according to institution policy.

VI. IMMOBILIZATION AND RESPIRATION

Motion obliterates recorded detail; consequently, it is essential that the radiographer be able to reduce patient motion as much as possible. Several means can be employed to reduce motion unsharpness, but good *patient communication* is required for any to be effective.

The single most important way to reduce *involuntary* motion is to use the *shortest possible exposure time.* Various types of *immobilization devices* can also be used to effectively reduce motion. Motion from muscular tremors as a result of anxiety or pain are involuntary and can be greatly minimized with good communication, a carefully placed positioning sponge or sandbag, and the use of the shortest exposure time possible.

Suspension of patient respiration for parts other than the extremities is an effective means of reducing *voluntary* motion; patient understanding and cooperation is required, thus making good *communication* the *most effective means of reducing voluntary motion.* The phase of respiration on which the exposure is made can be essential to the diagnostic quality of the radiographic image. Chest radiography, for example, normally requires that the exposure be made on inspiration (the second inspiration if the patient is of the hypersthenic type). Most abdominal examinations are exposed on expiration. The phase of respiration on which the exposure is made can also make a significant difference in the resulting radiographic density (discussed in Part IV).

Chapter Exercises

 Congratulations! *You have completed your review of this chapter. If you are able to answer the following group of comprehensive questions, you can feel confident that you have mastered this section. You are then ready to go on to "Registry-type" questions that follow. For greatest success, do not go to these multiple choice questions without first completing the short answer questions below.*

1. Discuss how knowledge of anatomy and pathologic conditions relates to positioning skills *(p. 73)*.

2. Identify the sagittal and midsagittal, coronal and midcoronal, and transverse (horizontal) planes *(p. 75)*.

3. List the four types of body habitus and provide physical characteristics of each *(p. 76)*.

4. Name, identify, and describe the quadrants and nine regions of the abdomen *(p. 77)*.

5. Identify anatomic localization points and their corresponding vertebrae *(p. 77)*.

6. Define and identify various skeletal movement terms *(p. 80)*.

7. Discuss the importance of establishing an orderly sequence of preparation for performing radiologic examinations *(pp. 80, 82)*.

8. Explain the importance of obtaining two views at right angles to each other for most radiologic examinations *(pp. 80, 82)*.

9. Discuss the inclusion of articulations in radiography of the extremities *(p. 82)*.

10. List the information that must be included on the radiographic image *(p. 82)*.

A&U Chapter Review Questions

1. Before bringing the patient into the radiographic room, the radiographer should:
   1. be certain the x-ray room is clean and orderly
   2. check that all necessary accessories are available in room
   3. check for clean x-ray table and fresh pillowcases
   (A) 1 only
   (B) 1 and 2 only
   (C) 2 and 3 only
   (D) 1, 2, and 3

2. The position of the asthenic gallbladder, as compared to the position of the hyper-sthenic gallbladder is more:
   (A) superior and lateral
   (B) superior and medial
   (C) inferior and lateral
   (D) inferior and medial

3. What is the relationship between the midsagittal and coronal planes?
   (A) parallel
   (B) perpendicular
   (C) 45°
   (D) 70°

4. The best way to control involuntary motion is:
   (A) immobilization
   (B) careful explanation
   (C) short exposure time
   (D) physical restraint

5. Prior to x-ray examinations of the skull and cervical spine the patient should remove
   1. dentures
   2. earrings
   3. necklaces
   (A) 1 only
   (B) 1 and 2 only
   (C) 2 and 3 only
   (D) 1, 2, and 3

6. Film identification markers should include:
   1. patient's name and/or ID number
   2. date
   3. a right or left marker
   (A) 1 only
   (B) 1 and 2 only
   (C) 1 and 3 only
   (D) 1, 2, and 3

7. The radiographer should be able to:
   1. take a short patient history prior to the exam
   2. give a preliminary diagnosis for stat exams
   3. evaluate patient condition and needs
   (A) 1 only
   (B) 1 and 2 only
   (C) 1 and 3 only
   (D) 1, 2, and 3

8. With the patient recumbent and head positioned at a higher level than the feet, the patient is said to be in the:
   (A) Trendelenburg position
   (B) Fowler's position
   (C) decubitus position
   (D) Sim's position

9. The plane that passes vertically through the body dividing it into equal left and right halves is termed the:
   (A) median sagittal plane
   (B) midcoronal plane
   (C) sagittal plane
   (D) transverse plane

10. The uppermost portion of the iliac crest is approximately at the same level as the:
    (A) costal margin
    (B) umbilicus
    (C) xiphoid tip
    (D) fourth lumbar vertebra

Answers and Explanations

1. (D) A patient will naturally feel more comfortable and confident if brought into a clean, orderly x-ray room that has been prepared appropriately for the examination to be performed. A disorderly, untidy room and a disorganized radiographer hardly inspire confidence; more likely, they will increase anxiety and apprehension.

2. (D) The position, shape, and motility of various organs can differ greatly from one body habitus to another. The position of the diaphragm, lungs, stomach, gallbladder, and large and small intestines vary greatly with body habitus. The large extreme (*hypersthenic*) will have structures *higher and more lateral*, while these structures in individuals of the small extreme habitus (*asthenic*) have structures *low and medial* (see Fig. 6–3).

3. (B) The *median sagittal*, or midsagittal, plane passes vertically through the midline of the body, dividing it into left and right halves. Any plane parallel to the MSP is termed a sagittal plane. *The midcoronal plane is perpendicular to the MSP* and divides the body into anterior and posterior halves. A *transverse* plane passes across the body, also perpendicular to a sagittal plane. These planes, especially the MSP, are very important reference points in radiographic positioning.

4. (C) Motion obliterates recorded detail; it is therefore essential that the radiographer be able to reduce patient motion as much as possible. Even the slightest movement can cause severe degradation of the radiographic image. The single most important way to reduce *involuntary* motion is to use the *shortest possible exposure time*. Suspension of patient respiration for parts other than the extremities is an effective means of reducing *voluntary* motion; patient understanding and cooperation is required, thus making good *communication* the most effective means of reducing *voluntary* motion.

5. (D) The patient must remove any metallic objects if they are within the area(s) of interest. Dentures, earrings, necklaces, and braided hair can obscure bony details in the skull or cervical spine. The radiographer must be certain the patient's belongings are cared for properly and returned following the examination (see Figs. 6–7 and 6–8).

6. (D) Correct and complete patient information on every radiograph is of paramount importance. Each radiograph must be accurately labeled with such patient information as *name or identification number, institution name, date of examination, and side marker.* Other information may be included according to institution policy.

7. (C) The acquisition of pertinent *clinical history* is one of the most valuable contributions to the diagnostic process. Because the diagnostic radiologist rarely has the opportunity to speak with the patient, this is a crucial responsibility of the radiographer. As the radiographer obtains a brief pertinent clinical history, the radiographer also *assesses the patient's condition* by observing and listening. In order to provide safe and effective care, the radiographer must be able to assess the severity of a trauma patient's injury, their degree of motor control, the need for support equipment or radiographic accessories. Providing a diagnosis from the radiographic images is not within the radiographer's scope of practice.

8. (B) When the patient is recumbent with his or her head *lower* than his or her feet, the patient is said to be in the *Trendelenburg* position. In the *Fowler's* position, the patient's head is positioned *higher* than his or her feet. The *decubitus* position is used to describe the patient as recumbent (prone, supine, or lateral) with the central ray directed horizontally. The *Sim's* position is the left anterior oblique (LAO) position assumed for enema tip insertion.

9. (A) The *median sagittal*, or midsagittal, plane passes vertically through the midline of the body, dividing it into left and right halves. Any plane parallel to the MSP is termed a sagittal plane. *The midcoronal plane is perpendicular to the MSP* and divides the body into anterior and posterior halves. A *transverse* plane passes across the body, also perpendicular to a sagittal plane. These planes, especially the MSP, are very important reference points in radiographic positioning.

10. (D) Surface landmarks, prominences, and depressions are very useful to the radiographer in locating anatomic structures not visible externally. The *costal margin* is about the same level as L3. The *umbilicus* is the same approximate level as the L3 to L4 interspace. The *xiphoid* tip is about the same level as T10. The fourth lumbar vertebra is at the same approximate level as the *iliac crest*.

Imaging Procedures, Including Anatomy, Positioning, and Pathology

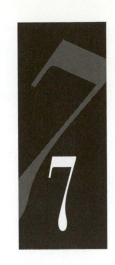

I. THE APPENDICULAR SKELETON

The *appendicular* skeleton (Fig. 7–1) is made of the *extremities* (appendages or limbs), the arms, shoulder girdle, legs, and pelvis. Most of these bones serve as *levers for attachment* of muscles, thereby making movement possible. Bones serve as a *reservoir for minerals* such as calcium and phosphorus, storing them until the body requires them. Bone tissue is osseous (*os* = bone), and there are two types of osseous tissue: *cancellous* (spongy) and *compact* (hard, cortical) (Fig. 7–2A).

Bones are classified as *long, short, flat,* and *irregular.* Many of the bones comprising the extremities are long bones. Long bones have a *shaft* and *two extremities* (ends). The shaft (or *diaphysis*) (Fig. 7–2B) of long bones is the *primary ossification center* during bone development. It is composed of compact tissue and is covered with a membrane called *periosteum.* Within the shaft is the *medullary cavity,* which contains *bone marrow* and is lined by a membrane called *endosteum.* In the adult, yellow marrow occupies the shaft and red marrow is found within the *proximal* and *distal* extremities of long bones. The *secondary ossification center,* the *epiphysis* (Figure 7–2B), is separated from the diaphysis in early life by a layer of cartilage, the *epiphyseal plate.* As bone growth takes place, the epiphysis becomes part of the larger portion of bone, the epiphyseal plate disappears but a characteristic line remains and is thereafter recognizable as the *epiphyseal line.* The articular ends of bones are covered with *articular (hyaline) cartilage.*

A. UPPER EXTREMITY AND SHOULDER GIRDLE

1. Hand, Fingers, and Thumb. The hand (Fig. 7–3) is composed of five *metacarpal* bones, which correspond to the palm of the hand, and 14 *phalanges,* the fingers. The second through fifth fingers have three phalanges each (proximal, middle, and distal rows) and the first finger or thumb has two phalanges (proximal and distal). The rows of phalanges articulate with each other forming proximal and distal *interphalangeal joints* (hinge type joints), which permit flexion and extension motion.

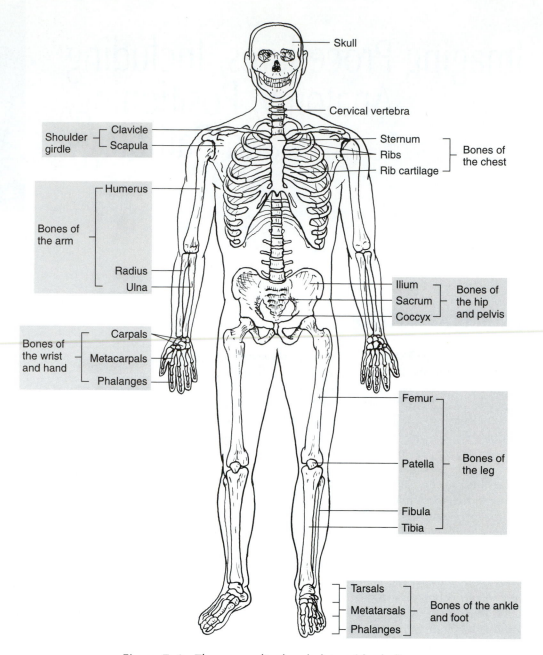

Figure 7–1. The appendicular skeleton (shaded).

The *bases* of the proximal row of phalanges articulate with the heads of the metacarpals to form the (condyloid) *metacarpophalangeal joints* (MPJ), which permit flexion and extension, abduction and adduction, and circumduction. The bases of the metacarpals articulate with each other and the distal row of carpals at the *carpometacarpal joints*. The first carpometacarpal joint (thumb) is a saddle joint, permitting flexion and extension, abduction and adduction, and circumduction.

Traumatic *fractures* of the metacarpals and phalanges are common. Fractures of the distal (ungual) phalangeal tufts usually occur from crushing injuries, such as being closed in car doors or struck with a hammer.

Articulations May be Classified as

Diathrotic: freely movable
Amphiarthrotic: partially movable
Synarthrotic: immovable

2. Wrist. The wrist (Fig. 7–3) is composed of eight carpal bones arranged in two rows (proximal and distal). The proximal row consists of, from lateral to medial, the *scaphoid*, the *lunate/semilunar,* the *triangular/triquetrum*, and the *pisiform*. The distal row, from lateral to medial, consists of the *greater multiangular/trapezium,* the *lesser multiangular/trapezoid,* the *capitate/os magnum* (the largest carpal), and the *hamate/unciform* (which has a hook-like process, the hamulus).

The joints of the wrist include the articulations between the carpals *(intercarpal joints)*, which provide a gliding motion, and the *radiocarpal joint* (between the distal radius and navicular), which provides flexion and extension, abduction and adduction.

Carpal tunnel syndrome is a painful condition of the wrist. If the anteroposterior (AP) diameter of the tunnel is diminished, the median nerve, which passes through the tunnel, is impinged upon, causing severe pain and disability in the affected hand and wrist. Surgical decompression of the carpal tunnel can provide significant relief.

3. Forearm. The bones of the forearm, or antebrachium (Fig. 7–4), consist of the *radius* (laterally) and *ulna* (medially), which participate in formation of the elbow joint proximally and the wrist distally.

The distal ulna presents a *head* and *styloid process* and articulates with the distal radius to form the *distal radioulnar joint*. The ulna is slender distally but enlarges proximally and becomes the larger of the two bones of the forearm. At its proximal end, the ulna presents the *olecranon process* (posteriorly) and *coronoid process* (anteriorly) that are joined by a large articular cavity, the *semilunar,* or

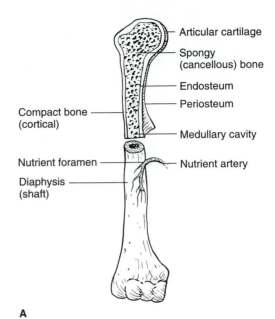

A

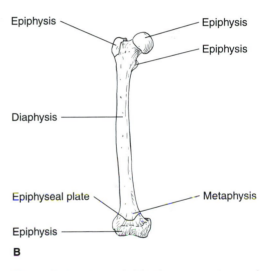

B

Figure 7–2. **(A)** and **(B)** Characteristics and ossification centers of long bones.

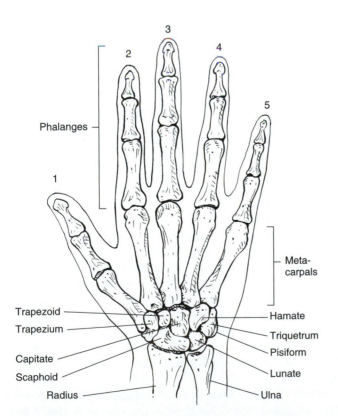

Figure 7–3. Dorsal aspect of the right hand and wrist. (PA projection)

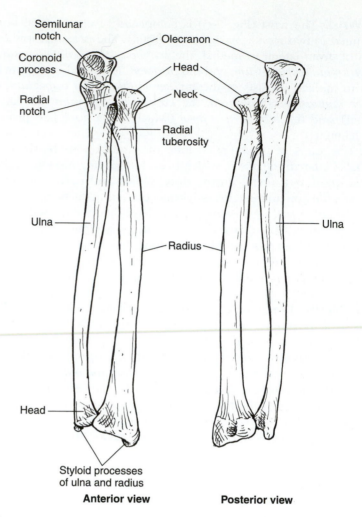

Figure 7–4. Bones of the left forearm.

Carpal Bones

Proximal Row, Lateral to Medial
Scaphoid
Lunate/semilunar
Triangular/triquetrum
Pisiform
Distal Row, Lateral to Medial
Greater multiangular/trapezoid
Lesser multiangular/trapezium
Capitate/os magnum
Hamate/cuneiform

---

trochlear, notch. The coronoid process fits into the humeral *coronoid fossa* during flexion and the olecranon process fits into the humeral *olecranon fossa* during extension. Just distal and lateral to the semilunar notch is the *radial notch,* which provides articulation for the radial head to form the *proximal radioulnar articulation.* Just as the ulna is the principal bone associated with the elbow joint, the radius is the principal bone associated with the wrist joint. Fracture of the distal radius is one of the most common skeletal fractures.

The distal radius presents a *styloid process* laterally; the *ulnar notch* is located medially, helping to form the *distal radioulnar articulation.* The distal surface of the radius (carpal articular surface) is smooth for accommodating the navicular and lunate in the formation of the *radiocarpal joint.* The proximal radius has a cylindrical *head* with a medial surface that participates in the *proximal radioulnar joint;* its superior surface articulates with the capitulum of the humerus.

Fractures of the radial head and neck frequently result from a fall onto an outstretched hand with the elbow *partially flexed.* Severe fractures are often accompanied by posterior dislocation of the elbow joint. *Colles' fractures* of the distal radius usually result from a fall onto an outstretched hand with the arm *extended*.

4. Elbow. The distal *humerus* articulates with the radius and ulna to form the elbow joint (Figs. 7–5 and 7–6). The lateral aspect of the distal humerus presents a raised, smooth, rounded surface, the *capitulum,* which articulates with the superior surface of the *radial head* (Fig. 7–4). The *trochlea* is on the medial aspect of the distal humerus and articulates with the semilunar notch of the ulna. Just proximal to the capitulum and trochlea are the *lateral* and *medial epicondyles;* the medial is more prominent and palpable.

Lateral epicondylitis (tennis elbow) is a painful condition caused by prolonged rotary motion of the forearm. The *olecranon fossa* is found on the posterior distal humerus and functions to accommodate the olecranon process with the elbow in extension (Fig. 7–7).

5. Humerus. The *deltoid tuberosity* is found on the anterolateral surface of the humeral shaft. The large, round *humeral head* is covered with hyaline cartilage and articulates with the scapula's glenoid fossa. The *anatomical neck* marks the location of the fused epiphyseal plate in the adult and separates the head and metaphysis. The proximal humerus presents two protuberances on its anterior surface; the *greater tubercle* is lateral and the *lesser tubercle* is medial. Between the tubercles is the *bicipital,* or *intertubercular, groove.* The humeral shaft narrows just distal to the tubercles at the point of the *surgical neck.* Humeral *fractures* usually involve the surgical neck or its distal end.

6. Shoulder. The shoulder (pectoral) girdle consists of the scapulae (Fig. 7–8) and clavicles (Fig. 7–9). The S-shaped *clavicle* (collar bone) is the last bone to completely ossify, at about age 21, and is one of the most commonly fractured bones in young people. Its medial end articulates with the sternum to form the *sternoclavicular joint;* it articulates laterally with the scapula's acromion process,

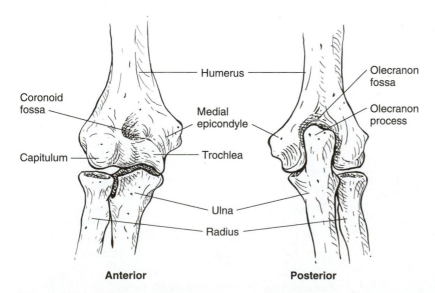

Figure 7–5. Anterior and posterior views of the bony articulation of the right elbow joint.

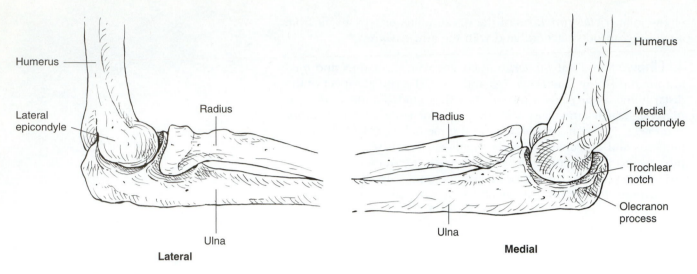

Figure 7–6. Medial and lateral views of the bony articulation of the right elbow joint.

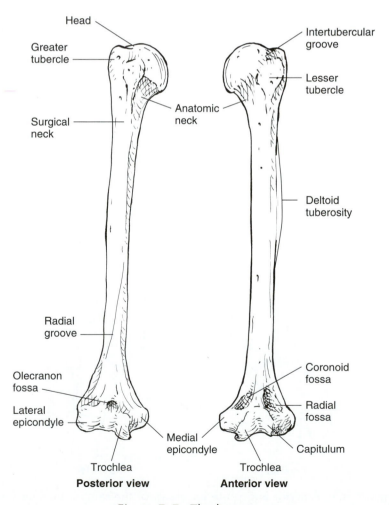

Figure 7–7. The humerus.

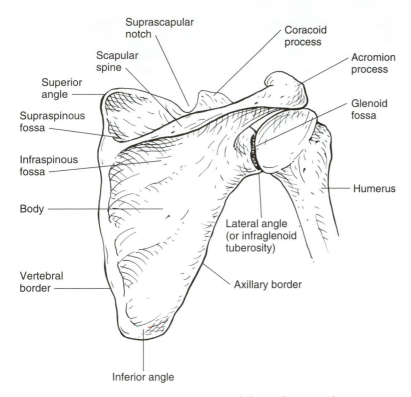

Figure 7–8. Posterior view of the right scapula.

forming the *acromioclavicular joint*. Superior *dislocation* of the *acromioclavicular joint* is a common athletic injury.

The *scapula* is a flat bone, shaped like an inverted triangle, with a *costal surface* that lies against the upper posterior rib cage. The scapula has a *superior border*, a *medial*, or *vertebral, border*, a *lateral*, or *axillary, border*, and an *inferior angle*, or *apex*. Its superior border presents a *scapular notch* and, projecting anteriorly just medial to the humeral head, the palpable *coracoid process*. The *scapular spine* divides the posterior surface into a *supraspinatus fossa* and *infraspinatus fossa;* the *acromion process* is the lateral extension of the scapular spine. The *glenoid fossa* is on the lateral aspect of the

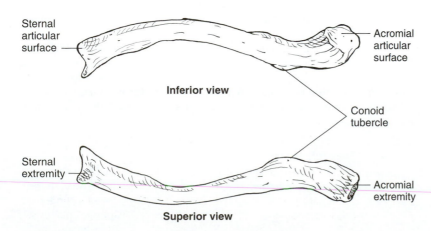

Figure 7–9. The right clavicle.

Articulation Summary: Upper Extremity and Shoulder Girdle

- Acromioclavicular
- Sternoclavicular
- Shoulder (glenhumeral)
- Elbow: three articulations:
  1) b/w humeral trochlea and semilunar/trochlear notch
  2) b/w capitulum and radial head
  3) proximal radioulnar joint
- Distal radioulnar
- Radiocarpal (distal radius w/scaphoid and lunate)
- Intercarpal
- Carpometacarpal
- Metacarpophalangeal
- Interphalangeal

scapula and, with its articulation with the humeral head, forms the (ball and socket) *shoulder joint*.

The *rotator cuff* is composed of a group of shoulder muscles. Rotator cuff injuries are a result of acute injury or chronic wear and tear. The articular capsule of the shoulder is loose, permitting a great range of movement but also making it susceptible to dislocation.

7. Positioning.

Positioning of the upper extremity and shoulder girdle requires a thorough knowledge of the anatomy concerned, an awareness of possible pathologic conditions, and their impact on positioning limitations and technical factors.

Radiopaque objects such as watches, bracelets, and rings should be removed whenever possible, because they can obscure important anatomic information. The patient must be instructed regarding the importance of remaining still, and immobilization devices such as sandbags or sponges should be used as required. The shortest possible exposure time should be employed, especially when involuntary motion can be a problem, as with trauma, pediatric, or geriatric patients.

Most upper-extremity examinations are more comfortably and accurately positioned with the patient seated at the end of the x-ray table, with the forearm and elbow resting on the table. Most can be performed tabletop (ie, without a Bucky grid); the humerus sometimes requires a grid, while the shoulder, clavicle, and scapula usually do. *Suspended respiration* is suggested for radiography of the proximal portion of the upper extremity and shoulder girdle. Patients should be adequately shielded.

The use of just a few important bony landmarks and their correct placement with respect to the film is the basis for accurate positioning. Rotation of the arm and placing the humeral epicondyles in correct relationship to the film is the foundation of forearm, elbow, and shoulder positioning. Positioning of the wrist and hand uses the radial and ulnar styloid processes, bending maneuvers (ie, radial and ulnar flexion), metacarpophalangeal joints (MPJ), and interphalangeal joints (IPJ).

The following tables provide a summary of routine and frequently performed special projections of the upper extremity and shoulder girdle.

HAND	POSITION OF PART:	CENTRAL RAY DIRECTED:	STRUCTURES INCLUDED/ BEST SEEN:
PA	Pronated, elbow flexed 90°, fingers extended and slightly spread	⊥ 3rd MPJ	PA carpals, metacarpals, phalanges and their articulations; see Fig. 7–10. Provides obl proj of thumb

This position is often performed to include the wrist for *bone age* studies; 30″ SID is sometimes recommended, with the CR entering ⊥ the head of the 3rd metacarpal.

OBL	Prone, elbow flexed 90°, hand and forearm obliqued 45°	⊥ 3rd MPJ	Obl proj carpals, metacarpals, phalanges and their articulations; use of a "finger sponge" places jts ‖ to film and opens jt spaces

(continued)

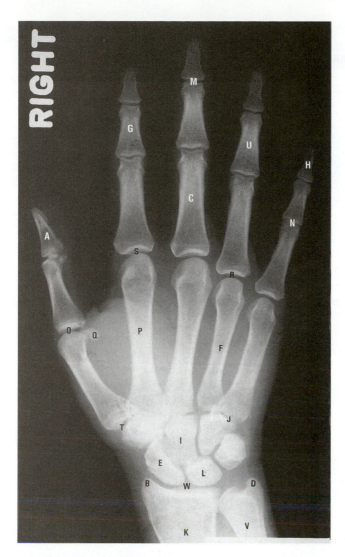

Figure 7–10. PA projection of the hand; note that an oblique projection of the first metacarpal and phalange is obtained. Review the skeletal anatomy of the hand and correctly identify each of the lettered structures. (Courtesy of Bob Wong, RT.)

List of Abbreviations and Symbols Used in the Following Tables

AC	acromioclavicular
$\angle$	angle
ASIS	anterior superior iliac spine
AP	anteroposterior
$\approx$	approximately (about)
b/w	between
CMC	carpometacarpal joint
CR	central ray
°	degrees
dist	distal
EAM	external auditory meatus
fx	fracture
>	greater than
"	inches
IOML	infraorbitomeatal line
IPJ	interphalangeal joint
jt	joint
kV	kilovoltage
lat	lateral
LAO	left anterior oblique
LPO	left posterior oblique
<	less than
MPJ	metacarpophalangeal *or* metatarsophalangeal joint
MSP	midsagittal plane
m/w	midway
OID	object-to-image-receptor distance
obl	oblique
OML	orbitomeatal line
$\parallel$	parallel to
$\perp$	perpendicular to
PA	posteroanterior
proj	projection
prox	proximal
RAO	right anterior oblique
RPO	right posterior oblique
SID	source-to-image receptor distance
w/	with
w/o	without

HAND (con't)	POSITION OF PART:	CENTRAL RAY DIRECTED:	STRUCTURES INCLUDED/ BEST SEEN:
LAT *in* *extension*	Elbow flexed 90°, fingers extended, wrist lateral, ulnar surface down	$\perp$ MPJs	*Superimposed* carpals, metacarpals, phalanges and their articulations. Decrease 10 kV for foreign body
LAT *in* *flexion*	Elbow flexed 90°, fingers slightly flexed and superimposed	$\perp$ MPJs	Superimposed carpals, metacarpals, phalanges and their articulations. *Shows anterior/ posterior fracture displacement*

A "fan lateral" with the fingers separated is often performed to better visualize each phalange.

FINGERS	POSITION OF PART:	CENTRAL RAY DIRECTED:	STRUCTURES INCLUDED/ BEST SEEN:
PA	Hand pronated and fingers extended, elbow flexed 90°	⊥ proximal IPJ	PA proximal, middle, and distal phalanges
LAT	Elbow flexed 90°, forearm lateral, finger(s) extended and ∥ film	⊥ proximal IPJ	Lat of proximal, middle, and distal phalanges. 2nd and 3rd digits are done *radial side down;* 4th and 5th done *ulnar side down*

THUMB	POSITION OF PART:	CENTRAL RAY DIRECTED:	STRUCTURES INCLUDED/ BEST SEEN:
AP	Dorsal surface adjacent and ∥ film	⊥ MPJ	
PA	Palmar surface ∥ film, *requires increase OID*	⊥ MPJ	
LAT	Lateral surface adjacent to film, fingers elevated and resting on sponge	⊥ MPJ	AP, PA, or lat projection of 1st digit. *3 articulations should be seen;* CMC, MPJ, and IPJ

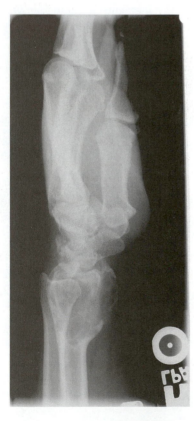

Figure 7–11. Lateral projection of wrist. Note large bone cyst on distal radius. (Courtesy of The Stamford Hospital.)

WRIST	POSITION OF PART:	CENTRAL RAY DIRECTED:	STRUCTURES INCLUDED/ BEST SEEN:
PA	Hand pronated w/MPJs slightly flexed, elbow flexed 90°	⊥ midcarpal region	PA carpals, prox metacarpals, dist radius and ulna. *Flexion of MPJs reduces OID*
LAT	Elbow flexed 90°, ulnar surface down, radius and ulna superimposed	⊥ midcarpal region	Lat carpals, superimposed prox metacarpals and dist radius and ulna; see Fig. 7–11
PA semi-pronation OBL	Elbow flexed 90°, wrist 45° w/film, ulnar surface down	⊥ midcarpal region	Useful for scaphoid, and other *lat carpals* (greater and lesser multangular) *and their interspaces*
AP semi-supination OBL	Arm extended, 45° w/film, ulnar surface down	⊥ midcarpal region	Useful for pisiform, triquetrum, and hamate *medial carpals and their interspaces*

(continued)

WRIST (con't)	POSITION OF PART:	CENTRAL RAY DIRECTED:	STRUCTURES INCLUDED/ BEST SEEN:
Ulnar Flexion/ Deviation	Position as PA wrist, evert hand (laterally) without moving forearm	⊥ scaphoid	Scaphoid and other *lat* carpal interspaces; *reduces foreshortening of navicular*
Radial Flexion/ Deviation	Position as PA wrist, move elbow toward body w/o moving hand/wrist	⊥ midcarpal region	*Medial* carpal interspaces; see Fig. 7–12
Scaphoid (Stecher)	Forearm a) Pronated *or* b) Pronated and elevated 20°	a) 20° toward elbow entering scaphoid *or* b) ⊥ scaphoid	Scaphoid w/o *foreshortening* and self- superimposition
Carpal Canal (Gaynor– Hart)	*Hyperextend* wrist w/palm vertical	25°–30° into long axis of hand	Carpal canal *(tunnel)*; trapezium, scaphoid, capitate, triquetrum, pisiform

FOREARM	POSITION OF PART:	CENTRAL RAY DIRECTED:	STRUCTURES INCLUDED/ BEST SEEN:
AP	Supinated and extended, epicondyles ∥ film; *shoulder and elbow on same plane*	⊥ mid- forearm	AP radius and ulna, including wrist and elbow joints; see Fig. 7–13, *arm must be supinated* to avoid overlap of radius and ulna
LAT	Elbow flexed 90°, epicondyles superimposed and ⊥ film, hand lateral; *shoulder and elbow on same plane*	⊥ mid- forearm	Radius and ulna superimposed distally, lat proj of radius and ulna, elbow and wrist joints

ELBOW	POSITION OF PART:	CENTRAL RAY DIRECTED:	STRUCTURES INCLUDED/ BEST SEEN:
AP	Extended, sup- inated; epicondyles ∥ film	⊥ elbow jt	AP elbow jt, proximal radius and ulna, distal humerus; radial head and tuberosity partially superimposed on ulna

(continued)

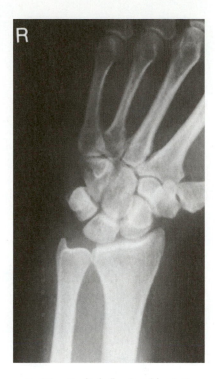

Figure 7–12. Radial flexion/deviation maneuver of left wrist. Radial flexion/deviation is used to better demonstrate the medial carpals (pisiform, triangular, hamate, and medial aspect of capitate and lunate).

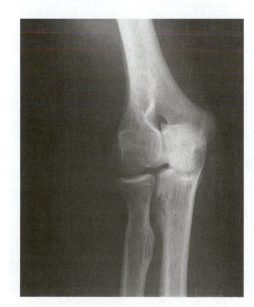

Figure 7–13. Lateral (external) oblique view of elbow. Note that the radial tuberosity is free of ulnar superimposition. The proximal radioulnar articulation is nicely shown at C. *Review the skeletal anatomy* of the elbow by correctly identifying each of the labeled structures.

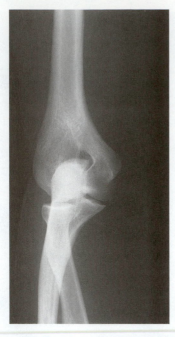

Figure 7–14. Medial (internal) oblique view of elbow; notice that coronoid process is seen free of superimposition.

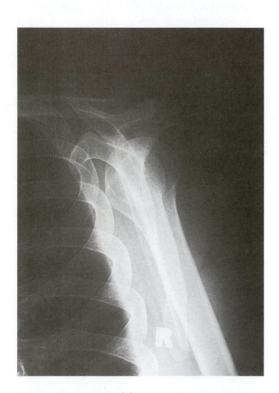

Figure 7–15. PA oblique projection, scapular Y view of the shoulder. Useful for demonstration of dislocations. Humeral head displaced inferior to coracoid process indicates *anterior dislocation,* while humeral head displaced inferior to acromion process indicates *posterior dislocation.*

ELBOW (con't)	POSITION OF PART:	CENTRAL RAY DIRECTED:	STRUCTURES INCLUDED/ BEST SEEN:
LAT	Flexed 90°, epicondyles ⊥ film, forearm and wrist lateral	⊥ elbow jt	Lat elbow jt, prox radius and ulna and distal humerus; radial head partially superimposed on ulna
Medial (internal) OBL	Arm extended, palm down, epicondyles 45° to film	⊥ elbow jt midway b/w epicondyles	Obl elbow jt; *coronoid process in profile;* see Fig. 7–14
Lateral (external) OBL	Forearm extended and rotated laterally, radial surface down, epicondyles 45° to film	⊥ elbow jt midway b/w epicondyles	Obl elbow jt; radial head, neck, and tuberosity free from superimposition of ulna; see Fig. 7–15

HUMERUS	POSITION OF PART:	CENTRAL RAY DIRECTED:	STRUCTURES INCLUDED/ BEST SEEN:
AP	Arm extended and supinated; epicondyles ‖ film	⊥ midhumerus	AP humerus, includes shoulder and elbow jts; *greater tubercle in profile;* epicondyles ‖ film
LAT	Elbow flexed 90°, epicondyles ⊥ film	⊥ midhumerus	Lat humerus including shoulder and elbow jts; *lesser tubercle in profile;* epicondyles superimposed

SHOULDER	POSITION OF PART:	CENTRAL RAY DIRECTED:	STRUCTURES INCLUDED/ BEST SEEN:
AP *rotational projections*	Arm extended and (1) supinated, w/epicondyles ‖ film (2) palm against thigh, epicondyles 45° to film (3) elbow slightly flexed, back of hand against thigh	⊥ coracoid process	(1) External rotation: true AP humerus, shows greater tubercle in profile; see Fig. 7–16 (2) neutral position: good for calcific deposits, trauma (3) internal rotation: lateral of humerus, shows lesser tubercle in profile

(continued)

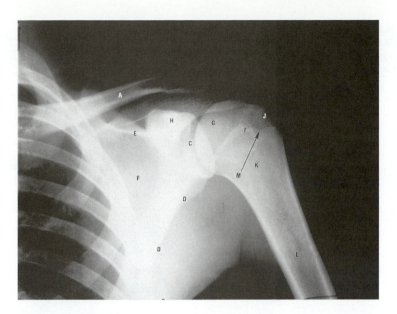

Figure 7–16. Shoulder in external rotation places humerus in a true AP position and places the greater tubercle (J) in profile. *Review the skeletal anatomy* of the shoulder by correctly identifying each of the labeled structures. (Courtesy of Bob Wong, RT.)

SHOULDER (con't)	POSITION OF PART:	CENTRAL RAY DIRECTED:	STRUCTURES INCLUDED/ BEST SEEN:
Trans-thoracic Lateral	Patient erect lateral w/ affected surgical neck centered to film; un-affected arm over head	⊥ affected surgical neck	Lateral shoulder and proximal humerus through thorax
PA Obl *scapular Y*	Affected shoulder centered with MCP 60° to film	⊥ shoulder joint	Oblique shoulder; especially good for *demonstration of dislocations* (Fig. 7–15)

CLAVICLE	POSITION OF PART:	CENTRAL RAY DIRECTED:	STRUCTURES INCLUDED/ BEST SEEN:
PA or AP	Patient recum-bent or erect; center affected clavicle to film; less OID in PA position	⊥ midshaft	Entire length of clavicle and articulations, best done PA erect or AP recumbent for patient comfort
PA Axial	Patient PA, af-fected clavicle centered to film	to supra-clavicular fossa 25 to 30° caudad	Axial projection of clavicle; can demonstrate fractures not seen in direct PA or AP

ACROMIO-CLAVICULAR JOINTS	POSITION OF PART:	CENTRAL RAY DIRECTED:	STRUCTURES INCLUDED/ BEST SEEN:
	Patient AP or PA *erect,* MSP to midfilm, arms at sides (always bilateral for comparison)	⊥ midline at level of AC jts	AP/PA projection of acromioclavicular jt and associated soft tissues; demonstrates *dislocation/ separation* when performed erect; often recommended that two exposures be made: one w/o and one w/weights (and properly identified)

SCAPULA	POSITION OF PART:	CENTRAL RAY DIRECTED:	STRUCTURES INCLUDED/ BEST SEEN:
AP	AP upright or recumbent; scapula centered w/arm abducted and elbow flexed	⊥ midscapula, ≈ 2″ inferior to coracoid process	AP scapula with lateral portion away from ribs; exposure may be made during quiet breathing to blur lung markings; see Fig. 7–17
LAT	Erect PA 45–60° obl w/affected side toward image receptor and (1) arm across chest foracromion and coracoid; *OR* (2) palpate scapular borders and rotate body to superimposed	⊥ to mid-vertebral border	Lateral scapula, (1) acromion and coracoid processes, (2) superimposed vertebral and axillary borders (Fig. 7–18) free of rib cage

B. LOWER EXTREMITY AND PELVIS

1. Foot and Toes. The bones of the foot (Fig. 7–18) include the seven *tarsal bones,* five *metatarsal bones,* and 14 *phalanges.* The *calcaneus* (os calsis), or heel bone, is the largest tarsal. It serves as attachment for the Achilles tendon posteriorly, articulates anteriorly with the *cuboid bone,* presents three articular surfaces superiorly for its articulation with the *talus,* and has a prominent shelf on its anteromedial edge called the *sustentaculum tali.*

The inferior surface of the talus *(astragalus)* articulates with the superior calcaneus to form the three-faceted *subtalar joint.* The talus also articulates anteriorly with the navicular. Articulating anteriorly with the navicular are the three *cuneiform bones:* medial/first, intermediate/

Tarsal Bones

calcaneus/os calsis
talus/astragalus
navicular
cuboid
first/medial cuneiform
second/intermediate cuneiform
third/lateral cuneiform

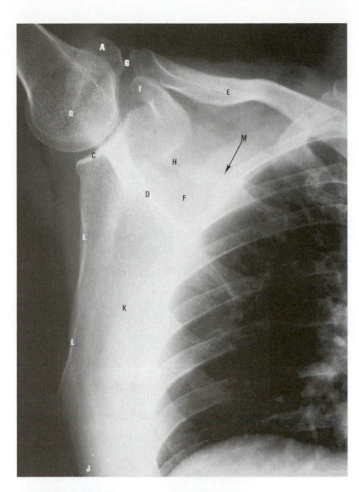

Figure 7–17. AP projection of scapula. Note that arm abduction moves scapula away from rib cage, revealing a greater portion of the scapular body. *Review the skeletal anatomy* of the scapula by correctly identifying each of the labeled structures. (Courtesy of Bob Wong, RT.)

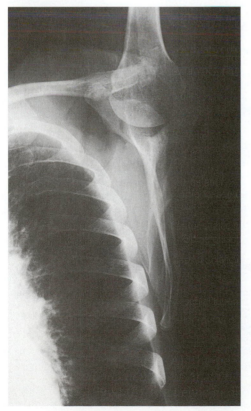

Figure 7–18. Lateral projection of scapula. Taken with arm elevated and forearm resting on head. Demonstrates scapular body with vertebral and axillary borders exactly superimposed. (Courtesy of The Stamford Hospital.)

second, and lateral/third. The navicular articulates laterally with the cuboid.

Fractures of the calcaneus can occur, especially as a result of a fall from a height directly onto the heel. The calcaneus can also be associated with painful *spur* formation.

The metatarsals and phalanges of the foot are similar to the metacarpals and phalanges of the hand. The bases of the fourth and fifth metatarsals articulate with the cuboid. The fifth (most lateral) metatarsal projects laterally and presents a large *tuberosity* at its base making it very susceptible to fracture. *Stress fractures* are common to the metatarsals (Fig. 7–19).

The first, or great, toe *(hallux)* has two phalanges; the second through fifth toes have three phalanges each. The phalanges of the toes are shorter than those of the fingers. Stubbing and crushing-type injuries are common causes of fractured phalanges. The articulations of the foot are named similarly to those of the hand.

2. Ankle. The ankle joint *(mortise)* is formed by the articulation of the talus and distal portions of the tibia and fibula (Fig. 7–20). The medial and lateral malleoli are the most frequently fractured components of the ankle joint; severe fractures can disrupt the integrity of the joint and lead to permanent instability and/or arthritis.

3. Lower Leg. The *tibia* and *fibula* (Fig. 7–21) compose the bones of the lower leg. The tibia is larger and is situated medially. It articulates superiorly with the femur and inferiorly with the talus to form a portion of the ankle joint. The tibia consists of a shaft and two expanded extremities. Its distal extremity has a prominence, the *medial malleolus,* which also participates in the formation of the ankle

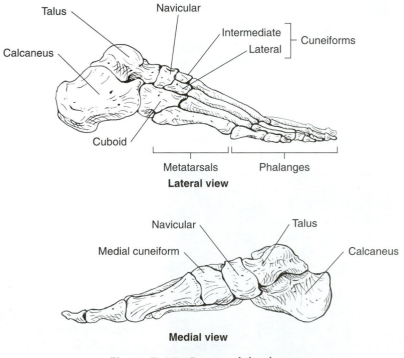

Figure 7–19. Bones of the foot.

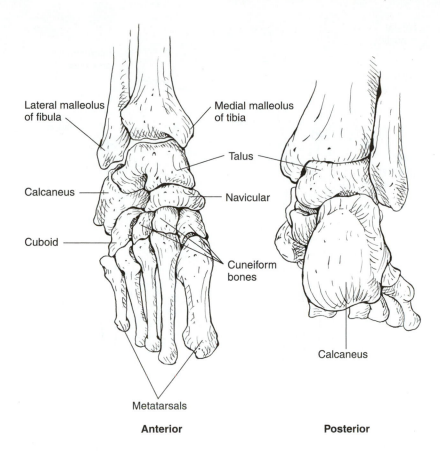

Figure 7–20. Ankle and foot: anterior and posterior views.

mortise. The fibular notch provides articulation for the fibula to form the *distal tibiofibular joint.*

The proximal end of the tibia presents a *medial* and a *lateral condyle,* on whose superior surfaces there are facets for articulation with the femur. The articular facets form a smooth surface called the *tibial plateau,* which provides attachment for the cartilaginous *menisci* of the knee joint. Between the two articular surfaces is a raised prominence, the *intercondylar eminence (tibial spine).* The proximal anterior surface of the tibia presents the *tibial tuberosity,* which provides attachment for the patellar ligament. *Osgood–Schlatter's disease* is a chronic *epiphysitis* of the tibial tuberosity that occurs in some active young adults. its symptoms include pain and tenderness and it is manifested radiographically by bony separation at the epiphysis.

The fibula is the slender, lateral non–weight-bearing bone forming the lower leg; it also consists of a shaft and two expanded extremities. The bulbous distal end is the *lateral malleolus* (projects more distally than the medial), which helps to form the ankle joint and has a facet for articulation with the tibia *(distal tibiofibular joint).* The expanded proximal portion of the fibula is the *head,* which articulates with the lateral tibial condyle, forming the *proximal tibiofibular joint.* A *styloid* process extends superiorly from the head of the fibula. The *neck* is the constricted portion just distal to the fibular head. The fibula is most commonly fractured at the malleolus, just above the ankle joint.

4. Knee.
The knee is formed by the proximal tibia, the patella, and the distal femur, which articulate to form the *femorotibial* and *femoro-*

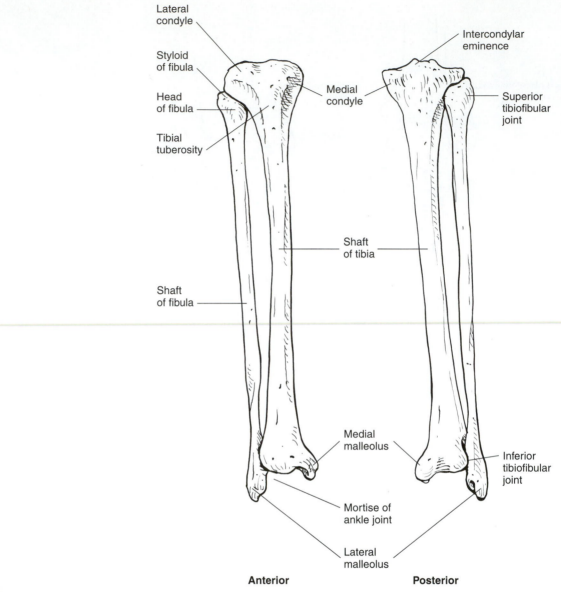

Figure 7–21. Right tibia and fibula.

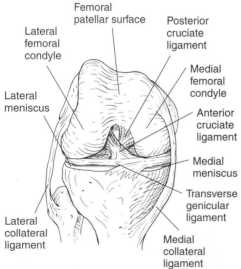

Figure 7–22. Ligaments of the knee joint.

patellar joints. The distal posterior femur presents two large *medial* and *lateral condyles* separated by the deep *intercondyloid fossa.* Two small prominences, the *medial* and *lateral epicondyles,* are just superior to the condyles. The femoral and tibial condyles articulate to form the *femorotibial joint.*

Semilunar cartilages, the *menisci,* lie medially and laterally between the articulating bones and, together with the *cruciate* and *collateral ligaments,* help to form the *articular capsule* of the knee (Fig. 7–22).

The *patella* is the largest *sesamoid* bone and, attached to the tibial tuberosity by the patellar ligament, glides over the patellar surface of the distal femur (femoropatellar joint) during flexion and extension of the knee. The *patella* is a triangular bone with its *base* superior and *apex* inferior.

The congenital anomaly, *bipartite patella,* can be misinterpreted as a fracture. Just opposite the *patellar surface,* on the posterior distal femur, is the smooth *popliteal surface,* which accommodates the popliteal artery.

5. Femur. The *femur* (Fig. 7–23) is the longest and strongest bone in the body. The femoral *shaft* is bowed slightly anteriorly and presents a long, narrow ridge posteriorly, called the *linea aspera.* The proximal end of the femur consists of a *head* that is received by the *accetabulum* of the pelvis. The femoral head has a small notch, the *fovea capitis femoris,* for ligament attachment. The *femoral neck,* which joins the head and shaft, angles upward approximately 120 degrees and forward (in *anteversion*) approximately 15 degrees. The *greater* (lateral) and *lesser* (medial) *trochanters* are large processes on the posterior proximal femur. The greater trochanter is a prominent positioning landmark that lies in the same transverse plane as the public symphysis and coccyx. The *intertrochanteric crest* runs obliquely between the trochanters; the *intertrochanteric line* runs anteriorly parallel to the crest. The femoral neck is the most commonly fractured portion of the femur (Fig. 7–24). Fractures of the femoral shaft are usually the result of a direct blow; fracture *displacement* is dependent on muscular pull and traumatic impact.

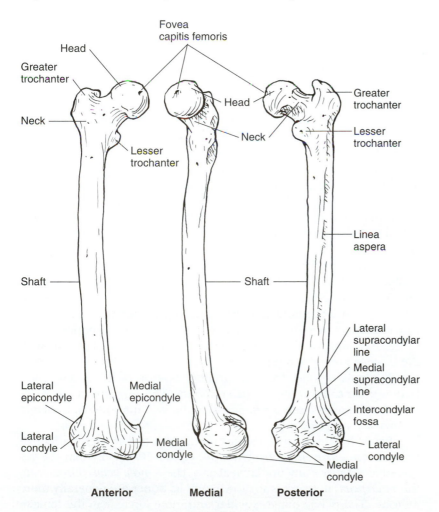

Figure 7–23. The right femur.

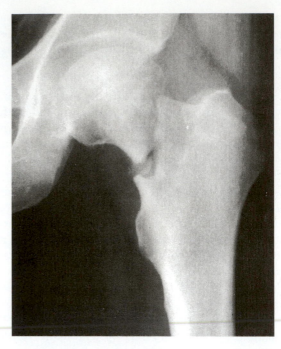

Figure 7–24. AP projection of the hip demonstrating fracture of the femoral neck. (From Way, LW, ed. *Current Surgical Diagnosis & Treatment,* 10th ed. East Norwalk, CT: Appleton & Lange, 1994, Figure 43–34; p 1044.)

Articulation Summary: Lower Extremity and Pelvic Girdle

- Sacroiliac
- Hip (femoral head w/acetabulum)
- Knee (femorotibial)
- Proximal tibiofibular
- Distal tibiofibular
- Ankle (distal tibia and fibula w/superior talus)
- Intertarsal
- Tarsometatarsal
- Metatarsophalangeal
- Interphalangeal

---

6. Pelvis. The pelvic girdle consists of two *innominate* (hip, or *coxal*) bones, one on each side of the sacrum. Each innominate bone consists of three fused bones, the *ilium, ischium,* and *pubis* (Fig. 7–25). Parts of these three bones contribute to the formation of the *acetabulum*—the socket articulation for the femoral head. The ilia are the large, superior bones whose medial *auricular* surface form the *sacroiliac joints* bilaterally. The broad, flat portion of each ilium is the *ala,* or wing; the upper part of the ala forms a ridge of bone called the *iliac crest,* which terminates in *anterior* and *posterior iliac spines.*

The ischium forms the posteroinferior portion of the pelvis. The posterior part of the ischium forms the major portion of the *greater* and *lesser sciatic notches* separated by the *ischial spine.* The most inferior portion is the *ischial tuberosity,* a large, rough prominence that provides attachment for posterior thigh muscles. The inferior *ramus* of the ischium extends medially from the tuberosities to unite with the inferior ramus of the pubis.

The public bones form the anterior portion of the pelvis. Their bodies unite to form the *public symphysis.* The superior ramus fuses with the ilium and inferior ramus with the ischium to form the large *obturator foramen.*

Pelvic fractures can cause disturbance of the urinary bladder or urethra; an *intravenous urogram/pyelogram* (IVU/IVP) may be required to diagnose any urinary leakage. The *female pelvis* differs from the *male pelvis* in that it is shallower and its bones are generally more delicate. The pelvic outlet is wider and more circular in the female;

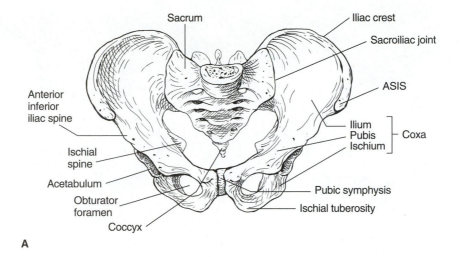

A

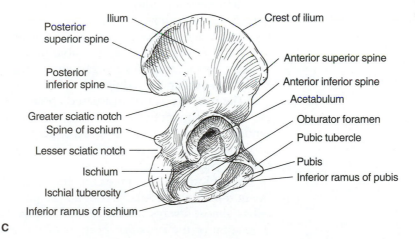

C

Figure 7–25. **(A)** The pelvis (anterior view). (Redrawn with permission from Martini, F. *Fundamentals of Anatomy and Physiology,* 2nd ed. Englewood Cliffs, NJ: Prentice-Hall, 1992.) **(B)** The pelvic girdle (posterior view). **(C)** The right hip bone (lateral view), showing the acetabulum.

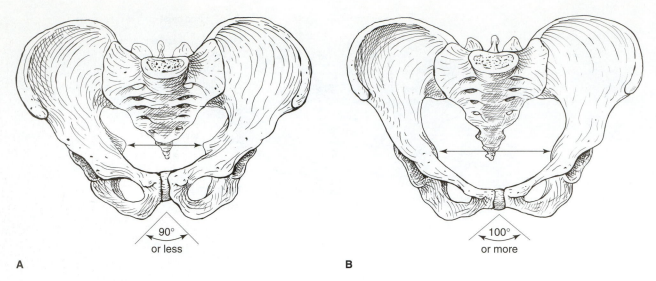

Figure 7–26. Architectural differences in the male (**A**) and female (**B**) pelves.

the ischial tuberosities and acetabula are further apart; the angle formed by the pubic arch is also greater in the female; all these bony characteristics facilitate the birth process (Fig. 7–26).

7. Positioning. Positioning of the lower extremity and pelvis requires a thorough knowledge of the skeletal anatomy, an awareness of possible pathologic conditions and their impact on positioning and technical factors.

Clothing with radiopaque objects such as buttons, snaps, or zippers should be removed whenever possible. Bulky or bunched clothing can produce undesirable radiographic artifacts and should therefore be removed whenever possible and replaced with a hospital dressing gown. Elastic-wasted garments can contribute to nonuniform density on abdominal radiographs.

The patient must be instructed about the importance of remaining still, and immobilization devices such as radioparent sponges, sandbags, or tape should be used as required. The shortest possible exposure time should be employed, especially when involuntary motion is a potential problem.

Many lower extremity examinations can be performed tabletop (ie, non-Bucky); the knee frequently requires a grid; femur, hip, and pelvis almost always do. *Suspended respiration* is suggested for radiography of the proximal portion of the lower extremity and the pelvis. Patients must be appropriately shielded.

Some of the lower leg examinations can be performed either AP or PA, depending on the condition and comfort of the patient. Lateral projections can be easily obtained using a horizontal (cross-table lateral) beam when extremity or patient movement is contraindicated.

The following tables provide a summary of routine and frequently performed special projections of the lower extremity and pelvis.

FOOT	POSITION OF PART:	CENTRAL RAY DIRECTED:	STRUCTURES INCLUDED/ BEST SEEN:
Dorso-plantar	Knee flexed ≈45°, plantar surface on cassette	⊥ or 10° toward heel to base of 3rd meta-tarsal	Tarsals (except cal-caneus and part of talus), metatarsals and phalanges with their articula-tions, in frontal projection
Medial Obl	Start as dorso-plantar, rotate medially 30°	⊥ base of 3rd metatarsal	Most tarsals and metatarsals (except the most medial) and their articula-tions, sinus tarsi, tuberosity of 5th metatarsal; see Fig. 7–27

Note: *Lateral oblique* foot demonstrates interspaces between the 1st and 2nd metatarsals and between the 1st and 2nd cuneiforms.

Lateral	Patient on affected side, patella ⊥ table-top, foot slightly dorsiflexed with plantar surface ⊥ cassette	⊥ base of 3rd metatarsal	Lateral foot and ankle joint; distal tibia and fibula; superimposed tarsals, tibia and fibula; see Fig. 7–28

Note: *Lateral weight-bearing feet* are occasionally requested to demonstrate the status of the *plantar arches.*

TOES	POSITION OF PART:	CENTRAL RAY DIRECTED:	STRUCTURES INCLUDED/ BEST SEEN:
Dorso-plantar	Knee flexed ≈45°, plantar surface on cassette	⊥ or 10° toward heel, to 2nd MPJ	Phalanges, their artic-ulations and distal metatarsals in frontal projection

(continued)

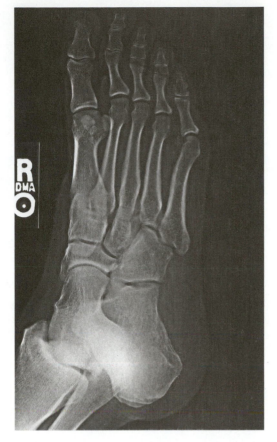

Figure 7–27. Medial oblique view of left foot demonstrates the articulations of the cuboid with the calcaneus, fourth and fifth metatarsals, and lateral cuneiform. The talonavicular articulation and sinus tarsi are also demonstrated. Note the fractured shaft of the fifth metatarsal. (Courtesy of The Stamford Hospital.)

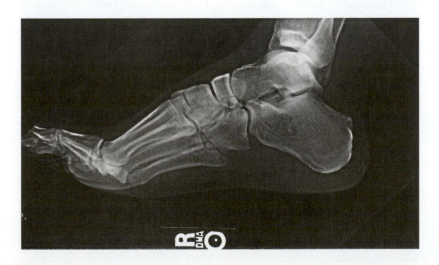

Figure 7–28. Lateral projection of foot dem-onstrates superimposed tarsals, metatarsals, and phalanges; a little more of the distal tibia and fibula should be visualized. (Courtesy of The Stamford Hospital.)

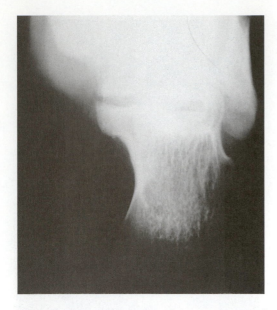

Figure 7–29. Plantodorsal projection of calcaneus; sustentaculum tali, trochlear process, and calcaneal tuberosity are well visualized. (Courtesy of The Stamford Hospital.)

TOES (con't)	POSITION OF PART:	CENTRAL RAY DIRECTED:	STRUCTURES INCLUDED/ BEST SEEN:
Medial Obl	Start as dorso-plantar, rotate medially 30 to 45°	⊥ 3rd MPJ	Oblique projection of phalanges, their articulations and distal metatarsals
LAT	Turn to side that brings affected toe(s) closest to film; unaffected toes may be taped back or occlusal film used for individual toes	⊥ proximal pip	Lateral projection of toe(s) and associated articulations

CALCANEUS	POSITION OF PART:	CENTRAL RAY DIRECTED:	STRUCTURES INCLUDED/ BEST SEEN:
Planto-dorsal	Patient seated on table with leg extended, plantar surface ⊥ tabletop (immobilize w/strip of tape held by patient)	40° cephalad to base of 3rd metatarsal	Axial projection of calcaneus; trochlear process, sustentaculum tali, talocalcaneal jt; see Fig. 7–29
Dorso-plantar	Patient prone, plantar surface ⊥ tabletop; cassette placed against plantar surface	40° caudally to level of base of 2nd metatarsal	Axial proj of calcaneus; trochlear process, sustentaculum tali, talocalcaneal jt
LAT	Patient on affected side, patella ⊥ tabletop, foot and ankle lateral	⊥ midcalcaneus	Lateral calcaneus, talus, navicular, ankle jt, and sinus tarsi; see Fig. 7–30

Figure 7–30. Lateral calcaneus; sinus tarsi is well visualized. (Courtesy of The Stamford Hospital.)

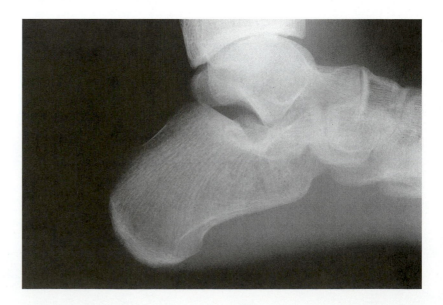

ANKLE	POSITION OF PART:	CENTRAL RAY DIRECTED:	STRUCTURES INCLUDED/ BEST SEEN:
AP	Leg extended AP, plantar surface ⊥ film	⊥ midway b/w malleoli thru tibiotalar jt	AP ankle jt, distal tibia/fibula, talus; see Fig. 7–31
LAT	Patient turned on-to affected side, patella ⊥ table-top, foot dorsi-flexed (≈90°)	⊥ ankle jt	Lateral distal tibia/fibula, ankle jt, talus, calcaneus, navicular
Medial Obl (*mortise view*)	Leg extended, plantar surface vertical w/leg rotated 15–20° medially so intermalleolar plane is parallel	⊥ ankle jt, midway between malleoli	Ankle mortise, oblique distal tibia/fibula and proximal talus; all 3 aspects of mortise jt seen in profile; see Fig. 7–32

LOWER LEG	POSITION OF PART:	CENTRAL RAY DIRECTED:	STRUCTURES INCLUDED/ BEST SEEN:
AP	Leg extended AP, no pelvic rotation, foot dorsiflexed	⊥ midshaft tibia	AP lower leg, both jts should be included

(continued)

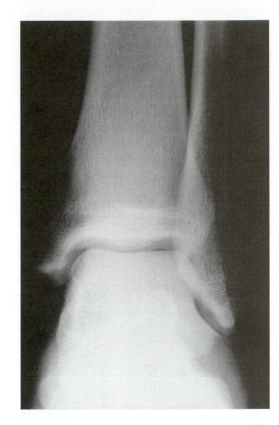

Figure 7–31. AP projection of the ankle joint. (Courtesy of The Stamford Hospital.)

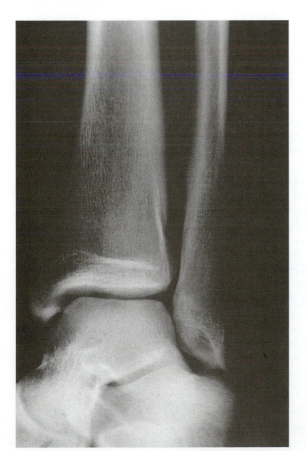

Figure 7–32. The 15 to 20° medial oblique projection of the ankle is used to demonstrate the ankle mortise. An oblique projection of the distal tibia/fibula, proximal talus, and their articular surfaces is also demonstrated. (Courtesy of The Stamford Hospital.)

LOWER LEG (con't)	POSITION OF PART:	CENTRAL RAY DIRECTED:	STRUCTURES INCLUDED/ BEST SEEN:
LAT	Patient on affected side, patella ⊥ table-top, ankle and foot lateral	⊥ midshaft	Lateral tibia/fibula, both jts should be included

KNEE	POSITION OF PART:	CENTRAL RAY DIRECTED:	STRUCTURES INCLUDED/ BEST SEEN:
AP	Leg extended AP, no pelvic rotation (leg may be rotated 3–5° internally)	to 1/2″ below patellar apex (knee jt); direction of CR depends on distance b/w ASIS and table-top: up to 19 cm (thin pelvis) ∡3–5° caudad; 19–24 cm ⊥ CR; >24 cm (thick pelvis) ∡3–5° cephalad	AP knee jt, distal femur, and proximal tibia/ fibula, patella seen thru femur
LAT	Patient on affected side, patella ⊥ tabletop, knee flexed 20–30°	5° cephalad to knee jt	Lateral proj of knee and patellofemoral jts; superimposed femoral condyles; *knee should not be flexed >10° with known or suspected patellar fx*; see Fig. 7–33
AP *weight bearing (bilateral)*	Patient AP erect against upright Bucky, weight evenly shared on legs	⊥ CR midway b/w knees at level of patellar apices	AP weight bearing knee joints particularly useful for evaluation of *arthritic conditions*

Note: The *proximal tibiofibular articulation* is best demonstrated in a 45° internal/medial oblique knee position.

Inter-condy-loid Fossa *(Camp-Coventry)*	Patient PA recumbent, knee flexed so tibia forms 40°∠ w/ tabletop and foot rested on support	CR 40° caudad (⊥ long axis of tibia) to knee jt	*PA axial* (supero-inferior) proj of intercondyloid fossa, tibial plateau, and eminences; "tunnel view"; see Fig. 7–34A&B
Inter-condy-loid Fossa *(Bècleré)*	Patient AP w/knee flexed ≈20–30° resting on supported cassette	∠ed cephalad (⊥ long axis of tibia) to knee jt	*AP axial* (infero-superior) proj of intercondyloid fossa, tibial plateau and eminences; "tunnel view"

Note: The *Holmblad* method of intercondyloid fossa is performed w/the patient in the kneeling position on the x-ray table. The affected knee is centered, CR forms a 20° angle w/femur (femur is 70° with table).

Figure 7–33. The knee should not be flexed more than 10° when transverse fracture of patella is known or suspected; flexion can cause pain, fragment separation, and fracture complication. CR angulation of 5° cephalad will superimpose the magnified medial femoral condyle on the lateral condyle and permit a better view of the joint space; angulation was not employed in this projection and the joint space is obscured by the magnified medial femoral condyle. (Courtesy of The Stamford Hospital.)

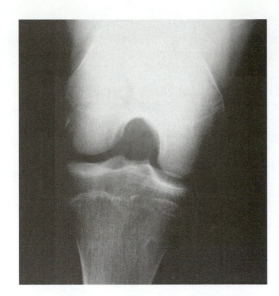

A

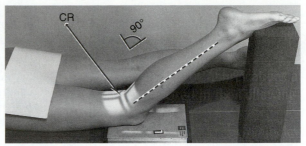

B

Figure 7–34. **(A)** Intercondyloid fossa, using the Camp–Coventry method. The tibial plateau and eminences are well visualized. (Courtesy of The Stamford Hospital.) **(B)** Patient and CR positioning for Camp–Coventry method. From Cornuelle et al. *Radiographic Anatomy and Positioning.* Stamford, CT: Appleton & Lange, 1998.)

PATELLA	POSITION OF PART:	CENTRAL RAY DIRECTED:	STRUCTURES INCLUDED/ BEST SEEN:
PA	Patient prone, leg rotated ≈5–10° laterally to place patella ‖ tabletop	⊥ patella (enters popliteal region)	PA patella, including knee jt; better detail than the AP position (less OID)
Tangential *(Hughston)*	Patient prone, knee flexed 50–60° with foot supported	45° cephalad through patellofemoral jt	Tangential proj of patella, patellofemoral articulation; useful for r/o patellar *subluxation*
Tangential *(Settegast)*	Patient prone or seated on x-ray table; knee flexed to place patella nearly ⊥ tabletop	Directed to patellar apex, exiting at its base	*Tangential* projection of the patella, patellofemoral articulation; useful for demonstrating *vertical* fx; *must not be attempted in known or suspected transverse fx of patella*

FEMUR	POSITION OF PART:	CENTRAL RAY DIRECTED:	STRUCTURES INCLUDED/ BEST SEEN:
AP	Patient supine, affected femur centered to midline of grid w/leg internally rotated 15°	⊥ midfemoral shaft (to include hip and possibly knee jt)	AP proj femur, including hip jt; leg rotation *overcomes anteversion* of femoral neck and places neck ‖ film
LAT	Patient recumbent lateral w/affected leg centered to grid; patella ⊥ tabletop	⊥ midshaft	Lateral proj femur, from knee jt up; may be performed w/horizontal beam if suspected fracture or pathologic disease

Note: If an orthopedic appliance is present, the radiograph should include the entire appliance and the articulation closest to it.

HIP	POSITION OF PART:	CENTRAL RAY DIRECTED:	STRUCTURES INCLUDED/ BEST SEEN:
AP	Patient supine, sagittal plane 2″ medial to ASIS centered to midline of grid, no pelvic rotation, leg rotated 15° internally	⊥ sagittal plane 2″ medial to ASIS at level of greater trochanter	AP hip jt, femoral neck and proximal femur; a portion of the pelvic bones is included. *The greater trochanter should be seen in profile.* Another method of hip localization is to bisect the ASIS and pubic symphysis: this is the peak of the femoral head. A point ≈2.5″ distal and ⊥ is the midpoint of the femoral neck

Note: *Leg inversion must never be forced and is contraindicated in cases of known or suspected fx or destructive disease.*

	POSITION OF PART:	CENTRAL RAY DIRECTED:	STRUCTURES INCLUDED/ BEST SEEN:
AP Oblique *(modified Cleaves)*	Patient supine, ASIS of affected side centered to grid, knee and hip acutely flexed, thigh(s) abducted 40°	⊥ the affected hip at a level 1″ above the pubic symphysis	AP oblique proj hip jt; lesser trochanter should be seen on the medial aspect of the femur; see Fig. 7–35; Note: Bilateral examination can be performed by positioning both hips and directing the CR to the MSP at a point 1″ above the pubic symphysis

Note: The above position must not be attempted when fracture is suspected.

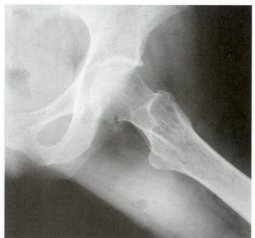

Figure 7–35. AP oblique (modified Cleaves) view of hip. The femoral neck and greater and lesser trochanters are well defined; the lesser trochanter is seen medially. (Courtesy of The Stamford Hospital.)

(continued)

HIP (con't)	POSITION OF PART:	CENTRAL RAY DIRECTED:	STRUCTURES INCLUDED/ BEST SEEN:
Axiolateral	Patient supine, unaffected leg elevated; leg rotated internally 15°, grid placed against thigh ∥ to femoral neck*	⊥ femoral neck* and grid	Lateral proj of proximal femur and its articulation with the acetabulum; *the lesser trochanter will be prominently seen on the posterior aspect of the femur*

Note: Leg inversion must never be forced and is contraindicated in cases of known or suspected fx or destructive disease.

*This position requires localization of the long axis of the femoral neck. First *mark* the midpoint between the ASIS and pubic symphysis of affected side; next *mark* a point 1″ distal to the prominence of the greater trochanter. A line between these 2 points parallels the long axis of the femoral neck.

PELVIS	POSITION OF PART:	CENTRAL RAY DIRECTED:	STRUCTURES INCLUDED/ BEST SEEN:
AP	Patient supine, MSP ⊥ tabletop, no pelvic rotation, legs rotated internally 15°	⊥ midline at a level 2″ above greater trochanter; top of cassette 1 to 2″ above iliac crest	AP proj pelvis and upper femora w/ femoral necks ∥ film and greater trochanters free of superimposition; see Fig. 7–36

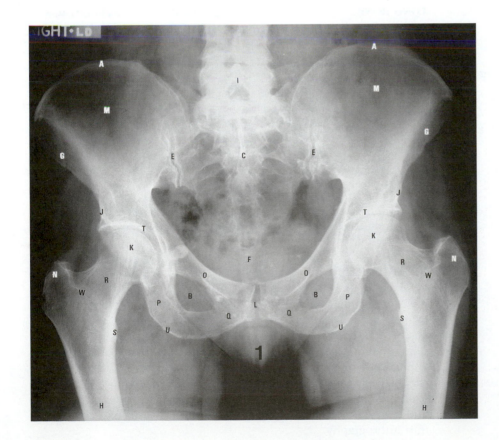

Figure 7–36. AP projection of the pelvis. The femoral necks are seen in their entirety: internal rotation of the feet/legs places them parallel to the film. *Review the skeletal anatomy* of the pelvis by correctly identifying each of the lettered structures. (Courtesy of Bob Wong, RT.)

ILIUM	POSITION OF PART:	CENTRAL RAY DIRECTED:	STRUCTURES INCLUDED/ BEST SEEN:
AP	Patient supine, sagittal plane passing through hip jt of affected side centered to grid, patient obliqued 40° toward affected side	⊥, enters the sagittal plane 2″ medial to ASIS at level m/w b/w crest and greater trochanter	AP proj of ilium, patient obliquity "opens" the ilium by placing it ∥ to the film

SACROILIAC JTS	POSITION OF PART:	CENTRAL RAY DIRECTED:	STRUCTURES INCLUDED/ BEST SEEN:
AP Obl (LPO and RPO)	Patient supine and obliqued 25–30° affected side up with sagittal plane passing 1″ me-dial to ASIS centered to grid	⊥ a point 1″ medial to ASIS	Sacroiliac (SI) jt of the *elevated side;* the opposite obl is similarly obtained; obliquity places SI jt ⊥ cassette

Note: Axial projection may be made with CR 20 to 25° cephalad.

> **To Locate Joints**
>
> **Hip:** Bisect the ASIS and pubic symphysis; center 1″ distal and lateral to that point
> **Knee:** Center immediately below the patellar apex
> **Ankle:** Center midway between the malleoli

8. Long-Bone Measurement. Accurate measurement of long bones, usually lower extremities, is occasionally required to evaluate abnormal growth patterns in children or lower back disorders in adults.

LONG BONE MEASURE-MENT	POSITION OF PART:	CENTRAL RAY DIRECTED:	STRUCTURES INCLUDED/ BEST SEEN:
AP (leg)	Patient supine, leg extended and centered to grid w/metal ruler taped alongside; one exposure each at hip, knee, and ankle jts (on one film)	⊥ hip, knee, ankle jts	Tightly collimated AP projections of hip, knee, and ankle jts with metallic ruler alongside

Note: For bilateral exam: ruler is placed between legs, there must be no rotation, and if one knee is somewhat flexed, the other must be identically flexed for the exposure.

9. Arthrography. *Arthrography* is a contrast examination performed to evaluate soft-tissue joint structures, such as articular cartilages, menisci, ligaments, and bursae. The examination is most often performed as *double* contrast, with a *positive contrast agent* (water-soluble iodinated) coating the structures and a *negative* contrast agent filling the joint cavity. Fluoroscopic images are made during the examination while applying various *stress maneuvers.* Overhead radiographs frequently follow. The knee is the most common joint to be examined in this way, although the hip, wrist, shoulder (Fig. 7–37A) and temporomandibular joint (TMJ) can also be evaluated with contrast arthrography.

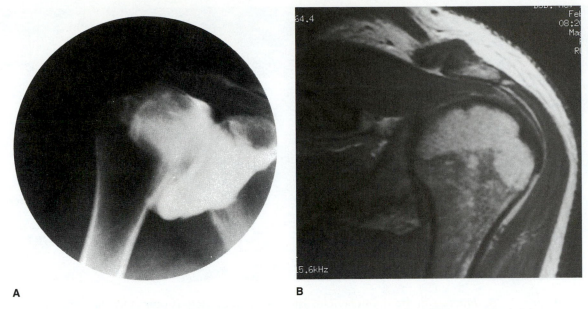

A   B

Figure 7–37. **(A)** A normal shoulder arthrogram. (Way, LW, ed. *Current Surgical Diagnosis & Treatment,* 10th ed. East Norwalk, CT: Appleton & Lange, 1994, Figure 43–18A; p 1026.) **(B)** MR image of the shoulder is accomplished noninvasively and provides visualization of structures having subtle differences in tissue density. (Courtesy of The Stamford Hospital.)

Many arthrographic procedures have been replaced by magnetic resonance imaging (MRI) studies, which have the advantage of being *noninvasive* and providing excellent soft-tissue diagnostic value (Fig. 7–37B).

10. Terminology and Pathology. Radiologically significant skeletal disorders or conditions of upper and lower extremities with which the student radiographer should be familiar are listed as follows.

Acromegaly
Battered child syndrome
Bone metastases
Bursitis
Carpal tunnel syndrome
Epicondylitis
Fracture (Fig. 7–24, 7–38, 7–41)
Gout
Osgood–Schlatter disease
Osteoarthritis
Osteochondroma

Osteomalacia
Osteomyelitis
Osteoporosis
Paget's disease (see Fig. 7–39)
Rickets
Slipped femoral capital epiphysis (see Fig. 7–40)
Subluxation
Talipes
Tendinitis

Some Conditions Requiring Adjustment in Exposure

Decrease In Exposure Factors	*Increase* In Exposure Factors
Arthritis	Acromegaly
Ewing's sarcoma	Chronic gout
Osteomalacia	Multiple myeloma
Osteoporosis	Osteochondroma
Rickets	Osteopetrosis
Thalassemia	Paget's disease (osteitis deformans)

11. Summary of Common Fracture Types

- Simple: an undisplaced fracture (fx)
- Compound: fractured end of bone has penetrated skin (open fx)
- Incomplete: fx does not traverse entire bone; little or no displacement
- Greenstick: break of cortex on one side of bone only; found in infants and children

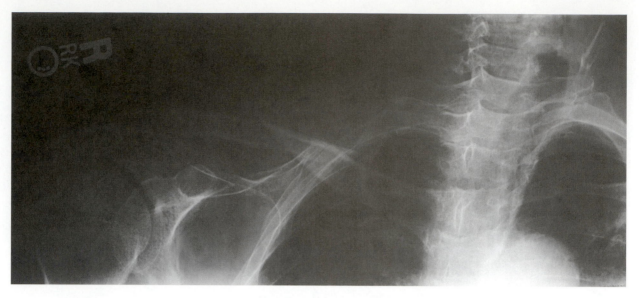

Figure 7–38. *Fracture* of the right clavicle. The S-shaped clavicle is one of the last bones to completely ossify, and is one of the most commonly fractured bones. Its medial end articulates with the sternum to form the *sternoclavicular joint;* it articulates laterally with the acromion process of the scapula, forming the *acromioclavicular joint.*

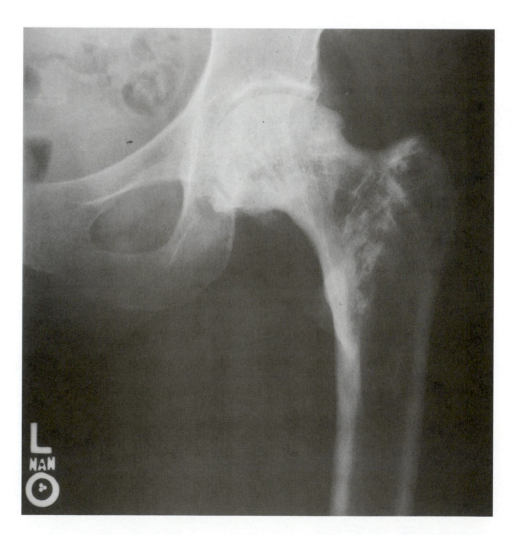

Figure 7–39. AP projection of the hip and proximal femur demonstrates *Paget's disease.* Early lytic changes are seen throughout the bone; observe the beginning of typical "cotton wool" appearance in the region of the head and trochanters. The hip is *well positioned,* the femoral neck is parallel to the image receptor (not foreshortened), the greater trochanter is seen in profile. (Courtesy of The Stamford Hospital.)

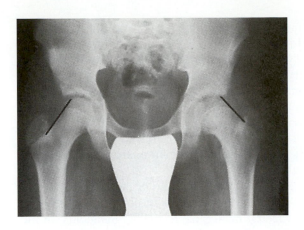

Figure 7–40. AP pelvis demonstrating left slipped femoral capital epiphysis. The growth plate is displaced. The femoral head remains within the acetabulum and the femoral neck moves anteriorly. *Note* correct placement of gonadal shield. (Reproduced with permission from Way LW, ed. *Current Surgical Diagnosis & Treatment,* 10th ed. East Norwalk, CT: Appleton & Lange, 1994.)

- Torus/buckle (see Fig. 7–41): greenstick fx with one cortex buckled/compacted and the other intact
- Stress/fatigue: response to repeated strong, powerful force (eg, jogging, marching)
- Avulsion: small bony fragment pulled from bony prominence as a result of forceful pull of the attached ligament or tendon (chip fracture)
- Hairline: faint undisplaced fx
- Comminuted: one fracture composed of several fragments

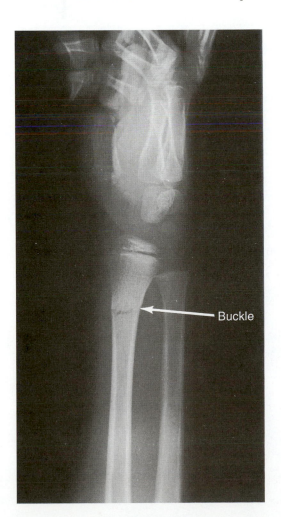

Buckle

Figure 7–41. Torus/buckle-type greenstick fracture. (From Simon, RS, Koenigsknecht, SJ. *Emergency Orthopedics: The Extremities,* 3rd ed. East Norwalk, CT: Appleton & Lange, 1995, Figure X-ray 32–X5, p 511.)

- Butterfly: comminuted fx with one or more wedge or butterfly-wing–shaped pieces
- Spiral: long fx encircling a shaft; result of torsion (twisting force); especially lower leg: distal tibia and proximal fibula
- Oblique: longitudinal fx forming an angle (approximately 45°) with the long axis of the shaft
- Transverse: fx occurring at right angles to long axis of bone
- Boxer's: fx just proximal to head of fifth metacarpal
- Monteggia: fx proximal third of ulnar shaft with anterior dislocation of radial head
- Colles' transverse fracture of distal third of radius with posterior angulation and associated avulsion fx of ulnar styloid process
- Trimalleolar: fx lateral malleolus, fx medial malleolus on medial and posterior surfaces
- Jones': fx base of fifth metatarsal
- Potts: fx distal tibia and fibula with dislocation of ankle joint
- Pathologic: fx of bone weakened by pathologic condition, for example, metastatic bone disease

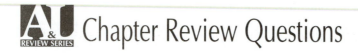 Chapter Review Questions

⭐ *Congratulations!* *You have completed a large portion of this chapter. You may go on to the "Registry-type" multiple-choice questions that follow. For greatest success, be sure to also complete the short answer questions found at the end of this chapter.*

1. A Colles' fracture involves the following:
   1. transverse fracture of the distal radius
   2. chip fracture of the ulnar styloid process
   3. posterior/backward displacement
   (A) 1 only
   (B) 1 and 2 only
   (C) 1 and 3 only
   (D) 1, 2, and 3

2. Which of the following projections will best demonstrate the carpal scaphoid?
   (A) lateral wrist
   (B) ulnar flexion/deviation
   (C) radial flexion/deviation
   (D) carpal tunnel

3. Which of the following projections requires that the humeral epicondyles be superimposed?
   1. lateral elbow
   2. lateral forearm
   3. lateral humerus
   (A) 1 only
   (B) 1 and 2 only
   (C) 1 and 3 only
   (D) 1, 2, and 3

4. An axial projection of the clavicle is often helpful in demonstrating a fracture not visualized using a perpendicular central ray. When examining the clavicle in the AP position, how is the central ray directed for the axial projection?
(A) cephalad
(B) caudad
(C) medially
(D) laterally

5. Which of the following should not be performed until a transverse fracture of the patella has been ruled out?
   1. AP knee
   2. lateral knee
   3. axial/tangential patella
(A) 1 only
(B) 1 and 2 only
(C) 2 and 3 only
(D) 1, 2, and 3

6. Which of the following best demonstrates the navicular, first and second cuneiforms and their articulations with the first and second metatarsals?
(A) lateral foot
(B) lateral oblique foot
(C) medial oblique foot
(D) weight-bearing foot

7. In which of the following positions or projections will the subtalar joint be visualized?
(A) dorsoplantar projection of the foot
(B) plantodorsal projection of the os calsis
(C) medial oblique position of the foot
(D) lateral projection of the foot

8. The proximal tibiofibular articulation is best demonstrated in which of the following positions?
(A) medial oblique
(B) lateral oblique
(C) AP
(D) lateral

9. In the medial oblique projection of the ankle, the:
   1. talofibular joint is visualized
   2. talotibial joint is visualized
   3. plantar surface should be vertical
(A) 1 only
(B) 1 and 3 only
(C) 2 and 3 only
(D) 1, 2, and 3

10. The scapular Y projection of the shoulder demonstrates:
    1. an oblique projection of the shoulder
    2. anterior or posterior dislocation
    3. a lateral projection of the shoulder
(A) 1 only
(B) 1 and 2 only
(C) 1 and 3 only
(D) 1, 2, and 3

Answers and Explanations

1. (D) A Colles' fracture is usually caused by a fall onto an outstretched (extended) hand, in order to "brake" a fall. The wrist then suffers an impacted transverse fracture of the distal inch of the radius with accompanied chip fracture of the ulnar styloid process. Because of the hand position at the time of the fall, the fracture is usually displaced backward approximately 30 degrees.

2. (C) The carpal scaphoid is somewhat curved, and consequently, is foreshortened radiographically in the posteroanterior (PA) projection. To better separate it from the adjacent carpals, the ulnar flexion maneuver is frequently employed. Radial flexion is used to better demonstrate the medial carpals. The scaphoid is superimposed on adjacent carpals in the lateral projection. The carpal tunnel/canal does not demonstrate the carpal scaphoid.

3. (D) The lateral elbow and lateral forearm must be flexed 90 degrees to superimpose the distal radius and ulna and humeral epicondyles. The lateral humerus can also be performed with the elbow flexed 90 degrees, but if the patient is unable to flex the arm, it may be left anteroposterior (AP) and a transthoracic lateral projection of the upper one-half to two-thirds of the humerus may be obtained. Because a coronal plane passing through the epicondyles is perpendicular to the film in this position, the epicondyles are superimposed.

4. (A) With the patient in the anteroposterior (AP) position, the central ray is directed cephalad. This serves to project the pulmonary apices away from the clavicle. The reverse is true when examining the clavicle in the posteroanterior (PA) position. Patients having clavicular pain are more comfortably examined in the PA erect or AP recumbent position.

5. (C) If a transverse fracture of the patella is present and the knee is *flexed,* there is danger of *separation* of the fractured segments. Because both a lateral knee and axial patella require knee flexion, they should be avoided until a transverse fracture is ruled out. When present, a transverse fracture may be seen through the femur on the anteroposterior (AP) projection. The axial ("sunrise") projection of the patella is generally used for demonstration of vertical patellar fractures.

6. (B) The lateral oblique projection of the foot demonstrates the navicular and first and second cuneiforms. To demonstrate the rest of the tarsals and intertarsal spaces, including the cuboid, sinus tarsi, and tuberosity of the fifth metatarsal, a medial oblique is required (plantar surface and film form a 30-degree angle). Weight-bearing lateral feet are used to demonstrate the longitudinal arches.

7. (B) The subtalar, or talocalcaneal, joint is a three-faceted articulation formed by the talus and os calsis (calcaneus). The plantodorsal and dorsoplantar projections of the os calsis should exhibit density sufficient to visualize the subtalar joint. If evaluation of the subtalar joint is desired, special views (such as Broden and Isherwood methods) would be required.

8. (A) With the femoral condyles of the affected side rotated *medially/internally* to form a 45-degree angle with the film, the *proximal* tibiofibular articulation is placed parallel with the film and the fibula is free of superimposition with the tibia. The lateral oblique completely superimposes the tibia and fibula. The anteroposterior (AP) and lateral projections superimpose enough of the tibia and fibula so that the tibiofibular articulation is "closed."

9. (D) The medial oblique projection (15- to 20-degree mortise view) of the ankle is valuable because it demonstrates the tibiofibular joint as well as the talotibial joint, thereby visualizing all the major articulating surfaces of the ankle joint. To demonstrate maximum joint volume, it is recommended that the plantar surface be vertical.

10. (B) The scapular Y projection requires that the coronal plane be about 60 degrees to the film, thus resulting in an oblique projection of the shoulder. The vertebral and axillary borders of the scapula are superimposed on the humeral shaft and the resulting relationship between the glenoid fossa and humeral head will demonstrate anterior or posterior dislocation. Lateral or medial dislocation is evaluated on the anteroposterior (AP) projection.

II. THE AXIAL SKELETON (FIG. 7–42)

A. VERTEBRAL COLUMN

The vertebral column (Fig. 7–43) is composed of 33 bones divided into cervical, thoracic, lumbar, sacral, and coccygeal regions, with each region having its own characteristic shape. *Intervertebral disks* between the vertebral bodies form *amphiarthrotic* joints. The cervical and lumbar regions form *lordotic* curves; the thoracic and sacral regions form *kyphotic* curves (Fig. 7–43, lateral). An exaggerated thoracic curve is called *kyphosis* ("hunchback"); an exaggerated lumbar curve is *lordosis* ("swayback"). Lateral curvature of the vertebral column is called *scoliosis*.

The typical vertebra has a *body* and a *neural arch* surrounding the *vertebral foramen*. The neural arch is composed of two *pedicles*, one on each side supporting a *lamina*. The laminae extend posteriorly to the midline and join to form the *spinous process* (lack of union, or malunion, results in *spina bifida*). Each pedicle has notches superiorly and inferiorly (*superior* and *inferior vertebral notches*) that form the *intervertebral foramina*, through which the spinal nerves pass. The neural arch also has lateral *transverse processes* for muscle attachment and *superior* and *inferior articular processes* for the formation of *apophyseal joints* (classified as diarthrotic). The vertebral

Neural Arch
Composed of:
Two pedicles
Two laminae
Encloses:
Vertebral foramen
Supports 7 processes:
Two superior articular processes
Two inferior articular processes
Two transverse processes
One spinous process

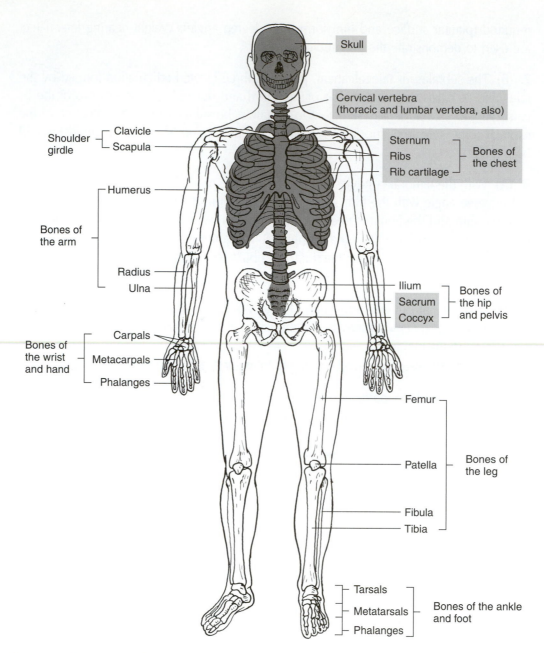

Figure 7–42. The axial skeleton. (Modified with permission from Rice, J. *Medical Terminology with Human Anatomy,* 3rd ed. East Norwalk, CT: Appleton & Lange, 1995.)

column permits flexion, extension, lateral, and rotary motions through its various articulations.

1. Cervical Spine. There are seven cervical vertebrae (Fig. 7–44). The *atlas* (C1) is a ring-shaped bone having no body and no spinous process; it is composed of an anterior and posterior arch, lateral masses, and transverse processes. Its superior articular processes articulate superiorly with the skull at the *atlantooccipital joint,* where flexion and extension occurs. The atlas articulates inferiorly with the *axis* (C2).

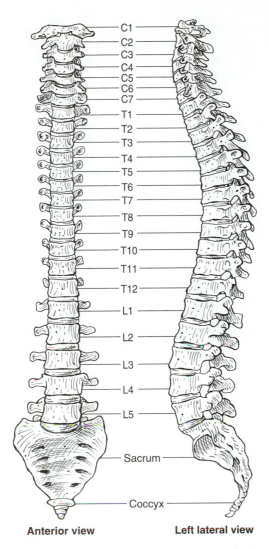

Anterior view   Left lateral view

Figure 7–43. AP and lateral views of the vertebral column.

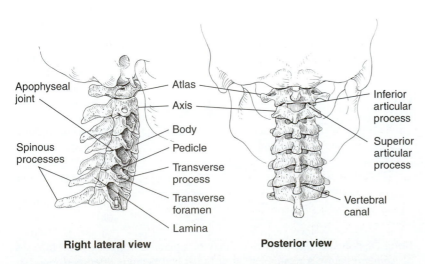

Right lateral view   Posterior view

Figure 7–44. Right lateral and posterior views of the cervical spine.

Articulation Summary: Vertebral

- Occipitoatlantal
- Atlantoaxial
- Costovertebral
- Costotransverse
- Lumbosacral
- Sacroiliac
- Sacrococcygeal
- Intervertebral
- Apophyseal/interarticular

The axis has a superior projection, the *dens,* or *odontoid process.* The axis articulates superiorly with the atlas at the *atlantoaxial joint,* a *pivot* joint where rotation takes place, and inferiorly with C3 at the apophyseal articulation.

The typical cervical vertebra is small and has a *transverse foramen* in each transverse process for passage of the vertebral artery. Cervical spinous processes are usually *bifid.* The spinous process of C7 *(vertebra prominens)* is not bifid, is larger, horizontal, and is a useful positioning landmark.

Fractures and/or dislocations of the cervical spine are usually due to acute *hyperflexion* or *hyperextension* as a result of indirect trauma. *Whiplash* injury is caused by a sudden, forced movement in one direction and then the opposite direction (as in rear-end automobile impacts). Whiplash symptoms frequently include neck pain and stiffness, headache, and pain and numbness of the upper extremities. Whiplash is often evidenced radiographically by straightening or reversal of the normal lordotic curve. Osteoarthritis is characterized in the cervical and lumbar spine by chronic, progressive degeneration of cartilage and *hypertrophy* of bone along the articular margins, characterized radiographically by narrowed joint spaces, and *osteophytes*. It can also be seen in the articulations of the fingers, toes, hips, and knees.

CERVICAL SPINE	POSITION OF PART:	CENTRAL RAY DIRECTED:	STRUCTURES INCLUDED/ BEST SEEN:
AP	Patient supine, MSP ⊥ table; adjust flexion so mastoid tip and occlusal plane are aligned	15 to 20° cephalad to thyroid cartilage	AP of *lower 5* cervical vertebrae and intervertebral disk spaces
AP *Atlas and Axis*	Patient supine, MSP ⊥ table, w/patient's mouth open, adjust flexion so mastoid tips and upper occlusal plane are aligned ⊥ cassette	⊥ center of opened mouth	AP proj of C1 and C2 (atlas and axis) (Fig. 7–45) and their articulations. *Too much flexion* superimposes teeth on odontoid; *too much extension* superimposes base of skull on odontoid
LAT	Patient erect w/L side adjacent to cassette, chin slightly elevated, shoulders depressed, MSP ‖ cassette centered, at level of C4	⊥ C4	Lat proj of all 7 vertebrae (Fig. 7–46). Shows intervertebral jt spaces, apophyseal jts, spinous processes, bodies; due to the unavoidable OID, a 72″ SID should be used

Note: Flexion and extension views may be obtained in this position in cases of *whiplash* injury. A recumbent lat w/horizontal beam is often performed recumbent w/a horizontal beam as the first radiograph in cases of suspected *subluxation*.

(continued)

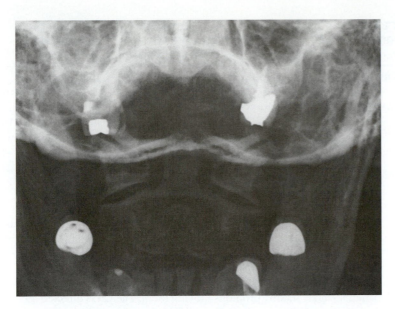

Figure 7–45.

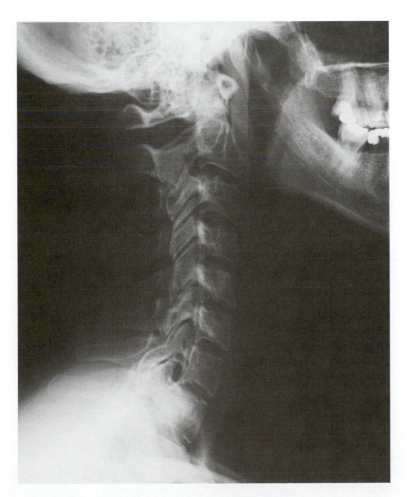

Figure 7–46.

CERVICAL SPINE (con't)	POSITION OF PART:	CENTRAL RAY DIRECTED:	STRUCTURES INCLUDED/ BEST SEEN:
OBL (*LAO and RAO*)	Patient PA erect, MSP 45° to cassette centered to C5 (1″ inferior to thyroid cartilage), chin slightly raised	15 to 20° caudad to center of cassette	Oblique cervical spine; best view of intervertebral foramina *closest* to cassette; a similar view can be obtained w/the patient *LPO* and *RPO,* CR ∠ed cephalad, and showing the foramina *farthest* from the cassette (see Fig. 7–47)

Note: Oblique cervical spine may be performed in the *recumbent position* on patients whose trauma prohibits moving them. The CR is directed 45° medially for one oblique and 45° laterally for the other.

LAT *cervicothoracic* (*"swimmer's lateral"*)	Patient erect (or recumbent) lat w/*midaxillary line* centered to grid, MSP ∥, arm adjacent to cassette over head, depress opposite shoulder farthest from grid	⊥ T2	Lateral proj of lower cervical and upper thoracic vertebrae; particularly useful for broad-shouldered individuals

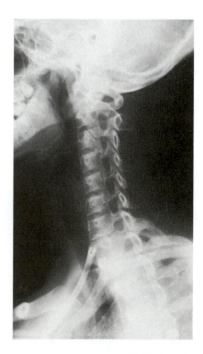
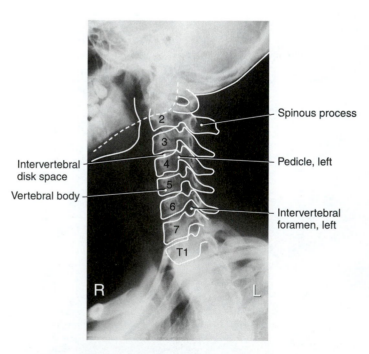

Figure 7–47. An RPO cervical spine. Locate and identify the bony structures shown particularly well in the oblique. (From Cornuelle et al. *Radiographic Anatomy and Positioning.* Stamford, CT: Appleton & Lange, 1998.)

2. Thoracic Spine. There are 12 thoracic vertebrae, which are larger in size than cervical vertebrae and which increase in size as they progress inferiorly toward the lumbar region. Thoracic spinous processes are fairly long and sharply angled caudally. The bodies and transverse processes have *articular facets* for the *diarthrotic* rib articulations (see Fig. 7–48).

A common metabolic bone disorder frequently noted in radiographic examinations of the thoracic spine is osteoporosis. *Osteoporosis* is characterized by bone demineralization and can result in compression fractures of the vertebrae. The condition is most common in sedentary and postmenopausal women.

THORACIC SPINE	POSITION OF PART:	CENTRAL RAY DIRECTED:	STRUCTURES INCLUDED/ BEST SEEN:
AP	Patient supine, MSP ⊥ tabletop, top of cassette 1″ above shoulders	⊥ T7	AP proj of thoracic vertebrae and intervertebral spaces; it is helpful to use the anode heel effect and/or compensating filtration to provide more uniform density

Note: To demonstrate *apophyseal joints, 70° obliques* are performed.

LAT	Patient L lat recumbent, midaxillary line centered to table, arms ⊥ long axis of body, top of cassette 1″ above shoulders	5 to 15° cephalad (⊥ long axis of spine)	Lateral proj of thoracic vertebrae, especially bodies, intervertebral spaces and foramina; a vertical beam may be used if the patient's MSP is adjusted to ‖ the tabletop

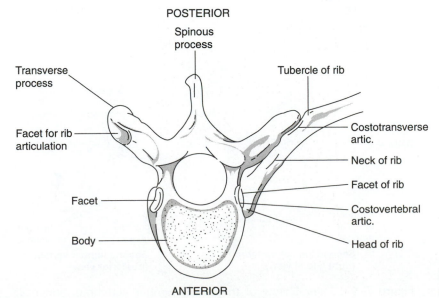

POSTERIOR

Spinous process

Transverse process

Tubercle of rib

Facet for rib articulation

Costotransverse artic.

Neck of rib

Facet of rib

Facet

Costovertebral artic.

Body

Head of rib

ANTERIOR

Figure 7–48. Thoracic vertebra and its articulation with rib (superior view).

3. Lumbar Spine. The five lumbar vertebrae are the largest of the vertebral column and increase in size toward the sacral region. The spinous processes are short, horizontal and serve as attachment for strong muscles (see Fig. 7–49). The causes of lumbar pain are numerous. Trauma, fracture, spasm of the paralumbar muscles, herniated intervertebral disk, and osteoarthritis are a few causes of low back pain. Disorders that may be detected radiographically include *osteoarthritis, spondylolysis, spondylolisthesis,* and *ankylosing spondylitis.* Myelography and MRI are used to evaluate *herniated intervertebral disks.*

LUMBAR SPINE	POSITION OF PART:	CENTRAL RAY DIRECTED:	STRUCTURES INCLUDED/ BEST SEEN:
AP	Patient supine, MSP ⊥ tabletop, knees flexed	⊥ to L3	AP proj of lumbar vertebrae L1–L4, intervertebral spaces, transverse processes; *flexion of the knees reduces lumbar curve and OID* (see Fig. 7–50)

(continued)

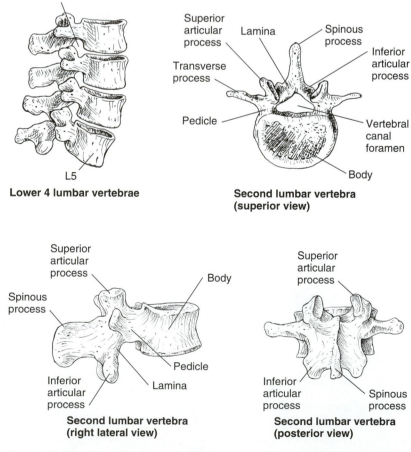

Lower 4 lumbar vertebrae

Second lumbar vertebra (superior view)

Second lumbar vertebra (right lateral view)

Second lumbar vertebra (posterior view)

Figure 7–49. Lateral view of the lower lumbar vertebrae. Superior, right lateral, and posterior views of L2.

LUMBAR SPINE (con't)	POSITION OF PART:	CENTRAL RAY DIRECTED:	STRUCTURES INCLUDED/ BEST SEEN:
AP (L5–S1)	Patient supine, MSP ⊥ tabletop, legs extended	To MSP at 30 to 35° cephalad to a point m/w b/w ASIS and pubic symph ⊥ L3	AP of lumbosacral articulation not seen on AP lumbar
OBL *(RPO and LPO)*	Patient AP recumbent, obliqued 45° w/spine centered to grid		Obl proj of lumbar vertebrae, especially for apophyseal articulations (L1–L4) of side *adjacent* to table; opposite obl is done to show opposite articulations (see Fig. 7–51A and B).

Note: *This proj demonstrates the characteristic "Scotty dogs"* (see Fig. 7–51A and B). Obl lumbar spine may also be performed in the PA position and demonstrates the apophyseal articulations *away* from the film.

Note: L5–S1 apophyseal articulations shown in 35° obl.

(continued)

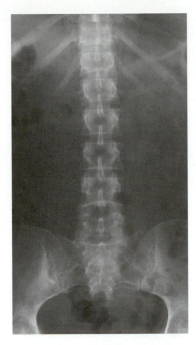

Figure 7–50. AP projection of the lumbar spine. Flexion of the knees reduces lumbar curve and OID; relieves strain on lower back muscles; patients are most comfortable with sponge or pillow support placed under knees. (From Cornuelle et al. *Radiographic Anatomy and Positioning.* Stamford, CT: Appleton & Lange, 1998.)

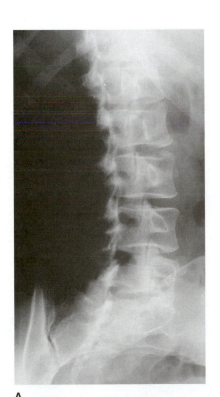

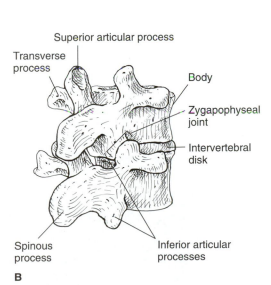

A   **B**

Figure 7–51. **(A)** Oblique lumbar spine, illustrating the lumbar apophyseal joints. Note "scotty dog" images. The scotty's "ear" corresponds to the *superior articular process,* his "nose" to the *transverse process,* his "eye" is the *pedicle,* his "neck" the *pars interarticularis,* his "body" is the *lamina,* and his "front foot" is the *inferior articular process.* (Courtesy of The Stamford Hospital.) **(B)** Forty-five degree posterolateral view of lumbar vertebrae. Note structures that form the classic "scotty dog." (From Cornuelle et al. *Radiographic Anatomy and Positioning.* Stamford, CT: Appleton & Lange, 1998.)

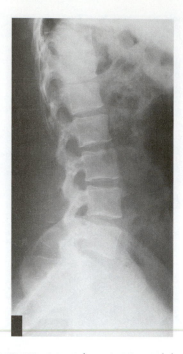

Figure 7–52. Lateral projection of the lumbar spine. If MSP is adjusted parallel to tabletop CR angulation is unnecessary. (From Cornuelle et al. *Radiographic Anatomy and Positioning.* Stamford, CT: Appleton & Lange, 1998.)

LUMBAR SPINE (con't)	POSITION OF PART:	CENTRAL RAY DIRECTED:	STRUCTURES INCLUDED/ BEST SEEN:
LAT	Patient L lateral recumbent, midaxillary line centered to grid	5 to 8° caudad L3	Lat proj, especially for vertebral bodies, interspaces, intervertebral foramina, spinous processes; if MSP adjusted ∥ tabletop, CR is vertical (see Fig. 7–52)
LAT (L5–S1)	Patient L lat recumbent, centerplane 1.5″ posterior to midaxillary line to grid, adjust MSP ∥ tabletop	⊥ coronal plane at level m/w b/w crest and ASIS	Lat proj L5–S1; if MSP not adjusted ∥ tabletop CR is ∠ed 5 to 8° caudad

4. Sacrum. There are five fused sacral vertebrae (Fig. 7–53); the fused *transverse processes* form the *alae*. The anterior and posterior *sacral foramina* transmit spinal nerves. The *sacrum* articulates superiorly with the fifth lumbar vertebra, forming the L5–S1 articulation and inferiorly with the *coccyx* to form the *sacrococcygeal joint*.

SACRUM	POSITION OF PART:	CENTRAL RAY DIRECTED:	STRUCTURES INCLUDED/ BEST SEEN:
AP	Patient AP supine, MSP ⊥ tabletop	15° cephalad to midline, to point m/w b/w pubic symphysis and ASIS	AP proj of sacrum; CR ∠ parallels sacral curve and provides less distorted visualization *(continued)*

Figure 7–53. Sacrum and coccyx. (Reproduced with permission from Chusid, JG. *Correlative Neuroanatomy & Functional Neurology,* 19th ed. East Norwalk, CT: Appleton & Lange, 1985.)

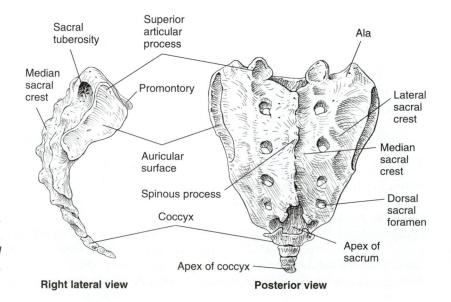

Right lateral view   **Posterior view**

SACRUM (con't)	POSITION OF PART:	CENTRAL RAY DIRECTED:	STRUCTURES INCLUDED/ BEST SEEN:
LAT	Patient L lat recumbent, 3.5" posterior to ASIS centered to grid	⊥ a point 3.5" post to ASIS	Lat proj of sacrum (see Fig. 7–54)

5. Coccyx. There are four or five fused coccygeal vertebrae (see Fig. 7–53). Fracture of the coccyx usually results from a fall onto it, landing in a seated position. Fracture displacement is fairly common and occasionally requires removal of the fractured fragment to relieve the painful symptoms.

COCCYX	POSITION OF PART:	CENTRAL RAY DIRECTED:	STRUCTURES INCLUDED/ BEST SEEN:
AP	Patient AP supine, MSP ⊥ tabletop	10° caudad to midline to point 2" above pubic symphysis	AP proj of coccyx; CR ∠ parallels coccygeal curve and provides less distorted visualization
Lat	Patient L lat recumbent, coronal plane 3.5" post to and 2" inf to ASIS centered to grid	⊥ a point 3.5" post to and 2" inf to ASIS at level of mid coccyx	Lat proj of coccyx and its articulation with the sacrum; (see Fig. 7–54)

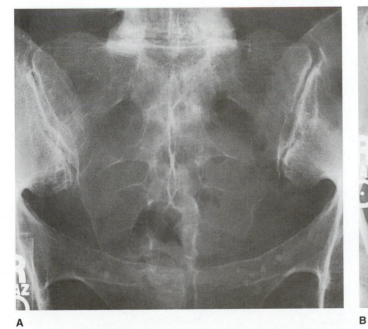

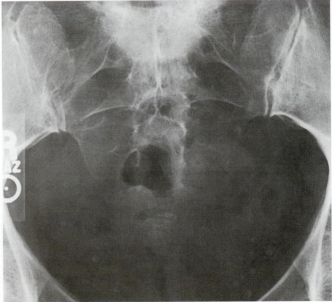

A

B

Figure 7–54. **(A)** AP projection of the sacrum. The CR is angled cephalad (because of the sacrum's kyphotic curve) to "open" the sacral foramina. (Courtesy of The Stamford Hospital.) **(B)** AP projection of the coccyx. The CR is angled caudad to overcome foreshortening of the coccyx. (Courtesy of The Stamford Hospital.)

6. Scoliosis Series

SCOLIOSIS SERIES	POSITION OF PART:	CENTRAL RAY DIRECTED:	STRUCTURES INCLUDED/ BEST SEEN:
	14″ × 17″ film of vertebrae to include 1″ of iliac crest/L5–S1	⊥ center of cassette	4 exposures made in this way: PA recumbent, PA erect, PA/bending L and R; *radiation dose is reduced when breast and thyroid shields are used and when examination is performed PA rather than AP*

B. THORAX

1. Sternum and Sternoclavicular Joints. The bones of the *thorax* (sternum, ribs, thoracic vertebrae; Fig. 7–55) function to protect the vital organs within (heart, lungs, major blood vessels). The *sternum* forms the anterior central portion of the thorax and is composed of three major divisions: the *manubrium, body,* and *xiphoid process.* Sternal fractures are uncommon; when they do occur, frac-

---

Articulation Summary: Thorax

- Sternoclavicular
- Sternochondral
- Costochondral
- Costovertebral
- Costotransverse

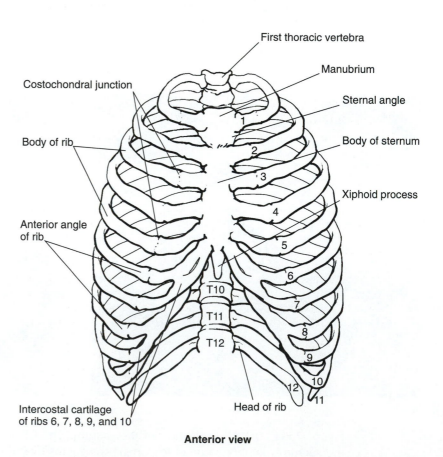

First thoracic vertebra
Manubrium
Sternal angle
Body of sternum
Xiphoid process
Costochondral junction
Body of rib
Anterior angle of rib
Intercostal cartilage of ribs 6, 7, 8, 9, and 10
Head of rib

Anterior view

Figure 7–55. The thoracic cage: anterior, posterior, and lateral views.

ture displacement is rare, but the possibility of traumatic injury to the heart must still be considered.

2. Ribs. The *rib* cage (see Fig. 7–55) consists of 12 pair of ribs. Ribs 1 to 7 articulate with thoracic vertebrae and the sternum, and are called "true ribs." Ribs 8 to 10 articulate with thoracic vertebrae and the superjacent costal cartilage to form the anterior costal margin, and are called *"false ribs."* The last two pairs of false ribs articulate only with thoracic vertebrae and are referred to as *"floating ribs."* *Rib fractures* are a common injury in thoracic trauma because of their relative thinness and exposed position. Their fracture may be complicated by *pneumothorax, hemothorax,* liver laceration (right lower ribs), or spleen laceration (left lower ribs).

STERNUM	POSITION OF PART:	CENTRAL RAY DIRECTED:	STRUCTURES INCLUDED/ BEST SEEN:
PA OBL (RAO)	Patient 15 to 20° RAO; greater obliquity for thin patients, sternum centered to midline of table	⊥ midsternum	Obl-frontal proj *RAO projects sternum into heart shadow for uniform density;* long exposure can be made during quiet breathing to blur pulmonary vascular markings
LAT	Patient erect L lat, shoulders rolled back, MSP vertical, cassette top 1.5″ above manubrial notch	⊥ midsternum	Lat proj of sternum free of superimposition of ribs; exposure made on deep inspiration to move sternum away from ribs

STERNO-CLAVICULAR JOINTS	POSITION OF PART:	CENTRAL RAY DIRECTED:	STRUCTURES INCLUDED/ BEST SEEN:
PA	Patient prone, MSP centered to grid, cassette centered at T3 (suprasternal notch)	⊥ T3	Bilateral PA proj of sternoclavicular jts visualized through superimposed vertebrae and ribs
PA OBL (LAO and RAO)	Patient prone, MSP centered to grid, rotate body ≈15° *affected side down*	⊥ affected joint	obl proj of sterno-clavicular jt *closest to film;* similar results can be obtained w/a ⊥ MSP and w/CR 15° toward midline from the affected side

---

Radiographically Significant Skeletal Disorders and Conditions of the Axial Skeleton

Achondroplasia
Ankylosing spondylitis
Cervical rib
Degenerative disk disease
Herniated disk
Hydrocephalus
Kyphosis
Lordosis
Osteophyte
Osteoporosis
Pectus excavatum
Scoliosis
Spina bifida
Spondylolisthesis
Spondylolysis
Transitional vertebra
Whiplash

RIBS	POSITION OF PART:	CENTRAL RAY DIRECTED:	STRUCTURES INCLUDED/ BEST SEEN:
AP	Patient supine or AP erect, MSP ⊥ midline of table, top of cassette 1″ above shoulder	⊥ center of cassette, about level of T7	AP proj, upper posterior ribs best delineated; do PA for better detail of anterior ribs
PA OBL (*LAO, RAO*)	Patient prone or erect PA, rotate 45°, *unaffected side down*	⊥ center of cassette, about level of T7 (at T10 to T12 for below diaphragm)	Obl shows *axillary* portions of ribs, RAO shows left ribs, LAO shows right ribs
AP OBL (*LPO, RPO*)	Patient supine or erect AP, rotate to 45° affected side toward the cassette	⊥ center of cassette, about level of T7 (at T10 to T12 for below diaphragm)	LPO shows *left* posterior ribs and their axillary portions, RPO shows *right* ribs and their axillary portions

Note: *Above-diaphragm* ribs are exposed on deep *inspiration* or during quiet breathing (long exposure). *Below-diaphragm* ribs are exposed on forced *expiration.*

C. HEAD AND NECK

1. Skull. The *skull* (Figs. 7–56 to 7–58) has 2 major parts: the *cranium,* which is composed of eight bones and houses the brain; and the 14 irregularly shaped *facial bones.* The eight cranial bones are the paired *parietal* and *temporal* bones and the unpaired *frontal, occipital, ethmoid* and *sphenoid* bones. The 14 facial bones include the paired *nasal, lacrimal, palatine, inferior nasal conchae, maxillae,* and *zygomatic* bones and the unpaired *vomer* and *mandible.*

The average shaped skull is termed *mesocephalic* (petrous pyramids and MSP from ≈47°), the broad skull is termed *brachycephalic* (petrous pyramids and MSP form ≈54°), and the elongated skull is termed *dolichocephalic* (petrous pyramids and MSP form ≈40°). These deviations are readily observable in axial CT and MR images. The inner and outer compact tables of the skull are separated by cancellous tissue called *diploë.* The internal table has a number of branching *meningeal grooves* and larger *sulci* that house blood vessels.

The bones of the skull are separated by immovable *(synarthrotic)* joints called *sutures.* The major sutures of the cranium are the *sagittal,* which separates the parietal bones; the *coronal,* which separates the frontal and parietal bones; the *lambdoidal,* which separates the parietal and occipital bones; and the *squammosal,* which separates the temporal and parietal bones (see Figs. 7–56 and 7–58). The articular surfaces of these bones have serrated-like edges with small projecting bones called *wormian* bones that fit together to form the articular sutures. The sagittal and coronal sutures meet at the *bregma,* which corresponds to the fetal anterior fontanel. The sagittal and lambdoidal sutures meet posteriorly at the *lambda,* which corresponds to the fetal posterior fontanel. The parietal, frontal, and sphenoid bones

---

Cranial Bones (8)

(1) Frontal
(2) Parietal
(2) Temporal
(1) Occipital
(1) Ethmoid
(1) Sphenoid

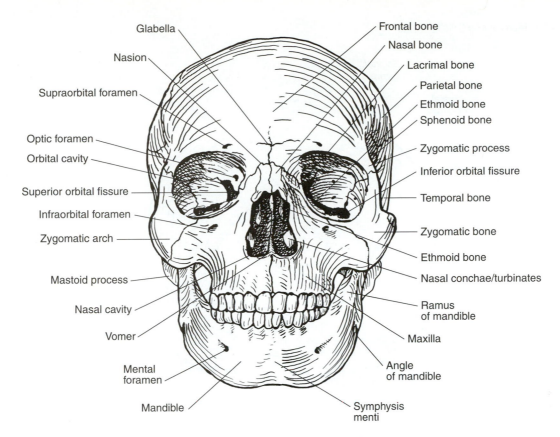

Figure 7–56. Anterior view of the skull, labeled.

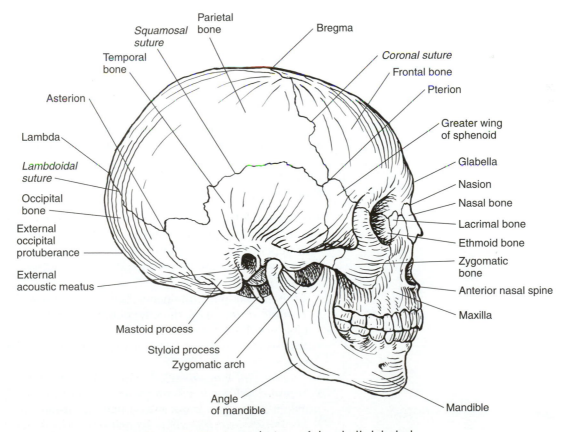

Figure 7–57. Lateral view of the skull, labeled.

137

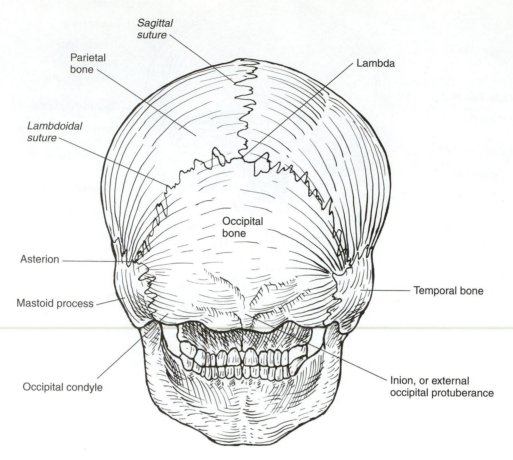

Figure 7–58. Posterior view of the skull.

meet at the *pterion* (see Fig. 7–57), the location of the anterolateral fontanel. The highest point of the skull is called the *vertex*.

a. Cranial Bones
Frontal Bone

- The frontal bone corresponds to the forehead region.
- *Orbital plates* (2): horizontal part of frontal bone; forms much of superior aspect of bony orbit.
- *Frontal eminences* (2): on anterior surface of frontal bone, lateral to MSP.
- *Glabella:* smooth prominence between eyebrows.
- *Frontal sinuses* (2): directly behind glabella, between the tables of the skull.
- *Superciliary arches/ridges* (2): ridge of bone under eyebrow region.
- *Supraorbital margins* (2): upper border/rim of bony orbit.
- *Supraorbital notches/foramina* (2): midportion of supraorbital margin; passage for artery and nerve to forehead.
- *Frontonasal suture:* where frontal bone articulates with nasal bones (corresponds exteriorly with *nasion*).

Parietal Bone

- Paired; form the vertex and part of lateral portions of cranium.
- Meet at midline to form sagittal suture; other borders help form coronal, squamosal, and lambdoidal sutures.
- *Parietal eminences:* rounded prominence on lateral surface of each parietal bone.

Ethmoid Bone (Figs. 7–57 and 7–60)

- Located between orbits; helps form parts of nasal and orbital walls.
- *Cribriform plate:* porous, passage for olfactory nerves; horizontal portion between orbital plates of frontal bone.
- *Crista galli:* extends superiorly from midportion of cribriform plate.
- *Perpendicular plate:* extends downward from crista galli to form major portion of nasal septum.
- *Superior and middle nasal turbinates/conchae:* cartilaginous; within nasal cavity, attached to perpendicular plate.
- *Ethmoidal labyrinths/lateral masses:* help form medial wall of orbit; ethmoidal sinuses within.

Sphenoid Bone (see Figs. 7–59 and 7–60)

- Wedge- or bat-shaped bone located between frontal and occipital bones.
- Anchor for eight cranial bones.
- Forms small part of lateral cranial wall and part of skull base.
- Consists of body, two lesser wings, two greater wings, two pterygoid processes and hamuli.
- *Body:* central portion; midline of skull base; anterior part joins ethmoid bone; contains the two sphenoid sinuses.
- *Lesser (minor) wings:* anterior portion, articulates with orbital plates; contain optic canals for passage of optic nerves and ophthalmic arteries.
- *Anterior clinoid processes:* formed by medial aspect of lesser wings.
- *Tuberculum sellae:* ridge of bone between anterior clinoid processes; anterior boundary of sella turcica.
- *Optic (chiasmic) groove:* horizontal depression crossing body of bone in front of sella turcica; where optic nerves cross.
- *Optic foramen and canal:* passage for optic nerve and ophthalmic artery at the orbit's apex.
- *Sella turcica:* deep depression in sphenoid bone; houses pituitary gland.
- *Dorsum sellae:* posterior boundary/wall of sella turcica.
- *Posterior clinoid processes:* extend laterally from dorsum sellae.
- *Clivus:* basilar portion; slopes down and posteriorly from dorsum sellae; articulates with basilar portion of occipital bone.
- *Superior orbital fissures:* large spaces between greater and lesser wings; for passage of four cranial nerves.
- *Greater (major) wings:* larger, posterior portion of sphenoid bone; contains the foramina rotundum, ovale, and spinosum for transmission of cranial nerves.
- *Pterygoid processes:* extend inferiorly from junction of body with great wing; each has a medial and lateral plate that articulates with posterior part of adjacent maxillae.

Types of Fractures

Linear fx
A skull fx, straight and sharply defined.

Depressed fx
A comminuted skull fx, with one or more portions pushed inward.

Hangman's fx
Fx of C2 with anterior subluxation of C2 on C3; result of forceful hyperextension.

Compression fx
Especially of spongy (cancellous) bone; diminished thickness or width as a result of compression-type force (eg, vertebral body).

Blowout fx
Fx of orbital floor as a result of a direct blow.

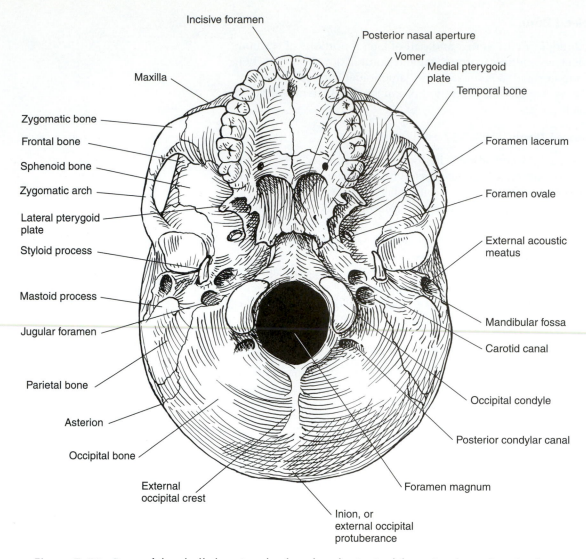

Figure 7–59. Base of the skull showing the fossal and principal foramina (superior view).

- *Inferior orbital fissures:* large openings, lie between the greater wings and the maxilla.

Occipital Bone (see Figs. 7–58 and 7–60)

- Forms part of posterior wall and inferior part of cranium.
- Upper portion of each side articulates with parietal bones to form lambdoidal suture.
- *Basilar portion:* articulates anteriorly with basilar portion (clivus) of sphenoid bone.
- *Lateral portions* (2): bilateral to foramen magnum; occipital condyles, hypoglossal canals, and jugular foramina located here.
- *Foramen magnum:* large opening; transmits inferior portion of brain (medulla oblongata), which is continuous with spinal cord.
- *Squamosal portion:* posterior, superior portion; presents the external occipital protuberance (inion, occiput).

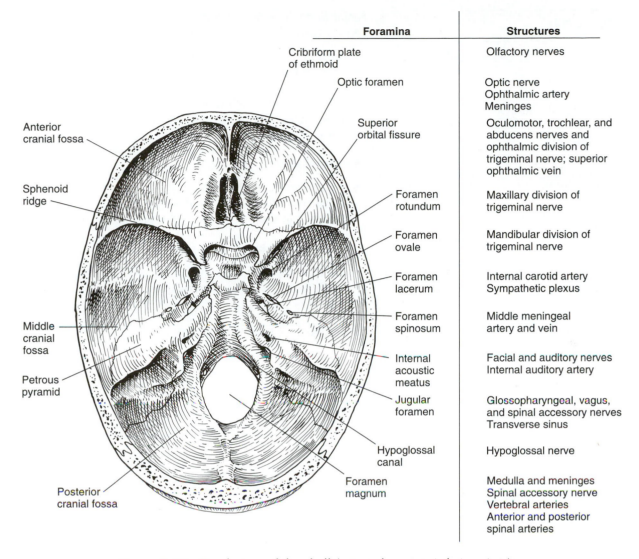

Foramina	Structures
Cribriform plate of ethmoid	Olfactory nerves
Optic foramen	Optic nerve Ophthalmic artery Meninges
Superior orbital fissure	Oculomotor, trochlear, and abducens nerves and ophthalmic division of trigeminal nerve; superior ophthalmic vein
Foramen rotundum	Maxillary division of trigeminal nerve
Foramen ovale	Mandibular division of trigeminal nerve
Foramen lacerum	Internal carotid artery Sympathetic plexus
Foramen spinosum	Middle meningeal artery and vein
Internal acoustic meatus	Facial and auditory nerves Internal auditory artery
Jugular foramen	Glossopharyngeal, vagus, and spinal accessory nerves Transverse sinus
Hypoglossal canal	Hypoglossal nerve
Foramen magnum	Medulla and meninges Spinal accessory nerve Vertebral arteries Anterior and posterior spinal arteries

Labels: Anterior cranial fossa, Sphenoid ridge, Middle cranial fossa, Petrous pyramid, Posterior cranial fossa

Figure 7–60. Basal view of the skull (external aspect, inferior view).

Temporal Bone (see Figs. 7–57 and 7–59)

- Irregularly shaped bone forming lateral aspects of cranium.
- Located between greater wings of sphenoid bone and occipital bone.
- Dense, **petrous portions** form ridges and contain the organs of hearing.
- Contain internal auditory meati and carotid canals.
- *Zygomatic processes:* extend from flat, squamous portion; articulate with zygomatic (facial) bones.
- *Mandibular fossae:* articulate with mandibular condyles to form temporomandibular joints (TMJs).
- *Temporal styloid processes:* sharp, slender processes extending anteriorly and inferiorly to mastoid processes.
- *External auditory meatus (EAM):* external openings of the ear canal.
- *Mastoid processes:* inferior to EAM; contain numerous air cells; communicate with tympanic cavity (middle ear) at mastoid antrum

Facial Bones (14)

(2) Nasal
(2) Lacrimal (smallest)
(2) Palatine
(2) Inferior nasal conchae
(2) Zygomatic
(2) Maxillae
(1) Vomer
(1) Mandible (largest; only movable)

b. Facial Bones (see Fig. 7–56)

Nasal Bone

- Small, rectangular.
- Form bridge of nose.
- Movable part of nose is composed of cartilage.
- Articulate with each other at midline to form **nasal suture.**
- Frontonasal suture: formed by articulation with frontal bone; corresponds to nasion externally.

Lacrimal Bones (see Fig. 7–56)

- Smallest of facial bones.
- Form part of medial orbital wall.
- Lacrimal groove: accommodates lacrimal (tear) duct.

Zygomatic (Malar) Bones (see Fig. 7–56)

- Inferior and lateral to outer canthus of eye; cheek bone.
- Have four processes: frontosphenoidal, orbital, temporal, and maxillary.

Maxillae (see Figs. 7–56 and 7–57)

- Second largest of facial bones.
- Articulate with each other to form most of upper jaw (hard palate).
- *Palatine processes:* plates of bone that articulate at midline to form two-thirds of the hard palate.
- Form most of roof of mouth **(hard palate)** and floor of nasal cavity.
- Contain the **maxillary sinuses** (maxillary antra; antra of Highmore) just superior to bicuspid teeth; the thin floor of the maxillary sinus is formed by the alveolar process.
- *Alveolar ridge/process:* contains sockets for teeth; spongy ridge of bone.
- *Anterior nasal spine:* corresponds to *acanthion* externally.
- *Infraorbital foramen:* located below orbit, lateral to nasal cavity.

Palatine Bones (Fig. 7–61)

- Small bones; form posterior one-third of hard palate.
- L-shaped; have vertical and horizontal processes.
- *Horizontal parts:* articulate with palatine processes of maxillae to complete the hard palate.
- *Vertical parts:* project superiorly from horizontal part to articulate with the sphenoid bones.

Inferior Conchae (nasal turbinates; see Fig. 7–56)

- Completely osseous.
- Placed inferiorly on each lateral wall of nasal cavity.

Vomer (see Fig. 7–56)

- Inferior to perpendicular plate of ethmoid bone.
- Forms posterior bony septum.
- *Choanae:* posterior opening into nasopharynx; separated by posterior portion of vomer.

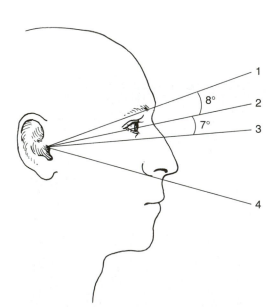

Figure 7–61. Four fundamental baselines are used in skull radiography: (1) the glabellomeatal (GML), (2) the orbitomeatal (OML, also known as canthomeatal or radiographic baseline), (3) the infraorbitomeatal (IOML), (4) the acanthiomeatal line. There is approximately a 7° difference between the OML and IOML and 8° between the OML and GML.

Mandible (see Figs. 7–56 and 7–57)

- U-shaped bone; largest facial bone.
- Only movable facial bone.
- *Mandibular symphysis:* where two halves fuse after birth.
- *Mental tubercles:* prominences at inferolateral margin of symphysis.
- *Mental protuberance:* protuberance at lower portion of symphysis.
- *Alveolar process/ridge:* spongy ridge of bone with sockets for teeth.
- *Body:* horizontal position.
- *Ramus:* posterior vertical portion.
- *Angle:* junction of vertical and horizontal parts: corresponds to external landmark: *gonion.*
- *TMJ:* articulation of head of condyle with mandibular fossa of temporal bone; only movable articulation in skull.
- *Coronoid process:* extends anterior and superior from ramus and has no articulation; serves as muscle attachment.
- *Mandibular notch:* deep notch between condyloid and coronoid processes.
- *Mental foramen:* small opening on outer surface of body, approximately below second premolar; passage for mandibular nerve.
- *Mandibular foramen:* opening on inner side of ramus for mandibular nerve.

SKULL (FIG. 7–62)	POSITION OF PART:	CENTRAL RAY DIRECTED:	STRUCTURES INCLUDED/ BEST SEEN:
PA	Patient prone, MSP ⊥ mid-table, OMI ⊥ cassette, see Fig. 7–62	⊥ nasion	PA proj of skull, *petrous pyramids should fill the orbits;* demonstrates frontal bone, lateral cranial walls, frontal sinuses, crista galli; see Fig. 7–62

The following variations of the basic true PA skull proj are used to demonstrate:

a) *General survey cranium*	CR ∠ed 15° caudad to nasion (ridges fill lower 1/3 orbits)
b) *Superior orbital fissures*	20 to 25° caudad to midorbits
c) *Foramina rotundum*	25 to 30° caudad to nasion (ridges below orbits)
d) *Sella turcica*	25° cephalad to a point 1.5″ above nasion (PA axial) *or* 10° cephalad to the glabella (PA proj)

Note: Similar projections of the same structures may be obtained in the AP position with the OML vertical if the CR is directed in the opposite direction. Anterior structures will be somewhat magnified and eye dose will be greater.

AP	Patient supine, MSP ⊥ mid-table, OML ⊥ cassette	⊥ nasion	AP proj of skull, *petrous pyramids should fill the orbits*

(continued)

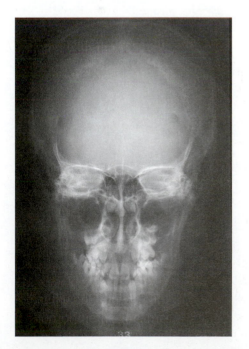

Figure 7–62. PA skull radiograph; the correct amount of flexion places the petrous pyramids within the orbits.

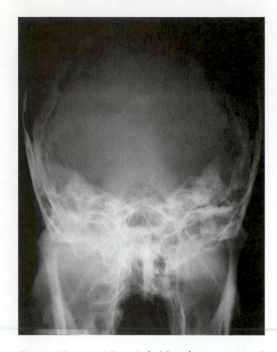

Figure 7–63. AP axial (Grashey position) projection of the skull; demonstrates the dorsum sella and posterior clinoid processes within the foramen magnum; useful for demonstration of the occipital bone. (Courtesy of the Stamford Hospital.)

SKULL (con't)	POSITION OF PART:	CENTRAL RAY DIRECTED:	STRUCTURES INCLUDED/ BEST SEEN:
AP Axial (*Towne/ Grashey*)	Patient supine, MSP ⊥ mid-table, OML vertical, top of cassette 1.5″ below vertex	30° caudad to a point ≈ 1.5″ above glabella (or 37° to IOML)	AP axial of skull, especially for *occipital bone,* symmetrical proj of petrous pyramids, projects dorsum sella and posterior clinoid processes within the foramen magnum (see Fig. 7–63)

Note: Excessive tube ∠ or neck flexion will project posterior arch of C1 in foramen magnum.

Note: A collimated proj of the *sella turcica* can be obtained in this proj; an AP axial of the *zygomatic arches* can be obtained by directing the CR to the glabella and decreasing the technical factors. Similar results can be obtained in the PA position (PA axial) with the CR ∠ed 25° cephalad to the OML. Particularly useful for hypersthenic or kyphotic patients although some magnification of the occipital bone must be expected.

LAT	Patient PA oblique w/skull MSP ‖ grid, interpupillary line vertical, IOML ‖ transverse axis of cassette	⊥ a point 2″ superior to EAM	Lateral proj of skull demonstrating superimposed cranial and facial structures; anterior and posterior clinoid processes and supraorbital margins should be superimposed
Basal Proj Submento-vertical (SMV)	Patient supine or seated AP, neck hyper-extended to place IOML ‖ film and ⊥ CR, MSP ⊥ cassette	⊥ IOML and film, enters MSP at level of sella	Full basal proj of skull, useful for many foramina (spinosum, ovale, carotid canals), sphenoid and maxillary sinuses, odontoid process seen through foramen magnum, symmetrical proj of petrous pyramids w/ mandibular condyles projected anterior to petrosae and symphysis superimposed on frontal bone (see Fig. 7–64)

Note: A decrease in 10 kVp will demonstrate a bilateral axial projection of the zygomatic arches (see Fig. 7–64B).

Vertico-submental (VSM)	Patient recumbent prone MSP ⊥ table, chin extended	Caudad and ⊥ IOML, pass through the sella	Similar to SMV with some magnification and distortion as a result of increased OID and direction of CR

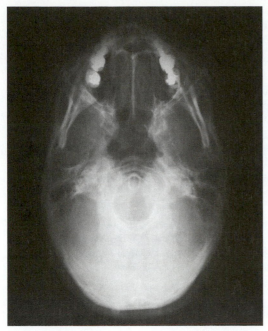

A

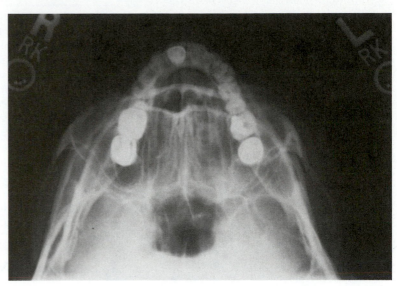

B

Figure 7–64. **(A)** Submentovertical (SMV) skull. The success of this projection depends on positioning the CR ⊥ the IOML and cassette. (Courtesy of The Stamford Hospital.) **(B)** SMV projection of the skull, collimated and exposure factors adjusted to demonstrate zygomatic arches. Note fracture of left zygomatic arch. (Courtesy of The Stamford Hospital.)

2. Sella Turcica

	POSITION OF PART:	CENTRAL RAY DIRECTED:	STRUCTURES INCLUDED/ BEST SEEN:
LAT	Patient PA oblique w/skull MSP ∥ grid, interpupillary line vertical, IOML ∥ transverse axis of cassette	⊥ a point 3/4″ anterior and superior to EAM	Lat proj of sella turcica, sphenoid sinus, superimposed supraorbital margins
AP Axial	See AP axial skull		
PA and PA Axial	See PA skull variations		

3. Orbits, Optic Foramen, Orbital Fissures

ORBIT

The orbital cavities are formed by seven bones (frontal, sphenoid, ethmoid, maxilla, palatine, zygoma/malar, and lacrimal). The orbital walls are fragile and the orbital floor is subject to traumatic **"blowout" fractures.** Orbital floor fractures can be demonstrated using the *parietoacanthial (Waters)* projection; conventional tomography and CT may be indicated for further evaluation.

OPTIC FORAMEN	POSITION OF PART:	CENTRAL RAY DIRECTED:	STRUCTURES INCLUDED/ BEST SEEN:
Parieto-orbital *(Rhese)*	Patient prone centered to table; skull resting on forehead, zygoma, chin w/MSP 53° to cassette and 37° to CR, acanthiomeatal line ⊥ cassette	⊥ through orbit adjacent to table	Parietoorbital proj of optic foramen (canal) in cross-section. Should be seen in lower outer quadrant of orbit: *longitudinal* displacement indicates incorrect baseline adjustment, *lateral* displacement indicates incorrect rotation

Note: This can be performed AP as the orbitoparietal projection with the MSP 53° to table and acanthiomeatal line vertical. CR passes through orbit farthest from film.

4. Facial Bones, Nasal Bones, Zygomatic Arches

FACIAL BONES	POSITION OF PART:	CENTRAL RAY DIRECTED:	STRUCTURES INCLUDED/ BEST SEEN:
Parieto-acanthial *(Waters)*	Patient PA, MSP ⊥ centered to grid, chin extended so OML is 37° to cassette	⊥ to parietal region, exiting at acanthion	Axial proj of facial bones, especially orbits, zygomas, and maxillae; best single proj for *facial bones;* see Fig. 7–65

Note: Patient should be upright to demonstrate air/fluid levels.

AP AXIAL *(Reverse Waters)*	Patient supine, MSP ⊥ mid-table, IOML ⊥ table, center cassette ≈3″ above inion	30° cephalad to lips	Axial, but *magnified,* proj of facial bones
LAT	Patient PA obl, MSP of skull ‖ table, inter-pupillary line ⊥, IOML ‖ to transverse axis of film	⊥ zygoma	Lat proj of super-imposed facial bones

NASAL BONES	POSITION OF PART:	CENTRAL RAY DIRECTED:	STRUCTURES INCLUDED/ BEST SEEN:
LAT	Patient recumbent prone, MSP of skull ‖ table, interpupillary line ⊥, IOML parallel to transverse axis of film	⊥ a point 3/4″ distal to nasion	Lat proj of superimposed nasal bones and their associated soft tissue; see Fig. 7–66

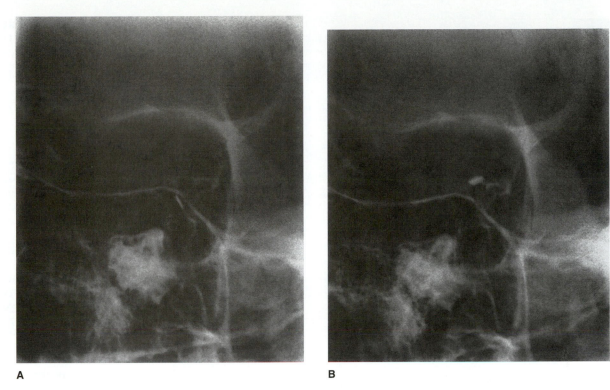

A   B

Figure 7–65. Right Optic Foramen (Rhese method) seen in lower outer quadrant of bony orbit. This exam was performed to demonstrate the presence of foreign body. Figure A was made after patient moved eye to look downward, Figure B after patient moved eye to look upward. (Courtesy of The Stamford Hospital.)

ZYGOMATIC ARCHES	POSITION OF PART:	CENTRAL RAY DIRECTED:	STRUCTURES INCLUDED/ BEST SEEN:
Tangential *(SMV)* *(Full Basal)*	See Skull: basal proj/SMV		

Note: In this projection, the skull may be rotated *15° toward the affected side* to better "open up" the zygomatic arches in individuals having flat cheekbones or a depressed fracture.

AP Axial	See Skull: AP axial (Towne/Grashey)		

5. Mandible, Temporomandibular Joints (TMJs)

MANDIBLE	POSITION OF PART:	CENTRAL RAY DIRECTED:	STRUCTURES INCLUDED/ BEST SEEN:
PA	Patient PA, nose and forehead on table, MSP ⊥, cassette centered to tip of nose	⊥ the lips	PA proj of mandible, especially body and rami

(continued)

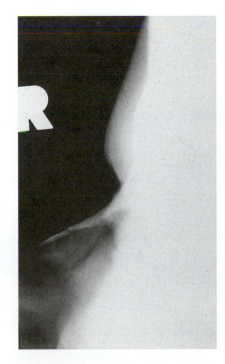

Figure 7–66. Lateral nasal bones demonstrating fracture. (Courtesy of The Stamford Hospital.)

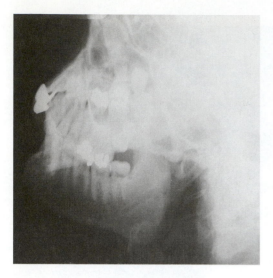

Figure 7–67. Axiolateral mandible, opening body and ramus for visualization.

MANDIBLE *(con't)*	POSITION OF PART:	CENTRAL RAY DIRECTED:	STRUCTURES INCLUDED/ BEST SEEN:
PA Axial	Patient PA, nose and forehead on table, MSP ⊥, cassette centered to glabella	20 to 25° cephalad to center of film	PA axial mandible, especially for rami and condyles
Axio-lateral	Patient PA, MSP of skull ∥ cassette centered 1/2″ anterior and 1″ inferior to the EAM	25° cephalad, enters at mandibular angle of unaffected side	Axiolateral mandible, especially for body and ramus; rotate MSP 15° forward to better demonstrate body (see Fig. 7–67)

TMJ	POSITION OF PART:	CENTRAL RAY DIRECTED:	STRUCTURES INCLUDED/ BEST SEEN:
AP Axial	Patient AP, MSP ⊥ midcassette, OML ⊥ table	30° caudad, enters ≈3″ above nasion	AP axial proj of condyloid processes and their articulations; unless contraindicated, another exposure is made with the *mouth open*
Infero-superior Trans-facial	Patient PA obl, skull MSP ≈ horizontal, interpupillary line ≈15° to vertical, cassette centered 1/2″ anterior and 1″ inferior to EAM	30° cephalad, exits TMJ adjacent to film	Obl lat TMJ; *both sides* examined in the open and closed-mouth positions unless contraindicated; see Fig. 7–68A and B

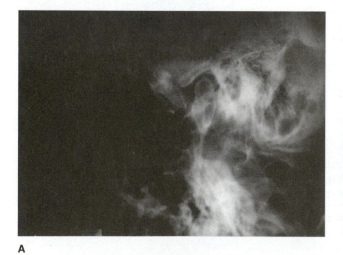

A

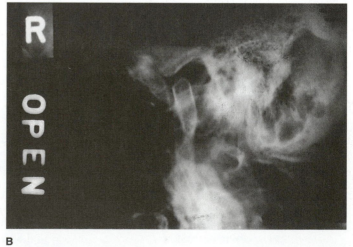

B

Figure 7–68. **(A)** Radiograph demonstrates the oblique lateral projection of the TMJ in the closed-mouth position. **(B)** The open-mouth position. (Courtesy of The Stamford Hospital.)

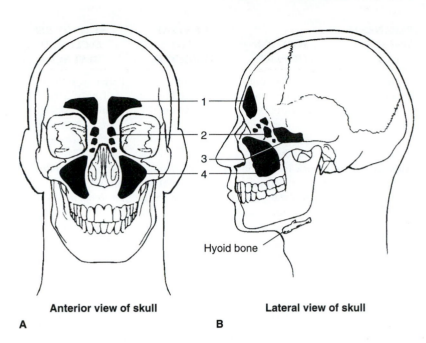

Anterior view of skull   **Lateral view of skull**

A   **B**

Hyoid bone

Figure 7–69. The paranasal sinuses, AP and lateral views.

6. Paranasal Sinuses. There are four paired *paranasal sinuses: frontal, ethmoidal, maxillary,* and *sphenoidal* (Fig. 7–69). The left and right frontal sinuses are usually asymmetrical. They are located behind the glabella and superciliary arches of the frontal bone. The frontal sinuses are not present in young children and reach their adult size in the 15th or 16th year. The ethmoidal sinuses are composed of 6 to 18 thin-walled air cells that occupy the bony labyrinth of the ethmoid bone. The ethmoidal sinuses of children are very small and do not fully develop until after the 14th year. The maxillary sinuses (antra of Highmore) are the largest of the paranasal sinuses and are located in the body of the maxillae. The *maxillary* sinuses are particularly prone to infection and collections of stagnant mucus. The maxillary sinuses reach their adult size around the 12th year. The sphenoidal sinuses are located in the body of the sphenoid bone and are usually asymmetrical. They generally reach adult size by the 14th year.

Radiography of the paranasal sinuses must be performed in the erect position so that any *fluid levels* may be demonstrated and to distinguish between fluid and other pathology such as *polyps.*

To demonstrate air and fluid levels *the CR must always be directed parallel to the floor,* even if the patient is not completely erect (just as in chest radiography). If the CR is angled to parallel the plane of the body, any fluid levels will be distorted or actually obliterated.

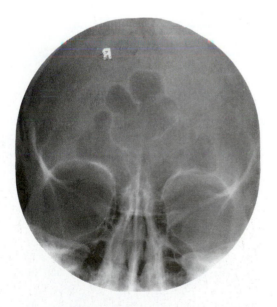

Figure 7–70. PA axial projection (Caldwell position) of the frontal and anterior ethmoid sinuses. The caudal angulation is somewhat excessive because the petrous pyramids are seen at the lowermost portion of the orbits. Correct angulation places the petrous pyramids in the lower one-third of the orbits. (Courtesy of The Stamford Hospital.)

PARANASAL SINUSES	POSITION OF PART:	CENTRAL RAY DIRECTED:	STRUCTURES INCLUDED/ BEST SEEN:
PA Axial *(Caldwell)*	Patient PA, skull MSP centered to grid, OML ⊥, grid, cassette centered to nasion	15° caudad to nasion	PA axial of *frontal* and *anterior ethmoid* sinuses, petrous pyramids are seen in the *lower one-third of the orbits;* see Fig. 7–70 *(continued)*

PARANASAL SINUSES (con't)	POSITION OF PART:	CENTRAL RAY DIRECTED:	STRUCTURES INCLUDED/ BEST SEEN:
Parieto-acanthial (Waters)	Patient PA, skull MSP centered to grid, OML 37° to cassette centered to acanthion	⊥, enters parietal region and exits acanthion	Parietoacanthial proj of *maxillary* sinuses projected *above petrous pyramids;* see Fig. 7–71

Note: Insufficient neck extension results in petrosa superimposed on floor of maxillary sinus); distorted projection of frontal and ethmoid.

Note: A modification of this projection made with the *mouth open* will demonstrate the *sphenoid sinuses* through the open mouth.

LAT	Patient PA obl, skull MSP ‖ to cassette centered 1″ posterior to outer canthus, inter-pupillary line vertical	⊥ mid-cassette, enters 1″ posterior to outer canthus	Lat proj of all paranasal sinuses; see Fig. 7–72
SMV (Basal)	Patient AP erect, neck hyper-extended to place IOML ‖ film and ⊥ CR, MSP ⊥ cassette	⊥ IOML and film, enters MSP at level of sella	Basal proj of sphenoid and ethmoid sinuses; mandibular symphysis should be superimposed on frontal bone

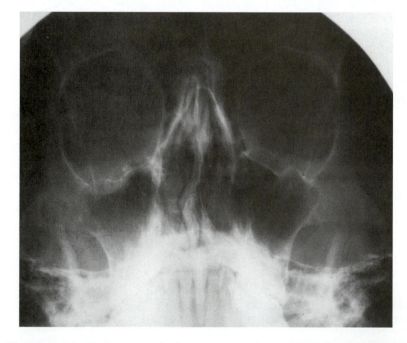

Figure 7–71. Parietoacanthial projection (Water's method). The sinuses are well collimated and centered to the image receptor. The chin is adequately extended and the petrous pyramids are seen below the floor of the maxillary sinuses. The parietoacanthial projection provides a foreshortened view of the frontal and ethmoid sinuses. In a modification of this projection, the sphenoid sinuses would be seen through the open mouth. (Courtesy of The Stamford Hospital.)

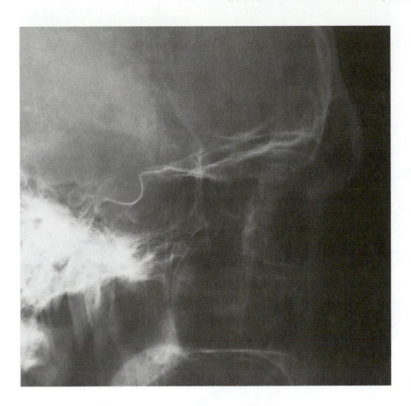

Figure 7–72. Lateral projection of the paranasal sinuses. (Courtesy of The Stamford Hospital.)

7. Temporal Bones: Mastoids and Petrous Portions

TEMPORAL BONE: MASTOIDS AND PETROUS PORTION
(see Fig. 7–73)

	POSITION OF PART:	**CENTRAL RAY DIRECTED:**	**STRUCTURES INCLUDED/ BEST SEEN:**
PA Trans-orbital	Patient PA, MSP centered to grid, OML ⊥ cassette, tightly collimated beam centered to nasion	⊥ nasion	PA internal auditory canals projected through the orbits
AP Axial	See Skull: AP axial (Towne/Grashey) and center to MSP so that CR passes through level of EAMs		
Axio-lateral (Laws)	Patient prone obl, interpupillary line ⊥ table, IOML ∥ cassette, MSP rotated forward to form 15° ∠ w/table, mastoid centered to table	15° caudad, entering ≈ 2″ posterior to and 2″ above upper EAM	Axiolateral proj of mastoid air cells, superimposed internal and external auditory meatus of side closest to film (see Fig. 7–74)

(continued)

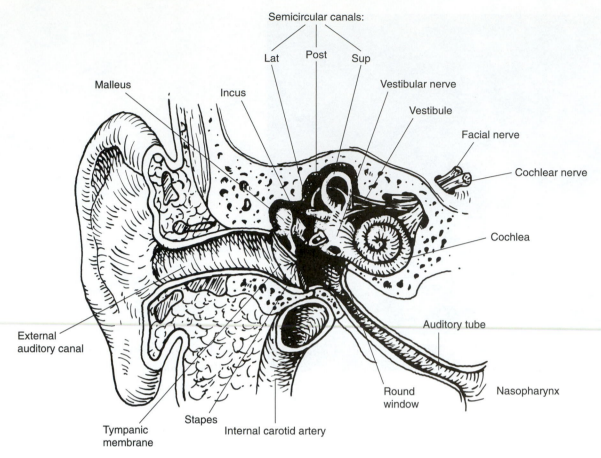

Figure 7–73. Temporal bone, demonstrating organs of hearing.

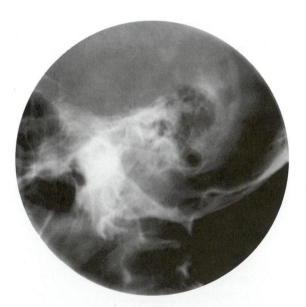

Figure 7–74. Axiolateral (Laws position) projection of right mastoid. (Courtesy of The Stamford Hospital.)

TEMPORAL BONE: MASTOIDS AND PETROUS PORTION

	POSITION OF PART:	CENTRAL RAY DIRECTED:	STRUCTURES INCLUDED/ BEST SEEN:
Posterior Profile *(Stenvers, axiolateral oblique)*	Patient PA, MSP 45°, head resting on forehead, zygoma, and nose, IOML ∥ transverse axis of film	12° cephalad exiting 1″ anterior to EAM closest to film	Pars petrosa projected in profile and parallel to film, mastoid process seen next to C1 and C2; middle ear, internal auditory canal, and bony labyrinth also demonstrated (see Fig. 7–75)
Anterior Profile *(Arcelin)*	Patient AP obl, MSP 45°, IOML ∥ transverse axis of film	10° caudad, entering 1″ anterior and 3/4″ above EAM away from film	Pars petrosa away from film projected in profile and parallel to film; internal auditory canal and bony labyrinth also demonstrated but somewhat magnified

Note: The Arcelin (anterior profile) method is the AP equivalent of the Stenvers. It requires a 10° caudal angle.

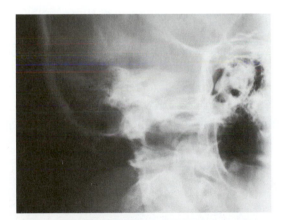

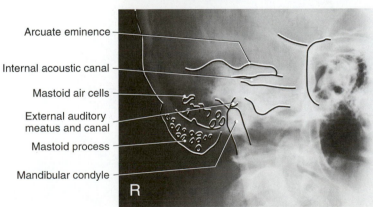

Arcuate eminence

Internal acoustic canal

Mastoid air cells

External auditory meatus and canal

Mastoid process

Mandibular condyle

R

Figure 7–75. Posterior profile projection, Stenvers method of petrous portions. The mastoid process is demonstrated in profile away from the bony structures of the skull and cervical spine. (From Cornuelle et al. *Radiographic Anatomy and Positioning.* Stamford, CT: Appleton & Lange, 1998.)

A&U Chapter Review Questions

⭐ *Congratulations!* You have completed a large portion of this chapter. You may go on to the "Registry-type" multiple-choice questions that follow. For greatest success, be sure also to complete the short answer questions found at the end of this chapter.

1. Which of the following positions requires that the orbitomeatal line be 37 degrees with the plane of the image recorder?
   A. PA axial/Caldwell
   B. AP axial/Townes
   C. parietoacanthial/Waters
   D. parietorbital/Rhese

2. All of the following statements regarding a PA projection of the skull, with central ray perpendicular to the film are true, EXCEPT:
   (A) orbitomeatal line is perpendicular to the film
   (B) petrous pyramids fill the lower third of the orbits
   (C) midsagittal plane (MSP) is perpendicular to the film
   (D) central ray exits at the nasion

3. Which of the following is demonstrated in a 25-degree RPO position and the central ray entering 1-inch medial to the elevated anterior superior iliac spine (ASIS)?
   (A) left sacroiliac joint
   (B) right sacroiliac joint
   (C) left ilium
   (D) right ilium

4. Which of the following is (are) demonstrated in the lateral projection of the cervical spine?
   1. intervertebral joints
   2. apophyseal joints
   3. intervertebral foramina
   (A) 1 only
   (B) 1 and 2 only
   (C) 2 and 3 only
   (D) 1, 2, and 3

5. The thoracic vertebrae are unique in that they participate in the following articulations:
   1. costovertebral
   2. costotransverse
   3. costochondral
   (A) 1 only
   (B) 1 and 2 only
   (C) 2 and 3 only
   (D) 1, 2, and 3

6.   With the body in the erect position, the diaphragm moves:
     (A) 2 to 4 inches higher than when recumbent
     (B) 2 to 4 inches lower than when recumbent
     (C) 2 to 4 inches superiorly
     (D) spasmodically

7.   Which of the following is a functional study used to demonstrate the degree of AP motion present in the cervical spine?
     (A) open-mount projection
     (B) moving mandible AP
     (C) flexion and extension laterals
     (D) right and left bending

8.   Which of the following statements is (are) correct regarding the parietoacanthial projection (Water's method) of the sinuses?
          1. patient should be examined erect
          2. OML is perpendicular to the film/image receptor
          3. petrosa should be projected below the maxillary antra
     (A) 1 only
     (B) 1 and 2 only
     (C) 1 and 3 only
     (D) 1, 2, and 3

9.   The intervertebral foramina of the thoracic spine are demonstrated with the:
     (A) coronal plane 45 degrees to the film/image receptor
     (B) midsagittal plane 45 degrees to the film/image receptor
     (C) coronal plane 70 degrees to the film/image receptor
     (D) midsagittal plane parallel to the film/image receptor

10. To better demonstrate the mandibular rami in the PA position, the:
     (A) skull is obliqued toward the affected side
     (B) skull is obliqued away from the affected side
     (C) central ray is angled cephalad
     (D) central ray is angled caudad

Answers and Explanations

1. (C) The *parietoacanthial projection/Waters position* requires that the orbitomeatal line be 37 degrees with the plane of the image recorder. This extension of the neck carries the petrous pyramids below the maxillary sinuses. The parietoacanthial projection/ Waters position is useful for demonstration of the maxillary sinuses (in the erect position) and provides the best single view of the facial bones. The posteroanterior (PA) axial/ Caldwell and anteroposterior (AP) axial/Townes both require that the orbitomeatal line (OML) be perpendicular to the image receptor. The parietorbital/Rhese is used to demonstrate the optic canals and does not utilize the OML.

2. (B) In the "true" PA projection of the skull with perpendicular central ray exiting the nasion, the petrous pyramids should *fill* the orbits. As the central ray (CR) is angled caudally, the petrous pyramids are projected lower in the orbits, and at approximately 25 to 30 degrees, they are below the orbits. The orbitomeatal line (OML) must be perpendicular to the image receptor, or the petrous pyramids will not be projected into the expected location in the angled projection. The midsaggital plane (MSP) must be perpendicular to the image receptor or the skull will be rotated.

3. (A) The sacroiliac joints angle posteriorly and medially 25 degrees to the midsaggital plane (MSP). Therefore, to demonstrate them with the patient in the anteroposterior (AP) position (RPO, LPO), the *affected* side must be elevated 25 degrees. This places the joint space perpendicular to the film and parallel to the central ray. When performed with the posteroanterior (PA) position (right anterior oblique [RAO], left anterior oblique [LAO], the *unaffected* side will be elevated 25 degrees.

4. (B) Intervertebral joints are well visualized in the lateral projection of all the vertebral groups. Cervical articular facets (forming apophyseal joints) are 90 degrees to the midsaggital plane (MSP) and are therefore well demonstrated in the lateral projection. The cervical intervertebral foramina lie 45 degrees to the MSP (and 15 to 20 degrees to a transverse plane) and are therefore demonstrated in the oblique position.

5. (B) There are 12 thoracic vertebrae, which are larger in size than cervical vertebrae and which increase in size as they progress inferiorly toward the lumbar region. Thoracic spinous processes are fairly long and are sharply angled caudally. The bodies and transverse processes have *articular facets* for the *diarthrotic* rib articulations (*see Fig. 7–48*). These structures form the *costovertebral* (head of rib with body of vertebra) and *costotransverse* (tubercle of rib with transverse process of vertebra) articulations. The *costochondral* articulation describes where the anterior end of the rib articulates with its costal cartilage.

6. (B) When the body is erect the diaphragm is more easily moved to a lower position during inspiration. For this reason, chest radiography is performed erect to allow maximum lung expansion. With the body in the supine position, the abdominal viscera exert greater pressure on the diaphragm and it usually assumes a position 2 to 4 inches higher than when erect.

7. (C) The degree of anterior and posterior motion is occasionally diminished with a "whiplash"-type injury. Anterior (forward, flexion) and posterior (backward, extension) motion is evaluated in the lateral position with the patient assuming flexion and extension as best as possible. Left and right bending films of the vertebral column are frequently obtained to evaluate scoliosis.

8. (C) The parietocanthial projection (Water's method) of the skull is valuable for the demonstration of facial bones or maxillary sinuses. The head is rested on extended chin so that the orbitomeatal line (OML) forms a 37-degree angle with the image receptor. This projects the petrous pyramids below the floor of the maxillary sinuses and provides an oblique frontal view of the facial bones.

9. (D) The thoracic *intervertebral foramina* are demonstrated in the lateral projection. The midsaggital plane (MSP) is parallel to the image receptor; the midcoronal plane (MCP) is perpendicular to the image receptor. The thoracic *apophyseal joints* are demonstrated in an oblique position with the coronal plane 70 degrees to the image receptor (MSP 20 degrees to the image receptor. The apophyseal joints closest to the image receptor are demonstrated in the posteroanterior (PA) (right/left anterior oblique [RAO/LAO]) oblique and those away from the image receptor in the anteroposterior (AP) (left/right posterior oblique [LPO/RPO]) oblique.

10. (C) The straight posteroanterior (PA) (0 degree) projection effectively demonstrates the mandibular body but the rami and condyles are superimposed on the occipital bone and petrous portion of the temporal bone. To better visualize the rami and condyles, the central ray is directed cephalad 20 to 30 degrees. This projects the temporal and occipital bones above the area of interest.

III. BODY SYSTEMS

A. RESPIRATORY SYSTEM

1. Introduction. The principle structures of the respiratory system are the lungs, which function to supply oxygen to the blood and relieve the body of carbon dioxide (Fig. 7–76). Pulmonary function depends upon the processes of *ventilation* and alveolar gas exchange. The right lung is shorter because the liver is below it; the left lung is narrower because the heart occupies a portion of the left side. The lungs have a somewhat conical shape; their narrow upper portion is called the *apex*, their wide *base* is defined by the *diaphragmatic surface*. Structures such as the mainstem bronchi and pulmonary artery and veins enter and leave the lungs at the *hilum*. The *right lung* has *three lobes;* the upper and middle lobes are separated by the horizontal fissure, the middle and lower lobes are separated by the oblique fissure. The *left lung* has *two lobes;* the upper and lower lobes are separated by the oblique fissure (Fig. 7–76).

The lungs are enclosed in a serous membrane, the *parietal pleura*. The *visceral/pleura* lines the inner thoracic wall and covers the superior surface of the diaphragm; the potential space between the two layers of pleura is the *pleural cavity*.

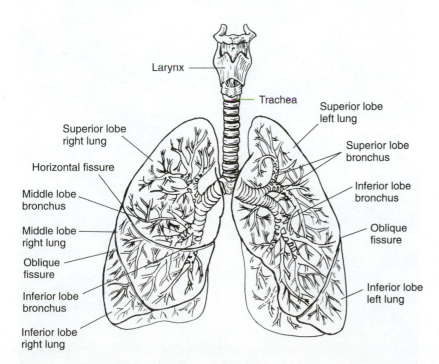

Figure 7–76. Trachea and bronchi (anterior view).

Pneumothorax is the presence of air in the pleural cavity. A large pneumothorax is usually accompanied by a partial or complete collapse of the lung (atelectasis). Radiographic indications of atelectasis include elevation of the *hemidiaphragm* of the affected side and an increase in (tissue) density of the collapsed lung. *Thoracentesis* is the procedure required to remove significant amounts of air, blood, or other fluids in the pleural cavity.

One of the most diagnostically useful and frequently performed radiographic examinations is the chest x-ray examination. During the course of their illness and recovery, patients often need successive chest examinations to monitor their progress, and reproduction of quality images is an important part of quality control. Accurate positioning and selection of technical factors is critical to the diagnostic value of the radiographic images. *Even slight rotation or leaning can cause significant distortion of the size and shape of the heart.* Consistent and accurate positioning is essential to radiographic quality.

The radiographer must take careful note of each patient's apparel, body type, and clinical information. Important considerations include removal of any radiopaque clothing and accessories, placing the cassette transversely for broad-chested individuals (in order to include the *costophrenic angles*—blunting of the costophrenic angles is often a result of pleural effusion), instructing female patients with large breasts to move them up and laterally for the PA projection, exposing on the second inspiration for hypersthenic individuals, and adjusting exposure factors for various pathologic conditions. Appropriate radiation protection measures must always be provided.

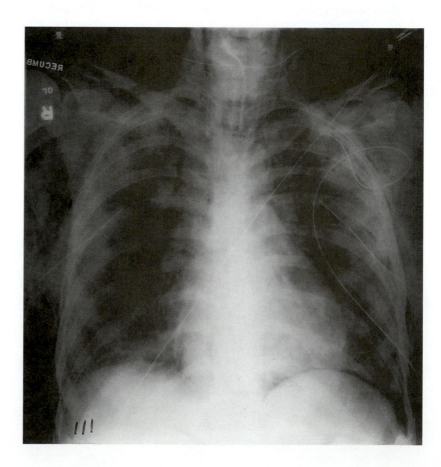

Figure 7–77. Mobile AP chest radiograph. Observe an endotracheal tube, ECG leads, one chest tube on the right and two on the left. The patient has extensive soft-tissue emphysema. Radiographers must exercise particular care when working around various patient tubes. (From the American College of Radiology Learning File. Courtesy of the ACR.)

Mobile chest radiography often brings the radiographer into contact with seriously ill patients. The radiographer must be very cautious when positioning these patients for there are often numerous tubes (eg, chest tubes, endotracheal tubes, electrocardiographic [ECG] leads, Swan–Ganz lines, urinary catheters) associated with maintaining the patient's airway or reinflating a collapsed lung, removing fluid or air from the pleural cavity, administering medications, measuring central venous pressure, or measuring urine output (Fig. 7–77).

The following tables provide a summary of routine projections and frequently performed special projections.

2. Chest; PA, Lateral, Obliques

CHEST	POSITION OF PART:	CENTRAL RAY DIRECTED:	STRUCTURES INCLUDED/ BEST SEEN:
PA	Patient erect PA, MSP exactly ⊥ cassette, shoulders depressed and rolled forward w/back of hands on hips, top of cassette 1.5 to 2″ above shoulders	⊥ T7	PA proj of thoracic viscera and skeletal anatomy; *inspiration* demonstrates air filled trachea and lungs, 10 posterior ribs; *expiration* shows pulmonary vascular markings; *inspiration and expiration* are done for pneumothorax, foreign body, diaphragm excursion, and atelectasis.

Note: Chest radiography is performed *erect* whenever possible to demonstrate air/fluid levels. The MSP must be exactly vertical; any *rotation can cause significant distortion* and misrepresentation of the visceral structures. *Rotation is detected on the PA radiograph by asymmetrical distance between the sternal ends of the clavicles and the lateral border of the thoracic vertebrae.* The shoulders are rolled forward to remove the scapulae from superimposition on the lung fields. Superiorly, the *pulmonary apices* must be seen; inferiorly the *costophrenic angles* must be seen in their entirety. *Inspiration must be adequate to demonstrate 10 posterior ribs.* A 72″ SID is recommended to decrease *magnification* of the heart. See Fig. 7–78.

LAT	Patient erect L lat, MSP ⊥ cassette, arms over head, top of cassette 1.5 to 2″ above shoulders	⊥ cassette, enters at level of T7	L lat proj of chest particularly useful for heart, aorta, L lung and its fissures, and other left-sided structures/pathology; L lat usually done to place heart closer to film

Note: The MSP must be *exactly vertical;* any lateral leaning can cause significant distortion and misrepresentation of the visceral structures. *Rotation* is detected on the lateral radiograph by superimposition of ribs on sternum or vertebrae. Pulmonary apices and angles must be visualized. See Fig. 7–79.

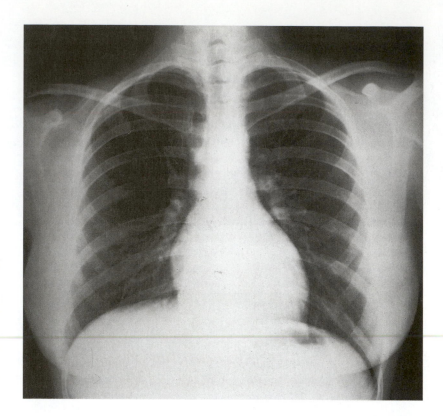

Figure 7–78. PA projection of the chest of a normal, healthy adult demonstrating the importance of positioning accuracy. Slight rotation has made the manubrium visible at the site of the right sternoclavicular joint, providing a density very similar to that created by a paraspinous or mediastinal mass. (From the American College of Radiology Learning File. Courtesy of the ACR.)

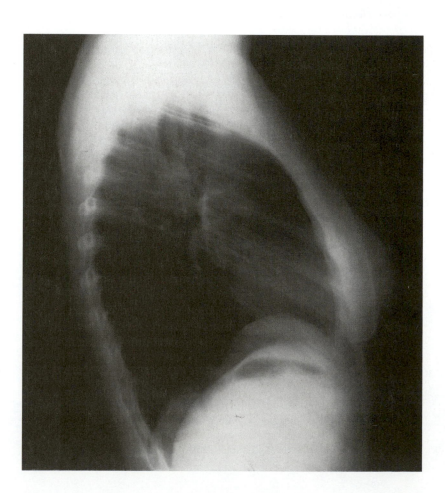

Figure 7–79. Lateral projection of the same chest as Figure 7–72 and without rotation. The sternum is seen free of superimposed ribs, the thoracic and lumbar vertebral spinous processes are seen. (From the American College of Radiology Learning File. Courtesy of the ACR.)

3. Chest; Axial and Decubitus

	POSITION OF PART:	CENTRAL RAY DIRECTED:	STRUCTURES INCLUDED/ BEST SEEN:
AP Axial (lordotic)	Patient erect AP, MSP ⊥ mid-cassette at level of T2	15 to 20° cephalad to T2	AP axial (lordotic) proj of pulmonary apices projected below clavicles (this position can also be done with patient leaning back and CR ⊥ film)
Decubitus (L and R Lat)	Patient recumbent lat on affected or un-affected side as indicated by hx; anterior or posterior surface adjacent to cassette. MSP ⊥ mid-cassette w/top 1.5″ above shoulders	⊥ mid-cassette	Frontal (AP or PA) proj of the chest useful for demonstration of air or fluid levels

Note: If free *air* is suspected, the affected side must be *up;* if *fluid* is suspected, the affected side must be placed *down*.

4. Airway. AP and lateral projections of the airway and larynx are occasionally required to rule out *foreign body, polyps, tumors,* or any other condition suspected of causing some airway obstruction.

The **AP** is positioned as for an AP cervical spine with the CR perpendicular to the *laryngeal prominence.* The lateral is positioned as for a lateral cervical spine and centered to the coronal plane passing through the trachea (anterior to the cervical spine) at the level of the laryngeal prominence. *Exposures are made on slow inspiration* to visualize air-filled structures.

Depending on the structure(s) of interest being examined, these positions may be performed with barium and/or during performance of the *Valsalva/modified Valsalva maneuver.* Tomograms may be performed during phonation of vowel sounds to demonstrate more superior structures such as the larynx and/or vocal cords.

5. Terminology and Pathology. The following is a list of radiographically significant conditions and devices with which the student radiographer should be familiar.

Asthma
Atelectasis
Bronchiectasis
Bronchitis
Central venous pressure line
Chest tube (see Fig. 7–77)
Chronic obstructive
   pulmonary disease
Cystic fibrosis
Emphysema (see Fig. 7–80)
Empyema

Endotracheal tube (see Fig. 7–77)
Hemothorax
Hickman catheter
Pleural effusion (see Fig. 7–81)
Pneumoconiosis
Pneumonia
Pneumothorax
Swan–Ganz catheter
Thoracentesis
Tuberculosis

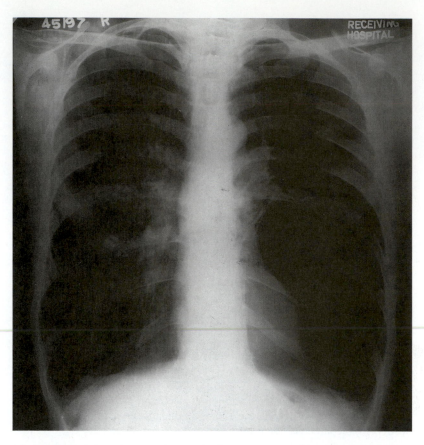

Figure 7–80. PA chest radiograph demonstrates the characteristic irreversible trapping of air found in emphysema, which gradually increases and overexpands the lungs, thus producing the characteristic flattening of the diaphragm and widening of the intercostal spaces. The increased air content of the lungs requires a compensating decrease in technical factors. (From the American College of Radiology Learning File. Courtesy of the ACR.)

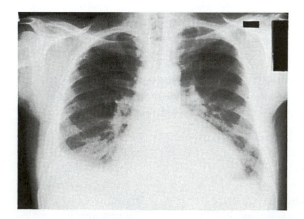

Figure 7–81. PA chest demonstrating pleural effusion secondary to heart failure. (Reproduced with permission from Way, LW, ed. *Current Surgical Diagnosis & Treatment,* 10th ed. East Norwalk, CT: Appleton & Lange, 1994.)

A&U Chapter Review Questions

⭐ *Congratulations! You have completed your review of a large portion of this chapter. You may go on to the "Registry-type" multiple-choice questions that follow. For greatest success, be sure also to complete the short answer questions found at the end of this chapter.*

1. Aspirated foreign bodies in older children and adults are most likely to lodge in the:
   - (A) right main bronchus
   - (B) left main bronchus
   - (C) esophagus
   - (D) proximal stomach

2. Which of the following is (are) important when positioning the patient for a PA projection of the chest?
   1. the patient should be examined erect
   2. shoulders should be depressed
   3. shoulders should be rolled forward
   - (A) 1 only
   - (B) 1 and 2 only
   - (C) 1 and 3 only
   - (D) 1, 2, and 3

3. Chest radiography should be performed using 72 inches SID whenever possible in order to:
   1. minimize magnification of the heart
   2. obtain better lung detail
   3. blur out vascular markings
   - (A) 1 only
   - (B) 1 and 2 only
   - (C) 1 and 3 only
   - (D) 1, 2, and 3

4. Blunting of the costophrenic angles seen on a PA projection of the chest can be an indication of:
   - (A) pleural effusion
   - (B) ascites
   - (C) bronchitis
   - (D) emphysema

5. Which of the following conditions is characterized by flattening of the hemidiaphragms?
   - (A) emphysema
   - (B) empyema
   - (C) atelectasis
   - (D) pneumonia

6. Inspiration and expiration projections of the chest may be performed to demonstrate:
    1. pneumothorax
    2. diaphragm excursion
    3. bronchitis
    (A) 1 only
    (B) 1 and 2 only
    (C) 1 and 3 only
    (D) 1, 2, and 3

7. Which of the following criteria are used to evaluate a good PA projection of the chest?
    1. 10 posterior ribs should be visualized
    2. sternoclavicular joints should be symmetrical
    3. scapulae should be outside the lung fields
    (A) 1 and 2 only
    (B) 1 and 3 only
    (C) 2 and 3 only
    (D) 1, 2, and 3

8. All of the following statements regarding respiratory structures are true, *except:*
    (A) the right lung has two lobes
    (B) the uppermost portion of the lung is the apex
    (C) each lung is enclosed in pleura
    (D) the trachea bifurcates into mainstem bronchi

9. To demonstrate the pulmonary apices below the level of the clavicles in the AP position, the CR should be directed:
    (A) perpendicular
    (B) 15 to 20 degrees caudad
    (C) 15 to 20 degrees cephalad
    (D) 40 degrees cephalad

10. With the body in the erect position, the diaphragm moves:
    (A) 2 to 4 inches higher than when recumbent
    (B) 2 to 4 inches lower than when recumbent
    (C) very little
    (D) intermittently

Answers and Explanations

1. (A) Because the right main bronchus is wider and more vertical, aspirated foreign bodies are more likely to enter it than the left main bronchus, which is narrower and angles more sharply from the trachea. An aspirated foreign body does not enter the esophagus or stomach, as they are digestive, not respiratory, structures.

2. (D) The chest should be examined in the erect position whenever possible to demonstrate any air or fluid levels. The shoulders should be relaxed and depressed to move the clavicles below the lung apices. The shoulders should be rolled forward to move the scapulae out of the lung fields.

3. (B) Chest radiographs are performed in the erect position at 72 inches SID whenever possible. The long source-to-image-receptor distance (SID) is easily achieved with a minimum patient exposure due to the low tissue densities being examined (ribs and lungs). The longer source-to-image-receptor distance minimizes magnification of the heart and provides better lung detail (also because of less magnification). Rather than blurring the pulmonary vascular markings, their details are also improved.

4. (A) Fluid in the thoracic cavity between the visceral and parietal pleura is called *pleural effusion*. In the erect position, fluid gravitates to the lowest point, settling in, and "blunting," the costophrenic angles. *Ascites* is an accumulation of serous fluid in the peritoneal cavity. *Bronchitis* is an inflammation of the bronchial tubes. Pulmonary *emphysema* is a chronic pulmonary disease characterized by increase beyond the normal in the size of air spaces distal to the terminal bronchiole, and with destructive changes in the walls of the bronchioles.

5. (A) *Emphysema* is characterized by irreversible trapping of air, which gradually increases and overexpands the lungs, thus producing the characteristic *flattening of the diaphragm* and *widening of the intercostal spaces* (see Fig. 7–80). The increased air content of the lungs requires a compensating *decrease in technical factors*. *Empyema* describes pus in the pleural cavity as a result of an infection of the lungs. *Atelectasis* is a collapsed or airless lung. *Pneumonia* is an inflammation of the lung; there are more than 50 causes of pneumonia.

6. (B) Phase of respiration is exceedingly important in thoracic radiography; lung expansion and the position of the diaphragm strongly influence the appearance of the finished radiograph. Inspiration and expiration radiographs of the chest are taken to demonstrate air in the pleural cavity (pneumothorax), to demonstrate degree of diaphragm excursion, or to detect the presence of foreign body. The expiration film will require a somewhat greater exposure (6 to 8 kVp [kilovoltage peak] more) to compensate for the diminished quantity of air in the lungs.

7. (D) To evaluate sufficient inspiration and lung expansion, 10 posterior ribs should be visualized. Sternoclavicular joints should be symmetrical; any loss of symmetry indicates rotation. Accurate positioning and selection of technical factors is critical to the diagnostic value of the radiographic images. Even slight rotation or leaning can cause significant distortion of the heart size and shape. To visualize maximum lung area, the shoulders are rolled forward to remove the scapulae from the lung fields.

8. (A) The trachea (windpipe) bifurcates into left and right mainstem bronchi, each entering its respective lung hilum. The left bronchus divides into two portions, one for each lobe of the left lung. *The right bronchus divides into three portions, one for each lobe of the right lung.* The lungs are conical in shape, consisting of upper pointed portions, termed the *apices* (singular = apex), and the broad lower portions (or *bases*). The lungs are enclosed in a double-walled serous membrane called the pleura.

9. (C) When the shoulders are relaxed, the clavicles are usually carried below the pulmonary apices. To examine the portions of lungs lying behind the clavicles, the CR is directed cephalad 15 to 20 degrees to project the *clavicles above the apices,* when the patient is examined in the AP position.

10. (B) When the body is erect the diaphragm is more easily moved to a lower position during inspiration. For this reason, chest radiography is performed erect to allow maximum lung expansion. With the body in the supine position, the abdominal viscera exert greater pressure on the diaphragm and it usually assumes a position 2 to 4 inches higher than when erect.

B. BILIARY SYSTEM

1. Introduction. The biliary tree consists of the left and right hepatic ducts, common hepatic duct, cystic duct, common bile duct, and the gallbladder (Fig. 7–82). The hepatic ducts leave the liver and join to form the *common hepatic duct*. The short *cystic duct* continues to the gallbladder. The common hepatic and cystic ducts unite to form the long *common bile duct,* which joints with the pancreatic duct to form the short *hepatopancreatic ampulla (of Vater).* The ampulla opens into the descending duodenum through the *duodenal papilla,* which is surrounded by the *hepatopancreatic sphincter (of Oddi).*

The *gallbladder* is located in a shallow fossa on the inferior surface of the liver between its right and quadrate lobes. Small gallstones are able to pass out the gallbladder through the cystic duct; those that are too large irritate the gallbladder mucosa, resulting in *cholecystitis. Gallstones* can also lodge in ducts. If a stone lodges in the cystic duct, cholecystitis without *jaundice* is the result, because bile can still drain into the duodenum. A stone lodged in the common bile duct will result in jaundice as well as cholecystitis. A "gallbladder attack" is the painful result of fatty chyme stimulating the release of *cholecystokinin,* which elevates pressure within the stone-laden gallbladder.

Radiographic examinations of the biliary system include *oral cholecystography, operative cholangiography, T-tube cholangiography,* and *endoscopic retrograde cholangiopancreatography (ERCP).* Each of these examinations requires the use of a contrast agent. With the

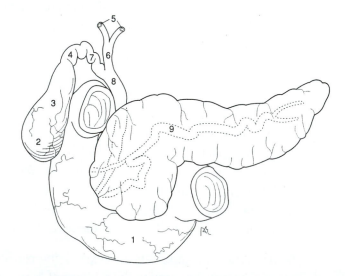

Figure 7–82. Illustrates the main hepatic and biliary ducts, gallbladder, and pancreas within the duodenal loop. Be able to identify the labeled structures.

exception of the ERCP, few of these exams are performed today, but rather are imaged via *sonography* (Fig. 7–83).

2. Patient Preparation.
For *oral cholecystograms* (OCG), iodinated tablets are taken the evening before the examination. The gallbladder stores and concentrates the contrast-laden bile, rendering the gallbladder radiopaque. The evening meal must be fat-free to prevent gallbladder contraction and subsequent release of the radiopaque bile. Oral cholecystography is used to evaluate the function of the biliary system as well as demonstrate the structure and contents of the gallbladder.

Operative cholangiography is used to examine the bile ducts and frequently follows a *cholecystectomy*. An iodinated contrast agent is introduced into the common bile duct to evaluate biliary patency and that of the hepatopancreatic ampulla. Any calculi can be detected and removed before completion of surgery.

Occasionally, a T-shaped tube is left in the common bile duct for postsurgical drainage. T-tube cholangiography is performed by injecting a contrast agent through the tube to detect any remaining calculi and evaluate the biliary tree patency.

ERCP is a specialized procedure used to evaluate suspected biliary and/or pancreatic conditions. An *endoscope* is passed through the mouth, esophagus, stomach, and into the descending duodenum to the orifice of the hepatopancreatic ampulla. Contrast material is injected into the common bile duct for evaluation of the biliary system.

3. Gallbladder.
An oral cholecystogram frequently begins with a prone 14 × 17-inch film of the abdomen to check *opacification* and location of the gallbladder as well as patient preparation and technical factors. Collimated recumbent PA and oblique, and erect or decubitus radiographs follow. In the absence of gallstones, a fatty meal may then be given the patient and another similar series of images taken 20 to 30 minutes later. The fatty meal is used to check gallbladder (GB) function: in the presence of fat the GB should contract and evacuate its bile. Fluoroscopic images may be taken in addition to, or in place of, the post fat radiographs. *The gallbladder of the average build patient is located between the 10th and 12th ribs on the right,* midway between the vertebral column and lateral border of the body. *Hypersthenic* individuals usually require centering about 2 inches higher and more laterally, while centering for *asthenic* individuals is usually 2 inches lower and more midline. In the *erect* position, the gallbladder of an asthenic patient can be as low as the iliac fossa.

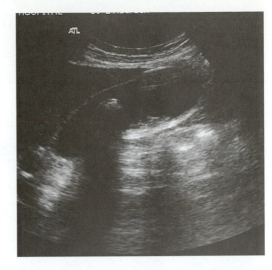

Figure 7–83. A sonogram of the gallbladder demonstrating the presence of gallstones.

OCG	POSITION OF PART:	CENTRAL RAY DIRECTED:	STRUCTURES INCLUDED/ BEST SEEN:
PA	Prone or PA erect, sagittal plane passing m/w b/w spine and R lat border of body, at level of 9th rib centered to grid (CR lower when done erect)	⊥ center of cassette	PA recumbent or erect proj of GB. *The erect position will demonstrate layering of any gallstones* (see Fig. 7–84)

(continued)

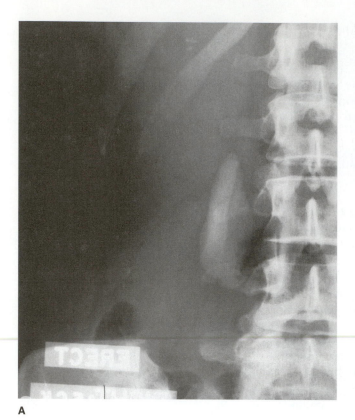

A

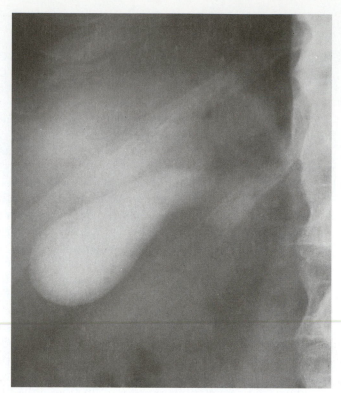

B

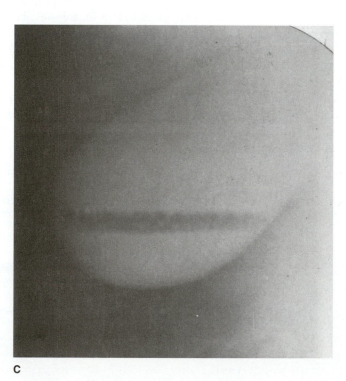

C

Figure 7–84. **(A)** Note the position of the gallbladder (GB) in the PA erect projection with respect to the vertebrae and iliac crest. Asthenic habitus patients will have a low and midline GB. **(B)** LAO of GB; no evidence of stones. Note normal position of GB in the sthenic habitus—between the 10th–12th ribs on the right. **(C)** The same patient as (B), but in the erect position, showing layering of gallstones. (From the ACR Learning File. Courtesy of the ACR.)

OCG (con't)	POSITION OF PART:	CENTRAL RAY DIRECTED:	STRUCTURES INCLUDED/ BEST SEEN:
OBL (LAO)	Recumbent LAO, sagittal plane passing m/w b/w spine and R lat border of body centered to grid at level of 9th rib	⊥ center of cassette	Obl GB, with less foreshortening and self-superimposition than in PA. *Greater obliquity (40°) for asthenic patients* than for hypersthenic (15°)
R Lat Decubitus	Patient recumbent R lat, posterior surface adjacent to upright grid and centered to level of gallbladder	⊥ center of cassette	R lat decubitus of gallbladder useful for *stratification* (layering) of gallstones (Fig. 7–84) and the GB free of superimposed bowel loops

4. OR/T-Tube

	POSITION OF PART:	CENTRAL RAY DIRECTED:	STRUCTURES INCLUDED/ BEST SEEN:
RPO	Patient supine with L side elevated 15 to 20°, R upper quadrant centered to grid	⊥ center of cassette	RPO of biliary tree and gallbladder area; to evaluate the hepatopancreatic ampulla and biliary tree for calculi or other pathology (following injection of contrast into common bile duct)

5. ERCP. Following *canalization* of the hepatopancreatic ampulla, fluoroscopic images are made in the AP (RPO) or PA (LAO) position. Filming procedure should immediately follow injection since, under normal conditions, contrast will empty from the biliary ducts in approximately 5 minutes (Fig. 7–85).

6. Terminology and Pathology. The following is a list of radiographically significant conditions with which the student radiographer should be familiar.

Cholecystitis	Hepatitis
Cholelithiasis	Jaundice
Cirrhosis	Pancreatitis

C. DIGESTIVE SYSTEM

1. Introduction. The digestive system (Fig. 7–86) consists of the *gastrointestinal tract (GI)* and accessory organs. The *gastrointestinal tract, or alimentary canal,* is a continuous tube of varying dimen-

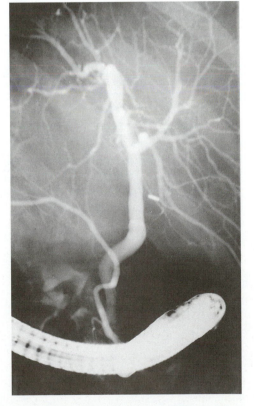

Figure 7–85. Fluoroscopic image of a normal ERCP. The pancreatic and common bile ducts are clearly delineated. (Courtesy of The Stamford Hospital.)

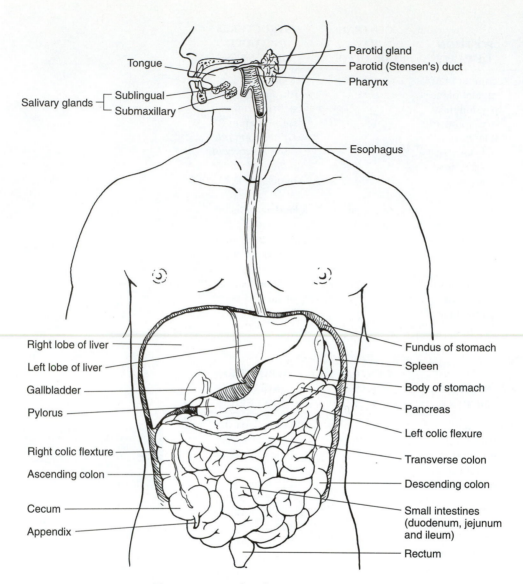

Figure 7–86. The digestive system.

sions consisting of the esophagus, stomach, and small and large intestines. The teeth, tongue, salivary glands, liver, gallbladder, and pancreas are accessory organs that aid in the mechanical and chemical breakdown of food. The major portion of the GI tract lies within the abdominopelvic cavity. Its principle functions are the chemical breakdown and absorption of nutrients.

The *esophagus* functions to propel a food bolus toward the stomach through *peristaltic* motion. The *cardiac sphincter* is located at the distal end of the esophagus. "Heartburn" is an inflammation of the esophagus *mucosa* as a result of gastric *reflux* of acidic material into the esophagus. *Esophageal varices* are dilated, *tortuous* veins directly beneath the esophageal mucosa. A hiatal hernia is a herniation of the stomach through the esophageal hiatus of the diaphragm, producing a sac-like dilatation above the diaphragm (Fig. 7–87). The presence of reflux, varices or herniation can be detected radiographically with the use of barium sulfate.

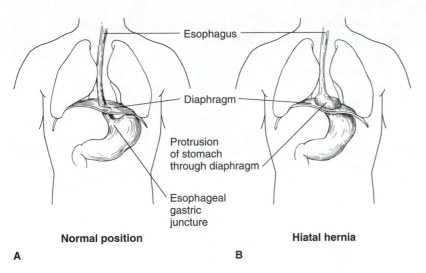

Figure 7–87. **(A)** Normal position of the stomach. **(B)** Note protrusion of stomach through esophageal hiatus (hiatal hernia).

The *stomach* is the dilated, sac-like portion of the GI tract. When the stomach is empty, its mucosal lining forms soft folds called *rugae* (Fig. 7–88). *Gastritis* is an inflammation of the gastric mucosa that can be caused by excessive secretion of acids or by ingestion of irritants such as aspirin or corticosteroids. Exteriorly, it presents a *greater curvature* on its lateral surface and a *lesser curvature* on its medial surface. The proximal opening of the stomach is the *cardiac sphincter*; the *pyloric sphincter* is located at its distal end. The portion of the stomach around the distal esophagus is called the *cardia*; that portion superior to the esophageal juncture is the *fundus*. The sharp angle (incisura) between the esophagus and fundus is the *cardiac notch*. The major portion of the stomach is the *body*; the distal portion is the *pylorus*. The *incisura angularis* is located on the

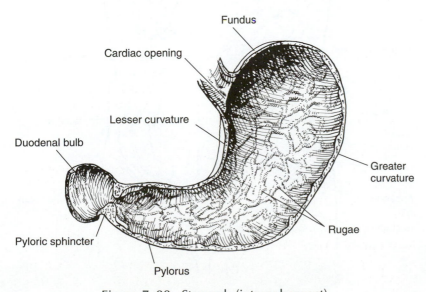

Figure 7–88. Stomach (internal aspect).

lesser curvature and marks the beginning of the pylorus. The distal portion of the pylorus is marked by the *pyloric sphincter.*

The *small intestine* is composed of the duodenum, jejunum, and ileum. The *duodenum* is the shortest portion. It begins just beyond the pyloric sphincter and is divided into four portions: the duodenal cap or bulb, descending duodenum, transverse duodenum, and ascending duodenum. These portions form a C-shaped loop *(duodenal loop)* that is occupied by the head of the pancreas. The descending portion receives the hepatopancreatic ampulla and duodenal papilla (see biliary section). The ascending portion terminates at the duodenojejunal flexure (angle of Treitz). While the position of the short (9 inches) duodenum is fixed, the *jejunum* (9 feet) and *ileum* (13 feet) are very mobile. Twisting of the small intestine is called *volvulus,* and can cause compression of blood vessels, leading to loss of blood supply, *ischemia,* and *infarct* of the affected area. The small intestine terminates at the *ileocecal valve.*

The approximately 5-foot-long *large intestine (colon)* (Fig. 7–89) functions in the formation, transport, and evacuation of feces. The colon begins at the terminus of the small intestine; its first portion is the dilated sac-like *cecum,* located inferior to the ileocecal valve (Fig. 7–90). Projecting posteromedially from the cecum is the short (approximately 3.5 inches) *vermiform appendix.* Its lumen is particularly narrow in adolescents and young adults and may become occluded by a fecalith and result in inflammation (appendicitis).

The *ascending colon* is continuous with the cecum and is located along the right side of the abdominal cavity. It bends medially and anteriorly in the right hypochondrium, forming the *right colic (hepatic) flexure.* The colon traverses the abdomen as the *transverse colon* and bends posteriorly and inferiorly in the left hypochondrium, forming the *left colic (splenic) flexure.* The *descending colon* contin-

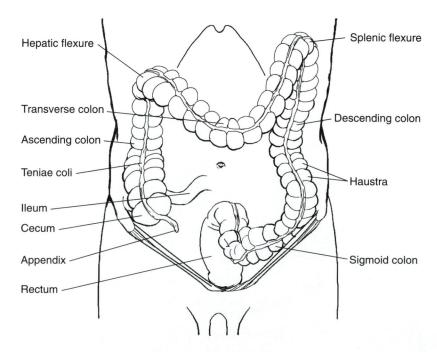

Figure 7–89. The colon.

ues down the left side of the abdominal cavity and, at about the level of the pelvic brim, the colon moves medially to form the S-shaped *sigmoid colon*. The *rectum* is that part of the large intestine, approximately 5 inches in length, between the sigmoid and the anal canal.

Diverticula are small saccular protrusions of intestinal mucosa through the intestinal wall (Fig. 7–91). They are most commonly associated with the sigmoid colon and can become occluded by fecaliths and subsequently inflamed (diverticulitis). If an inflamed diverticulum perforates, it can result in severe bleeding and peritonitis.

2. Patient Preparation.

Preliminary patient preparation is generally required of patients undergoing radiographic examinations of various portions of the digestive system. The upper GI tract (stomach and small intestine) must be empty and the lower tract (large intestine) must be cleansed of any gas and fecal material. Patients should be questioned about their preparation and a preliminary "scout" film taken to check abdominal contents and for any radiopaque (eg, gallstones, residual barium) material.

To make up for the lack of subject contrast, radiography of the digestive system most often requires the use of artificial contrast media in the form of barium sulfate suspension of water-soluble iodine and, frequently, air. *Double-contrast studies* of the stomach and large intestine are frequently performed. Barium sulfate functions to coat the organ with radiopaque material, while air inflates the structure. This permits visualization of the shape of the structure as well as *visualization of pathology within its lumen*. Thus, conditions such as *polyps* can be seen projecting within the air-filled lumen. A barium-filled *lumen* would make visualization of anything but the organ shape virtually impossible.

The speed with which barium sulfate passes through the alimentary canal depends on patient habitus (hypersthenic usually fastest) and the concentration of the barium suspension.

When performing examinations on patients suspected or known to have stomach or intestinal perforation, *water-soluble* iodinated

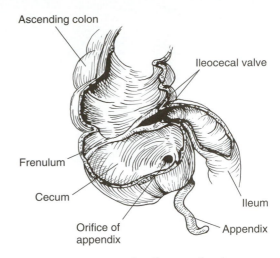

Figure 7–90. The ileocecal valve.

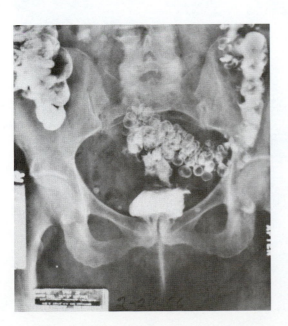

Figure 7–91. Barium enema roentgenogram showing multiple diverticula of the colon. (From Way, LW, ed. *Current Surgical Diagnosis Treatment,* 10th ed. East Norwalk, CT: Appleton & Lange, 1994.)

contrast media should be used instead of barium sulfate. If the water-soluble medium leaks through a perforation into the peritoneal cavity, it will simply be absorbed and excreted by the kidneys. Water-soluble contrast media are excreted more rapidly than are barium sulfate preparations.

These studies are far from pleasant for patients and the radiographer should make every effort to fully explain the procedure while endeavoring to expedite the examination and make the patient as comfortable as possible.

With the increased use of digital fluoroscopy, fewer "overhead" radiographs are done today. A summary of the most frequently performed projections follows.

3. Abdomen

	POSITION OF PART:	CENTRAL RAY DIRECTED:	STRUCTURES INCLUDED/ BEST SEEN:
AP	Supine, MSP centered to grid, cassette centered to iliac crest; see Fig. 7–92	⊥ to midline at level of crest	AP proj often used as "scout" film preliminary to contrast studies; shows size and shape of kidneys, liver, and spleen, psoas muscles, as well as any calcifications or masses

(continued)

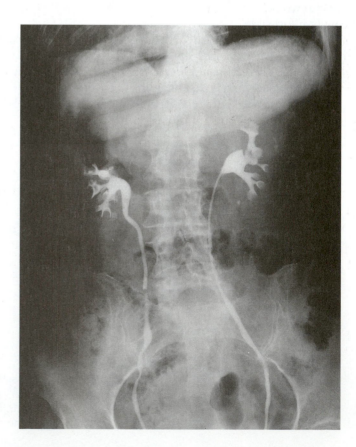

Figure 7–92. When positioning the abdomen, it is important to position the patient's hands at his or her side or resting high on the chest. Note the position of the patient's right hand in this retrograde urogram. (From the American College of Radiology Learning File. Courtesy of the ACR.)

	POSITION OF PART:	CENTRAL RAY DIRECTED:	STRUCTURES INCLUDED/ BEST SEEN:
Erect	AP erect, MSP centered to grid, cassette centered ≈2″ above iliac crest	⊥ to mid-cassette	AP erect proj used to demonstrate air/fluid levels; both hemidiaphragms should be included; see Fig. 7–93

(continued)

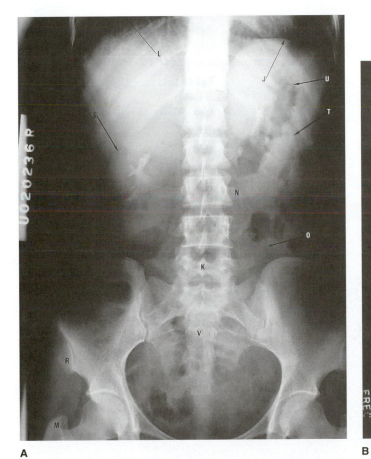

A

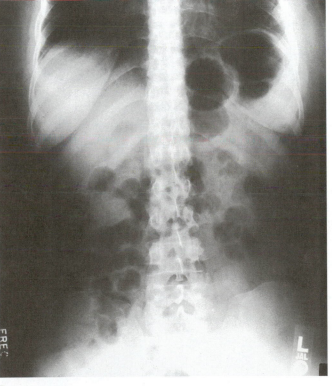

B

Figure 7–93. Observe the difference between these two radiographs. **(A)** Part of an intravenous urogram (IVU) examination taken in the recumbent position. **(B)** Part of an abdominal survey taken in the erect position. Observe the change in appearance and radiographic density, especially of the lower abdomen, as the patient is moved erect and the abdominal viscera assume a lower position; the lower abdomen essentially becomes "thicker" and radiographic density decreases. Both hemidiaphragms must be observed on the erect abdomen. (**(A)** courtesy of Bob Wong, RT. **(B)** from the American College of Radiology Learning File. Courtesy of the ACR.)

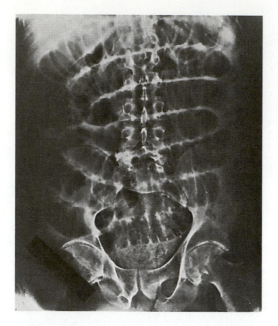

Figure 7–94. Small-bowel obstruction indicated by the dilated bowel loops having a *ladder-like* pattern. Patient is recumbent; therefore air/fluid levels are not demonstrated. (From Way, LW, ed. *Current Surgical Diagnosis & Treatment,* 10th ed. East Norwalk, CT: Appleton & Lange, 1994.)

	POSITION OF PART:	CENTRAL RAY DIRECTED:	STRUCTURES INCLUDED/ BEST SEEN:
LAT Decubitus	Patient lat recumbent, (AP or PA) MSP ⊥ and centered to upright grid, cassette centered ≈2″ above iliac crest	Horizontal and ⊥ mid-cassette	Usually *left* lat decubitus of abdomen to demonstrate air/ fluid levels in patients unable to assume the erect position; both hemidiaphragms should be included

Note: A "three-way abdomen" study is often performed to evaluate possible obstruction or free air and fluid within the abdomen and usually consists of AP recumbent, AP erect, and L lat decubitus projections of the abdomen (Fig. 7–94).

4. Esophagus

	POSITION OF PART:	CENTRAL RAY DIRECTED:	STRUCTURES INCLUDED/ BEST SEEN:
AP	Supine, MSP centered and ⊥ table, cassette top 1 to 2″ above shoulders, patient swallowing barium during (<0.1 sec) exposure	⊥ midcassette, ≈T6–T7	Barium-filled esophagus in AP proj
RAO	Prone obl, 35–40° RAO, cassette top 1 to 2″ above shoulders, patient swallowing barium during exposure	⊥ midcassette, ≈T6–T7	Barium-filled esophagus in RAO proj, demonstrated b/w vertebrae and heart; best single proj of barium filled esophagus; see Fig. 7–95
LAT (L or R)	Recumbent lat, MCP centered to grid, cassette top just above shoulders, patient swallowing during exposure	⊥ midcassette	Barium-filled esophagus in lat proj

Note: Esophagus for demonstration of *varices* must be performed in the *recumbent* position; table slightly Trendelenburg and/or performance of the Valsalva maneuver is also helpful. Exposure times of 0.1 sec or less should be used in order to avoid motion; however, respiration normally stops during and shortly after the act of swallowing, so that patients need not be instructed to stop breathing.

5. Stomach and Small Intestine. Radiologic examination of the stomach and/or small bowel generally begins with fluoroscopic examination. The fluoroscopist observes the swallowing mechanism, mucosal lining (rugae) of the stomach, and the filling and emptying mechanisms of the stomach and proximal small bowel in various positions. The patient is turned and rotated in various positions so that all aspects of the stomach and any abnormalities such as hiatal hernia (see Fig. 7–101) can be visualized. Double-contrast examinations of the upper GI system are performed frequently. Occasionally glucagon or another similar drug will be given the patient (IV or IM) prior to the examination to relax the GI tract and permit more complete filling. Various images will be made by the fluoroscopist and the radiographer may take supplemental "overhead" projections. *Small-bowel series* examinations require that successive films be made of the abdomen at specified intervals; an additional fluoroscopic image is made when barium reaches the *ileocecal valve.*

Contrast material (usually water soluble) may occasionally be instilled through a gastrointestinal (GI) tube for visualization of the GI tract. GI tubes can be used therapeutically to siphon gas and fluid from the GI tract or diagnostically, using contrast agent, to locate the site of obstruction or pathology.

	POSITION OF PART:	CENTRAL RAY DIRECTED:	STRUCTURES INCLUDED/ BEST SEEN:
LPO	Supine, obliqued ≈40° to left, centered midway b/w vertebrae and L abdominal wall at level of L1	⊥ midcassette (at level of L1)	Barium-filled fundus good position for *double contrast* of body, pylorus, and duodenal bulb; see Fig. 7–96

Note: As the fundus is the most posterior portion of stomach, it readily fills w/barium in AP position and moves more superiorly.

(continued)

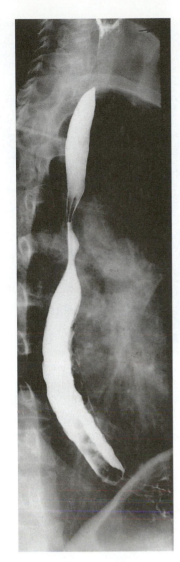

Figure 7–95. RAO of a barium-filled esophagus. The esophagus has three normal constrictions at the levels of the cricoid cartilage, the left bronchus, and the esophageal hiatus of the diaphragm. (Courtesy of The Stamford Hospital.)

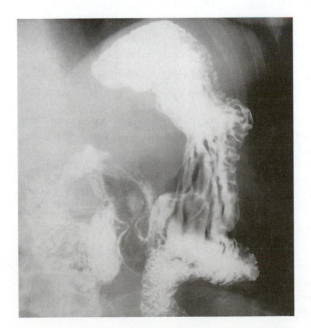

Figure 7–96. LPO of the stomach. In this position, air replaces the barium that drains from the duodenal bulb and pylorus, thus providing double-contrast visualization of these structures. (Courtesy of The Stamford Hospital.)

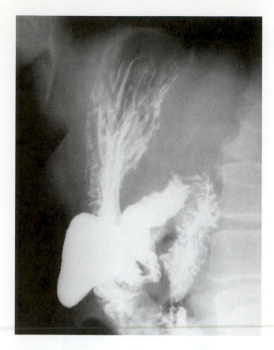

Figure 7–97. Lateral projection demonstrates the anterior and posterior stomach surfaces and the retrogastric space. (Courtesy of The Stamford Hospital.)

	POSITION OF PART:	CENTRAL RAY DIRECTED:	STRUCTURES INCLUDED/ BEST SEEN:
LAT	Recumbent lat (usually R), center m/w b/w MCP and anterior abdominal wall to cassette at level of L2	⊥ midcassette (at level of L2)	Lat stomach and prox small bowel demonstrating anterior and posterior aspects of stomach, retrogastric space, pyloric canal, duodenal loop; see Fig. 7–97

Note: This projection provides the best visualization of the pyloric canal and duodenal bulb in the hypersthenic patient.

	POSITION OF PART:	CENTRAL RAY DIRECTED:	STRUCTURES INCLUDED/ BEST SEEN:
RAO	Recumbent PA obliqued 40 to 70°, centered m/w b/w vertebrae and lat abdominal wall at level of L2	⊥ midcassette (at level of L2)	Right PA obl proj of stomach barium-filled pyloric canal and duodenal loop; demonstrates stomach's emptying mechanism, because *peristaltic activity is greatest in this position*
PA	Prone, MSP centered to grid, at level of L2	⊥ midcassette (at level of L2)	PA proj of transversely spread stomach, demonstrating contours, greater and lesser curvatures

Note: Hypersthenic patients frequently have high, transverse stomachs with indistinguishable curvatures. The adult hypersthenic stomach can be "opened" and its contours made readily visible by angling the CR 35 to 45° cephalad. The top edge of a lengthwise 14″ × 17″ cassette is placed level with the patient's chin and the CR directed to mid-cassette.

	POSITION OF PART:	CENTRAL RAY DIRECTED:	STRUCTURES INCLUDED/ BEST SEEN:
AP/ Small Bowel	Patient supine, MSP centered to grid, cassette centered to level of L2	⊥ midcassette (at level of L2)	AP proj of distal esophagus area, stomach, and proximal small bowel; demonstrates hiatal hernias w/ patient in Trendelenburg position

Note: This position is used to record progress of the barium column in *small bowel* examinations. The first radiograph is usually made 15 min after ingestion of the barium drink and centered at level of L2. Subsequent radiographs are made at 15- to 30-min intervals (and centered at level of crest), according to the individual patient and how quickly or slowly the barium progresses. Spot films are usually taken when the barium column reaches the ileocecal valve.

6. Large Intestine. The lower GI tract is most often examined by *retrograde* filling with barium sulfate and, frequently, air. The fluoroscopist observes filling of the large bowel in various positions and makes images as indicated. Much of the barium is then drained from the intestine, and air is introduced. The objective is to coat the bowel with barium, then distend its lumen with air. The double-contrast method is ideal for demonstration of intraluminal lesions, such as polyps.

The success of the barium enema examination depends on several factors, but without proper patient preparation a diagnostic examination is often impossible. *Poor preparation resulting in retained fecal material in the colon can mimic or conceal pathologic conditions.*

The barium enema is most easily tolerated and retained by the patient if it is cool or actually cold (≈40° to 45°F). There is probably no radiographic examination that causes more embarrassment and anxiety than the barium-enema and air-contrast procedure. The radiographer must be sensitive to the concerns and needs of the patient by providing a complete explanation of the procedure and by providing for the patient's modesty as much as possible.

The following table summarizes frequently performed projections taken following the fluoroscopic procedure.

	POSITION OF PART:	CENTRAL RAY DIRECTED:	STRUCTURES INCLUDED/ BEST SEEN:
AP	Supine, MSP centered to cassette at level of iliac crest	⊥ midcassette	AP proj of entire contrast-filled large intestine

Note: The large intestine of *hypersthenic* patients is high and around the periphery of the abdomen, hence they may require that the AP and PA be done on (2) 14″ × 17″-inch films placed crosswise in the Bucky tray. In contrast, the colon of the *asthenic* patient is low, redundant, and more midline.

	POSITION OF PART:	CENTRAL RAY DIRECTED:	STRUCTURES INCLUDED/ BEST SEEN:
PA	Prone, MSP centered to cassette at level of iliac crest	⊥ midcassette	PA proj of entire contrast-filled large intestine; AP or PA *erect* may be used to demonstrate double-contrast *flexures*
PA Axial	Prone, MSP centered to cassette at level of pubic symphysis	35° caudad to midline at level of ASIS	PA axial proj of *sigmoid colon;* angulation opens the length of the S-shaped colon; see Fig. 7–98

Note: AP axial may be performed to show similar structures; CR is directed 35° cephalad.

	POSITION OF PART:	CENTRAL RAY DIRECTED:	STRUCTURES INCLUDED/ BEST SEEN:
RAO	PA, obl ≈40°, centered to midline, cassette centered to level of iliac crest	⊥ midcassette	Right PA obl proj of the colon, demonstrates *ascending colon and hepatic flexure;* see Fig. 7–99
LAO	PA obl ≈40°, centered to midline, cassette centered to level of iliac crest	⊥ midcassette	Left PA obl proj of the colon, demonstrates *descending colon and splenic flexure*

Note: *RPO* will demonstrate *descending colon and splenic flexure; LPO* will demonstrate *ascending colon and hepatic flexure.*

(continued)

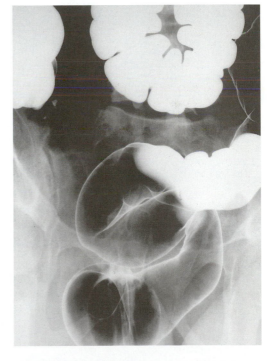

Figure 7–98. Double-contrast PA axial projection of the rectum and sigmoid. The caudal tube angulation serves to "open" the redundant S-shaped sigmoid colon. Similar results may be obtained in the AP position with a cephalad tube angle. (Courtesy of The Stamford Hospital.)

	POSITION OF PART:	CENTRAL RAY DIRECTED:	STRUCTURES INCLUDED/ BEST SEEN:
LAT	Lat recumbent, MCP centered to grid, cassette centered at level of ASIS	⊥ midcassette	L or R lat proj, especially for *rectum* and *rectosigmoid* area
LAT Decubitus (R and L)	Lat recumbent, (AP or PA), MSP ⊥ and centered to upright grid at level of iliac crest	Horizontal and ⊥ midcassette	Air rises to provide double-contrast delineation of *lateral walls of colon;* both decubitus are routinely performed; see Fig. 7–100

7. Terminology and Pathology. The following is a list of radiographically significant abdominal and digestive conditions and devices with which the student radiographer should be familiar.

Achalasia
Appendicitis
Ascites
Colostomy
Crohn's disease
Diverticulitis
Diverticulosis
Dysphagia
Enteritis
Esophageal reflux
Esophageal varices
Gastritis

Gastroenteritis
Hiatal hernia (see Fig. 7–101)
Ileostomy
Intussusception
Irritable-bowel syndrome
Peptic ulcer
Peritonitis
Polyp
Pyloric stenosis
Ulcerative colitis
Volvulus

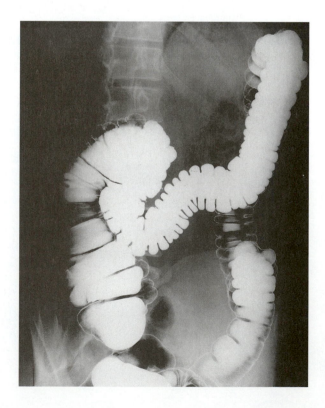

Figure 7–99. RAO of the barium and air-filled large bowel. Note that the hepatic flexure is "opened" for better visualization. An LPO would provide similar results. The opposite obliques (LAO, RPO) are used to demonstrate the splenic flexure and descending colon. (Courtesy of The Stamford Hospital.)

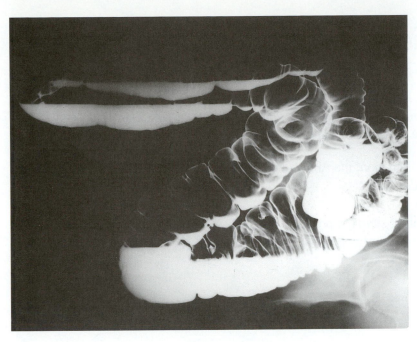

Figure 7–100. Right lateral decubitus view of the air and barium-filled colon. The heavier barium sulfate moves toward the dependent side, while air rises to fill the remainder of the barium-coated lumen. Thus, the *right lateral decubitus demonstrates double contrast of the "left-sided walls" of the ascending and descending colons* (ie, lateral side of descending colon and medial side of ascending colon). (Courtesy of The Stamford Hospital.)

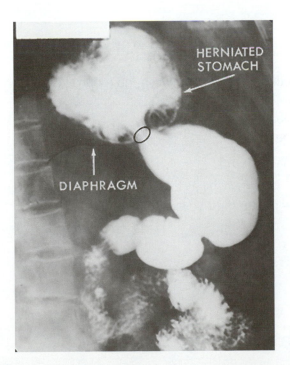

Figure 7–101. Large hiatal hernia extending up through the (circled) diaphragmatic esophageal hiatus. (From Way, LW. *Current Surgical Diagnosis & Treatment*, 10th ed. East Norwalk, CT: Appleton & Lange, 1994.)

A&U Chapter Review Questions

⭐ *Congratulations! You have completed a large portion of this chapter. You may go on to the "Registry-type" multiple-choice questions that follow. For greatest success, be sure also to complete the short answer questions found at the end of this chapter.*

1. During a gastrointestinal examination, the AP recumbent projection of a stomach of average shape will usually demonstrate:
   1. barium-filled fundus
   2. double contrast of distal stomach portions
   3. barium-filled duodenum and pylorus
   (A) 1 only
   (B) 1 and 2 only
   (C) 1 and 3 only
   (D) 1, 2, and 3

2. The salivary gland associated with Stenson's duct is the:
   (A) parotid
   (B) submaxillary gland
   (C) sublingual gland
   (D) Wharton's gland

3. Which of the following projections of the abdomen should be used to demonstrate air or fluid levels when the erect position cannot be obtained?
   (A) AP Trendelenburg
   (B) AP supine
   (C) lateral decubitus
   (D) lateral recumbent

4. Which of the following best describes the relationship between the esophagus and trachea?
   (A) esophagus is posterior to the trachea
   (B) trachea is posterior to the esophagus
   (C) esophagus is lateral to the trachea
   (D) trachea is lateral to the esophagus

5. To demonstrate esophageal varices, the patient must be examined in the:
   (A) recumbent position
   (B) erect position
   (C) anatomic position
   (D) Fowler's position

6. The usual preparation for an upper GI series is:
   (A) clear fluids 8 hours prior to exam
   (B) npo after midnight
   (C) enemas until clear before exam
   (D) light breakfast day of the exam

7. Which of the following positions would best demonstrate a double contrast of the hepatic and splenic flexures?
   (A) left lateral decubitus
   (B) AP recumbent
   (C) right lateral decubitus
   (D) AP erect

8. In which of the following positions are a barium-filled pyloric canal and duodenal bulb best demonstrated during a GI series?
   (A) RAO
   (B) left lateral
   (C) recumbent PA
   (D) recumbent AP

9. What position is frequently used to project the GB away from the vertebrae in the asthenic patient?
   (A) RAO
   (B) LAO
   (C) left lateral decubitus
   (D) PA erect

10. Which of the following barium/air-filled anatomic structures is best demonstrated in the RAO position?
    (A) splenic flexure
    (B) hepatic flexure
    (C) sigmoid colon
    (D) iliocecal valve

Answers and Explanations

1. (B) With the body in the anteroposterior (AP) recumbent position, barium flows easily into the fundus of the stomach, displacing it somewhat superiorly. The fundus, then, is filled with barium, while the air that had been in the fundus is displaced into the gastric body, pylorus, and duodenum, illustrating them in double-contrast fashion. Air-contrast delineation of these structures allows us to see through the stomach to retrogastric areas and structures. Barium-filled duodenum and pylorus is best demonstrated in the right anterior oblique (RAO) position.

2. (A) There are three groups of salivary glands. The largest are the parotid glands, which lie below and anterior to the ear and are emptied by Stenson's duct. The submaxillary glands are located near the angle of the mandible and are emptied by Wharton's duct. The sublingual gland, as its name implies, is located under the tongue; a group of ducts (of Rivinus) empty the gland. The largest of these is Bartholin's duct.

3. (C) Air or fluid levels will be clearly demonstrated only if the central ray is directed parallel to them. Therefore, to demonstrate air or fluid levels, erect or decubitus positions should be used. A "three-way abdomen" study is often performed to evaluate possible obstruction or free air or fluid within the abdomen and usually consists of anteroposterior (AP) recumbent, AP erect, and left lateral decubitus projections of the abdomen.

4. (A) The trachea (windpipe) is a tube-like passageway for air that is supported by C-shaped cartilaginous rings. The trachea is part of the respiratory system and is continuous with the main stem bronchi. The esophagus, part of the alimentary canal, is a hollow tube-like structure connecting the mouth and stomach, and lies posterior to the trachea. If one inadvertently aspirates food or drink into the trachea, choking occurs.

5. (A) Esophageal varices are tortuous dilatations of the esophageal veins. They are much less pronounced in the erect position and must always be examined with the patient recumbent. The recumbent position affords more complete filling of the veins, as blood flows against gravity.

6. (B) The upper gastrointestinal (GI) tract must be empty for best x-ray evaluation. Any food or liquid mixed with the barium sulfate suspension can simulate pathology. Preparation therefore is to withhold food and fluids for 8 to 9 hours before the exam, typically after midnight, as fasting exams are usually performed first thing in the morning.

7. (D) To demonstrate structures via double contrast, the barium must be moved away from the area and replaced with air. The *anteroposterior (AP) erect position* will accomplish that for both the colic flexures. The erect position allows barium to move downward, while air rises to fill the flexures. The decubitus positions are useful to demonstrate the lateral and medial walls of the ascending and descending colon.

8. (A) The right anterior oblique (RAO) position affords a good view of the pyloric canal and duodenal bulb. It is also a good position for the barium-filled esophagus, projecting it between the vertebrae and heart. The left lateral projection of the stomach demonstrates the left retrogastric space; the recumbent posteroanterior (PA) is used as a general survey of the gastric surfaces, and the recumbent anteroposterior (AP) with a slight left oblique affords a double contrast of the pylorus and duodenum.

9. (B) There are four types of body habitus. Listed from largest to smallest they are hypersthenic, sthenic, hyposthenic, and asthenic. The position, shape, and motility of various organs can differ greatly from one body type to another. The typical asthenic gallbladder (GB) is situated low and medial, often very close to the midline. To move the GB away from the midline, left anterior oblique (LAO) position is used. The GB of hypersthenic individuals occupies a high lateral, and transverse position.

10. (B) In the prone oblique positions (right/left anterior oblique [RAO/LAO]) the flexure disclosed is the one closer to the film. Therefore, the RAO position will open up the hepatic flexure. The anteroposterior (AP) oblique positions (right/left posterior oblique [RPO/LPO]) demonstrate the side away from the film.

D. Urinary System

1. Introduction. Two of the functions of the urinary system (Fig. 7–102) are to *remove wastes from the blood* and *eliminate it in the form of urine.* The tiny units within the renal substance that perform these functions are called *nephrons.* The major components of the urinary system are the *kidneys, ureters, and bladder.*

The paired *kidneys* are *retroperitoneal,* and embedded in adipose tissue between the vertebral levels of T12 and L3. The right kidney is usually 1 to 2 inches lower than the left because of the presence of the liver on the right. The kidneys move inferiorly 1 to 3 inches when the body assumes an erect position; they move inferiorly and superiorly during respiration. The slit-like openings on the medial renal surface is the *hilum,* which opens into a space called the *renal sinus* (Fig. 7–103). The renal artery and vein pass through the hilum. The upper, expanded portion of the ureter is called the *renal pelvis,* or *infundibulum,* and also passes through the hilum; it is continuous with the major and minor calyces within the kidney.

Within each kidney, the renal *parenchyma* is divided into two parts: the outer *cortex* and inner *medulla.* The cortex is compact and has a grainy appearance as a result of the many *glomeruli* within is tissues. The medulla contains 10 to 14 *renal pyramids* with a characteristic striated appearance that is due to the *collecting tubules* within (see Fig. 7–103).

The proximal portion of each *ureter* is at the renal pelvis. As the ureter passes inferiorly, three normal constrictions can be observed: at the ureteropelvic junction, at the pelvic brim, and at the ureterovesicular junction. Urine is carried through the ureters by peristaltic activity. If a ureter is obstructed by a kidney stone, *hydronephrosis* occurs. The ureters enter the *urinary bladder* posteroinferiorly (Fig. 7–104). The base of the bladder rests on the pelvic floor. The triangular-shaped area formed by the *ureteral* and *urethral orifices* is called the *trigone.* Micturition is the process of emptying the urinary bladder of its contents through the *urethra.* The male urethra is about

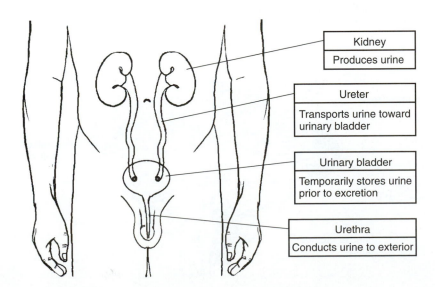

Figure 7–102. Components of the urinary system.

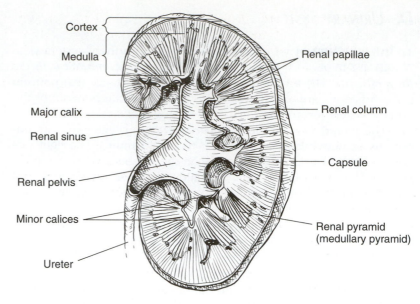

Figure 7–103. Section through the left renal pelvis.

7 to 8 inches long and is divided into prostatic, membranous, and penile portions. The female urethra is about 1.5 inches in length.

A common complication of regional enteritis or diverticular disease is the formation of a *fistula* between the urinary bladder and small or large intestine. Fistulous tracts may often be evaluated radiographically with contrast media.

Routine radiographic procedures of the urinary system are generally performed via the intravenous route. When performed in the retrograde manner, *cystoscopy* is required.

Routine intravenous procedures are most correctly referred to as *intravenous urography* (IVU), or *excretory urography,* although they are still commonly referred to as intravenous *pyelography* (IVP) (*pyel* refers only to renal *pelvis*). Intravenous procedures demonstrate *function* of the urinary system. Retrograde studies demonstrate only the *structure* of the part and are generally performed to evaluate the lower urinary tract (lower ureters, bladder, and urethra).

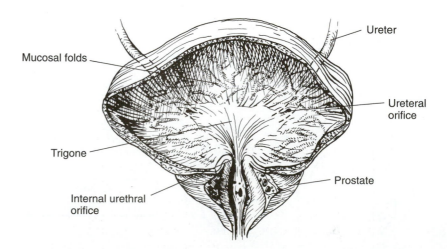

Figure 7–104. Bladder trigone (anterior portion of bladder removed).

2. Patient Preparation. Investigation of the urinary tract requires patient preparation sufficient to rid the intestinal tract of gas and fecal material. Typical preparation usually begins the evening before the examination with a light dinner, a gentle laxative, and nothing to eat or drink (npo; nothing per os [by mouth]) after midnight. Immediately before beginning the IVU, the patient must be instructed to empty his or her bladder; this prevents dilution of opacified urine in the bladder. If the patient has a urinary catheter, it is generally clamped just before the injection and unclamped before the postvoid radiograph. The IVU is preceded by a preliminary scout film of the abdomen to evaluate patient preparation and reveal any calcifications (renal or gallstones), position of kidneys, and accuracy of technical factor selection (Fig. 7–105).

Because the urinary structures have so little subject contrast, artificial contrast material must be employed for better visualization of these structures. Contrast agents used for urographic procedures can have unpleasant, and (rarely) even lethal, side effects. Intravenous injection of contrast frequently produces a warm, flushed feeling, a bitter or metallic taste, or mild nausea. These side effects are of short duration and usually pass as quickly as they come. More serious side effects include *urticaria,* respiratory discomfort and distress and rarely, *anaphylaxis.* An *antihistamine* is appropriate treatment for simple side effects, but the radiographer must always be prepared to deal quickly and efficiently with patients experiencing more serious reactions. *Nonionic* contrast agents are far less likely to produce side effects. Contrast agents and their side effects are more thoroughly discussed in Chapter 1.

The selected contrast agent is injected intravenously and successive radiographs are made at specified intervals. A time-interval marker must be included on each radiograph to indicate the postinjection time elapsed. Injection and postinjection protocol varies with the institution, radiologist, patient condition, and diagnosis. The contrast may be rapidly injected in a *bolus* to obtain a 30-second *nephrogram.* Radiographs collimated to the kidneys (11 × 14 inches crosswise) may be required at 1, 3, and 5 minutes to evaluate a diagnosis of renal hypertension. Both obliques and tomograms may be required to evaluate a suspected tumor or lesion. AP and oblique kidney, ureter, and bladder films (KUBs) are usually required at 10 to 15 minutes after injection. Maximum concentration of the contrast material usually occurs at 15 to 20 minutes after injection, but varies with degree of patient hydration. A prone KUB is frequently requested at 20 minutes. Because the ureters lie in a plane anterior to the kidneys, *ureteral filling* with contrast media is best achieved using the PA projection (see Fig. 7–106).

3. Types of Examinations. Compression over the distal ureters (delaying contrast or urine travel to bladder) may be required to more completely fill the kidneys with contrast medium or to visualize the contrast-filled kidneys for a longer period of time (Fig. 7–106). *Tomograms* are often useful to remove superimposed shadows from kidneys and better evaluate the renal collecting system. Patients having a condition interfering with renal function will often require delayed films to demonstrate the collecting system and/or ureters. Since the lower poles of the kidneys and the ureters are more anterior structures, the prone position is often used to demonstrate filling of these

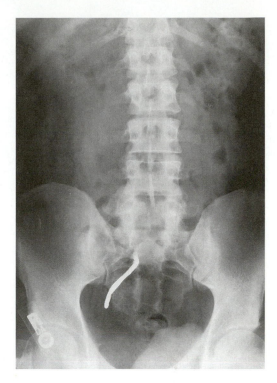

Figure 7–105. A preliminary or scout film of the abdomen is taken before the start of an IVU. The radiograph is checked for residual barium from previous contrast studies, patient preparation (including barium from previous studies; note residual barium in patient's appendix), location of kidneys, technical factors, and any calcifications. (Courtesy of The Stamford Hospital.)

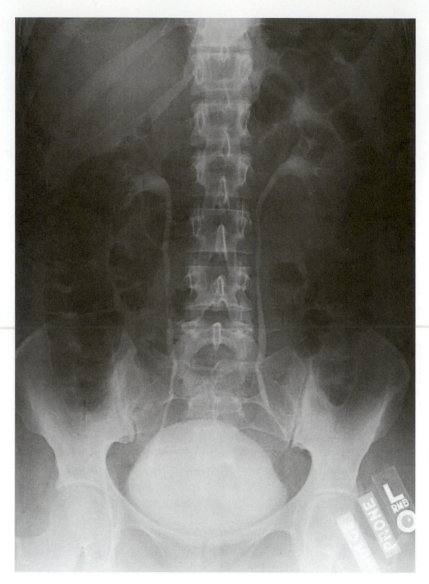

Figure 7–106. PA projection of IVU, demonstrating contrast-filled ureters. Since the ureters lie in a plane which is anterior to that of the kidneys, they are best demonstrated as contrast-filled structures in the *PA position.* The contrast material, which is heavier than urine, gravitates to fill the anterior ureters. (Courtesy of The Stamford Hospital.)

structures. An erect radiograph is occasionally requested to demonstrate renal mobility and ureteral tortuosity. An AP postvoid bladder film is usually required to detect any *residual urine* in the evaluation of tumor masses or enlarged prostate glands.

Retrograde urograms require catheterization of the ureter(s). Radiographs that include the kidney(s) and ureter(s) in their entirety are made after retrograde filling of the structures. A cystogram or (voiding) *cystourethrogram* requires urethral catheterization only. Radiographs are made of the contrast-filled bladder and frequently of the contrast-filled urethra during voiding. *Cystoscopy* is required for location and catheterization of the vesicoureteral orifices.

Excretory and retrograde urography involve accurate positioning of the abdomen to include the kidneys, ureters, and bladder. If these structures cannot fit on a single film, a second radiograph is generally taken for the bladder. The following is a review of abdomen KUB positioning and an overview of bladder positioning.

4. KUB (Kidney, Ureter, and Bladder)

POSITION OF PART:	CENTRAL RAY DIRECTED:	STRUCTURES INCLUDED/ BEST SEEN:
Patient supine, MSP ⊥ centered to grid, cassette centered to iliac crest	⊥ to midline at level of crest	AP proj of abdomen shows size and shape of kidneys, liver, spleen, psoas muscles, and, any calcifications or masses; should include from top of kidneys through symphysis pubis (see Fig. 7–107); obliques may be performed at 30°

Note: The PA projection will best demonstrate contrast-filled ureters (Fig. 7–106).

Note: The 30° oblique KUB places the kidney of the up side *parallel* to the image receptor; and the ureter of the side *down* parallel to the image receptor. Fig. 7–108 is a RPO that places the left kidney and right ureter parallel to the image receptor.

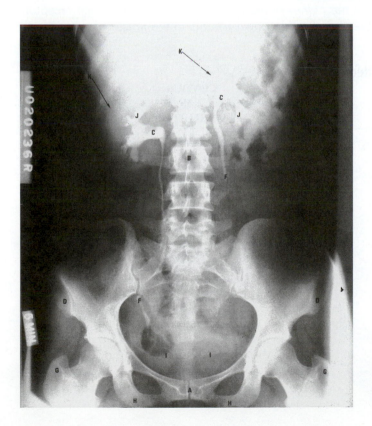

Figure 7–107. This KUB is a 5-min IVU film. Good collimation is evident and the kidneys, ureters, and bladder are included in their entirety. *Review the contents of the abdominal cavity* by correcting identifying each of the lettered structures. (Courtesy Bob Wong, RT.)

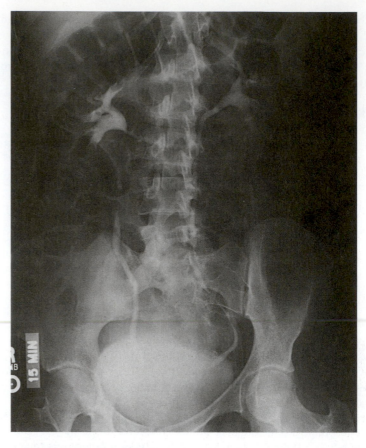

Figure 7–108. 15 minute RPO during IVU, demonstrating the left kidney and right ureter parallel to the image receptor. The 30° oblique KUB places the *kidney* of the *up* side *parallel* to the image receptor, and the *ureter* of the side *down parallel* to the image receptor.

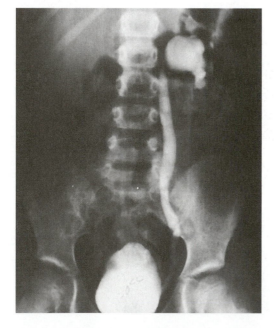

Figure 7–109. AP projection of voiding cystourethrogram demonstrating complete left vesicoureteral reflux. Because pediatric voiding disorders are frequently associated with vesicoureteral reflux, it is often necessary to include most of the abdomen in the radiograph. (Reproduced with permission from Way, LW, ed. *Current Surgical Diagnosis & Treatment,* 10th ed. East Norwalk, CT: Appleton & Lange, 1994.)

5. Bladder

	POSITION OF PART:	CENTRAL RAY DIRECTED:	STRUCTURES INCLUDED/ BEST SEEN:
AP	Patient supine, MSP ⊥ centered to grid, lower edge of cassette just below pubic symphysis	⊥ to center of cassette	AP proj shows contrast-filled or postvoid bladder
AP *(Voiding Studies)*	Patient supine, MSP ⊥ centered to grid, cassette centered to pubic symphysis	⊥ to midline at level of pubic symphysis	AP projection of bladder and proximal urethra; used for voiding cystourethrograms (see Fig. 7–109); a 5° caudal angle may be used to project bladder neck and urethra below pubis; obl proj are obtained at 40 to 60°

6. Terminology and Pathology. The following is a list of radiographically significant urinary conditions and devices with which the student radiographer should be familiar.

Cystitis	Polycystic kidney
Double-collecting system	Prostatic hypertrophy
Double ureter	Pyelonephritis
Fistula	Renal calculi
Foley catheter	Renal hypotension
Horseshoe kidney	Staghorn calculus (see Fig. 7–109)
Hydronephrosis	Supernumerary kidney
Hydroureter	(see Fig. 7–110)
Incontinence	Uremia
Nephroptosis	Ureteral stent
Nephrostomy tube	Ureterocele
Pelvic kidney	Vesicoureteral reflux

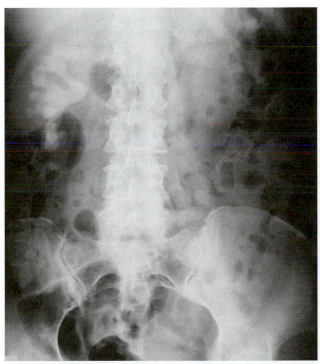
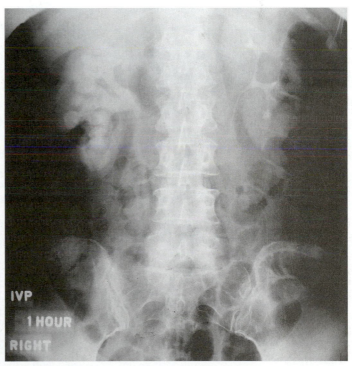

A   B

Figure 7–110. Although radiograph (**A**) may appear to be part of an IVU examination, no urine-filled ureter or bladder is associated with the opaque right kidney; the opaque area is associated with formation of a *staghorn calculus*. Radiograph (**B**) is a 1-hr IVU demonstrating both collecting systems. Staghorn calculi are usually associated with chronic infection and alkaline urine. They may be associated with a single calyx or an entire renal pelvis, and may be unilateral or bilateral. Whenever possible, staghorn (named for their shape, resembling a stag's antlers) calculi are removed because they can cause partial obstruction of the calyces and/or ureteropelvic junction. (From the American College of Radiology Learning File. Courtesy of the ACR.)

E. FEMALE REPRODUCTIVE SYSTEM

1. Introduction. The female reproductive system consists of the ovaries, oviducts, and uterus. The broad, suspensory, round, and ovarian ligaments are all associated with support of the reproductive organs.

The *ovaries* are the female gonads that function to release ova (female reproductive cells) during ovulation and produce various female hormones including estrogen and progesterone. The *oviducts,* or Fallopian tubes, are 3 to 5 inches long, arise from the uterine cornu (angles) and extend laterally to arch over each ovary. The oviduct lateral extremities are broader than their medial ends and are bordered by motile *fimbriae* (see Fig. 7–111). The fimbriae sweep over the ovary and function to collect the liberated ovum. *Fertilization* of the ovum usually occurs in the outer portion of the oviducts. Ova are propelled through the oviduct by peristaltic motion. *Salpingitis* is possibly the most common cause of female sterility; if fertilization does occur, the zygote is unable to traverse the oviduct due to its scarred or narrowed condition. Occasionally, a fertilized ovum will become implanted in the oviduct, a condition known as ectopic, or tubal, pregnancy. This condition is a gynecologic emergency because, if left untreated, the patient can die from internal hemorrhage.

The most superior, arched, portion of the *uterus* is the fundus. The angle on each side is the cornu, and marks the point of entry of the oviducts. The *body* is the large central region and the narrow inferior portion is the *cervix.*

2. Hysterosalpingogram. The most commonly performed radiologic examination of the reproductive system is hysterosalpingography, which is employed for evaluation of the uterus, oviducts, and ovaries of the female reproductive system. The procedure serves to delineate the position, size, and shape of the structures and demonstrate pathology such as *polyps, tumors,* and *fistulas.* However, it is most often used to demonstrate *patency* of the oviducts in cases of *infertility,* and is sometimes therapeutic in terms of opening a blocked oviduct.

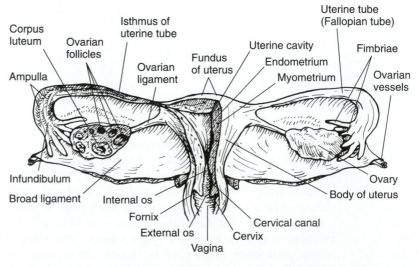

Figure 7–111. Uterus, uterine tubes (oviducts), and ovaries.

Hysterosalpingograms should be scheduled about 10 days after the start of menstruation. This is the time just *before* ovulation, when there should be little chance of irradiating a newly fertilized ovum.

After the cervical canal is cannulated, an iodinated organic contrast agent is injected via the cannula into the uterine cavity. If the oviducts are patent, contrast will flow through them and into the peritoneal cavity. Fluoroscopy is performed during injection and spot films are taken. Overhead radiographs may be performed following the fluoroscopic procedure.

	POSITION OF PART:	CENTRAL RAY DIRECTED:	STRUCTURES INCLUDED/ BEST SEEN:
AP	Patient supine, MSP centered to grid, and a point 2″ above the pubic symphysis centered to the cassette	⊥ midcassette	AP proj of uterus and oviducts; 30° obliques may be taken as required; see Fig. 7–112

3. Terminology and Pathology.

The following is a list of radiographically significant reproductive conditions with which the student radiographer should be familiar.

Bicornuate uterus	Leiomyoma
Ectopic pregnancy	Pelvic inflammatory disease
Endometriosis	Placenta previa
Infertility	Salpingitis

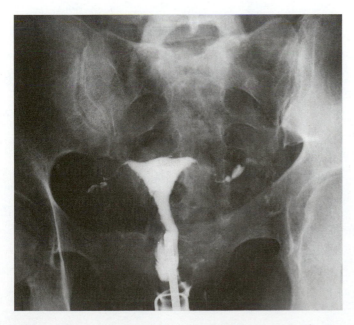

Figure 7–112. AP projection of hysterosalpingogram study. Contrast-filled uterus and oviducts are shown. (Courtesy of The Stamford Hospital.)

Chapter Review Questions

⭐ **Congratulations!** *You have completed your review of a large portion of this chapter. You may go on to the "Registry-type" multiple-choice questions that follow. For greatest success, be sure also to complete the short answer questions found at the end of this chapter.*

1. In what order should the following radiographs be performed?
   1. barium enema
   2. intravenous pyelogram
   3. upper GI
   (A) 3, 1, 2
   (B) 1, 3, 2
   (C) 2, 1, 3
   (D) 2, 3, 1

2. Which of the following will best demonstrate the size and shape of the liver and kidneys?
   (A) lateral abdomen
   (B) AP abdomen
   (C) dorsal decubitus abdomen
   (D) ventral decubitus abdomen

3. Which of the following examinations require(s) restriction of the patient's diet?
   1. GI series
   2. abdominal survey
   3. pyelogram
   (A) 1 only
   (B) 1 and 2 only
   (C) 1 and 3 only
   (D) 1, 2, and 3

4. During IV urography, the prone position is generally recommended to demonstrate:
   1. filling of obstructed ureters
   2. the renal pelvis
   3. the superior calyces
   (A) 1 only
   (B) 1 and 2 only
   (C) 1 and 3 only
   (D) 1, 2, and 3

5. Which of the following examinations require(s) catheterization of the ureters?
   1. retrograde urogram
   2. cystogram
   3. voiding cystogram
   (A) 1 only
   (B) 1 and 2 only
   (C) 2 and 3 only
   (D) 1, 2, and 3

6. Some common mild side effects of intravenous administration of water-soluble iod-inated contrast agents include:
   1. flushed feeling
   2. bitter taste
   3. urticaria
   (A) 1 only
   (B) 1 and 2 only
   (C) 1 and 3 only
   (D) 1, 2, and 3

7. Hysterosalpingograms may be performed for the following reason(s):
   1. demonstration of fistulous tracts
   2. investigation of infertility
   3. demonstration of tubal patency
   (A) 1 only
   (B) 1 and 2 only
   (C) 1 and 3 only
   (D) 1, 2, and 3

8. A postvoid radiograph of the urinary bladder is usually requested at the completion of an IVP, and may be helpful in demonstrating:
   1. residual urine
   2. prostate enlargement
   3. ureteral tortuosity
   (A) 1 only
   (B) 1 and 2 only
   (C) 1 and 3 only
   (D) 1, 2, and 3

9. During routine intravenous urography, the oblique position demonstrates the:
   (A) kidney of the side *up* parallel to the film
   (B) kidney of the side *up* perpendicular to the film
   (C) urinary bladder parallel to the film
   (D) urinary bladder perpendicular to the film

10. To better demonstrate contrast-filled distal ureters during intravenous urography, it is helpful to:
    1. use a 15-degree AP Trendelenburg position
    2. apply compression to the proximal ureters
    3. apply compression to the distal ureters
    (A) 1 only
    (B) 2 only
    (C) 1 and 2 only
    (D) 1 and 3 only

Answers and Explanations

1. (C) When scheduling patient examinations it is important to avoid the possibility of residual contrast medium covering areas of interest on later exams. The intravenous pyelogram (IVP) should be scheduled first because the contrast medium used is excreted rapidly. The barium enema (BE) should be scheduled next. The gastrointestinal (GI) series is scheduled last. Any barium remaining from the previous BE should not be enough to interfere with the stomach or duodenum, though a preliminary scout film should be taken in each case.

2. (B) The anteroposterior (AP) projection provides a survey of the abdomen, showing the size and shape of the liver, spleen, and kidneys. When performed erect, it should demonstrate both hemidiaphragms. The lateral projection is sometimes requested and is useful for evaluating the prevertebral space occupied by the aorta. Ventral and dorsal decubitus positions provide a lateral view of the abdomen useful for demonstration of air-fluid levels.

3. (C) A patient having a gastrointestinal (GI) series is required to be npo (nothing by mouth) for at least 8 hours prior to the exam; food or drink in the stomach can simulate disease. A patient scheduled for a pyelogram must have the preceding meal withheld so as to avoid the possibility of aspirating vomitus in case of allergic reaction. An abdominal survey does not require the use of contrast medium and no patient preparation is required.

4. (B) The kidneys lie obliquely in the posterior portion of the trunk, with their superior portions angled posteriorly and their inferior portions and ureters angled anteriorly. Therefore, to facilitate filling of the most anteriorly placed structures, the patient is examined in the prone position. Opacified urine then flows to the most dependent part of the kidney and ureter—the ureteropelvic region, inferior calyces, and ureters.

5. (A) Retrograde urograms require catheterization of the urethra and/or ureter(s). Radiographs that include the kidney(s) and ureter(s) in their entirety are made after retrograde filling of the structures. A cystogram or (voiding) cystourethrogram requires *urethral* catheterization only. Radiographs are made of the contrast-filled bladder and frequently of the contrast-filled urethra during voiding. Cystoscopy is required for location and catheterization of the vesicoureteral orifices.

6. (B) Because the urinary structures have so little subject contrast, artificial contrast material must be employed for better visualization of these structures. Contrast agents used for urographic procedures can have unpleasant, and (rarely) even lethal, side effects. Intravenous injection of contrast frequently produces a warm, flushed feeling, a bitter or metallic taste, or mild nausea. These side effects are of short duration and usually pass as quickly as they come. More serious side effects include urticaria, respiratory discomfort/distress and, rarely, anaphylaxis. An antihistamine is appropriate treatment for simple side effects, but the radiographer must always be prepared to deal quickly and efficiently with patients experiencing more serious reactions. Nonionic contrast agents are far less likely to produce side effects.

7. (D) The most commonly performed radiologic examination of the reproductive system is hysterosalpingography, which is employed for evaluation of the uterus, oviducts, and ovaries of the female reproductive system. The procedure serves to delineate the position, size, and shape of the structures and demonstrate pathology such as polyps, tumors, and fistulas. However, it is most often used to demonstrate *patency* of the oviducts in cases of *infertility,* and is sometimes therapeutic in terms of opening a blocked oviduct.

8. (B) An anteroposterior (AP) postvoid bladder film is usually required to detect any *residual urine* in the evaluation of *tumor masses* or *enlarged prostate glands*. An erect radiograph is occasionally requested to demonstrate renal mobility and ureteral tortuosity.

9. (A) During intravenous urography, both oblique positions are generally obtained. The 30-degree oblique KUB (kidney, ureters, bladder) places the kidney of the side *away* from the film *parallel* to the film. The kidney closer to the film is placed perpendicular to the film. The oblique positions provide an oblique projection of the urinary bladder.

10. (A) A 15- to 20-degree anteroposterior (AP) Trendelenburg position during intravenous (IV) urography is often helpful in demonstrating filling of the distal ureters and the area of the vesicoureteral orifices. In this position, the contrast-filled urinary bladder moves superiorly, encouraging filling of the distal ureters and superior bladder, and provides better delineation of these areas. The central ray should be directed perpendicular to the cassette. Compression of the *distal* ureters is used to prolong filling of the renal pelvis and calyces. Compression of the *proximal* ureters is not advocated.

F. Central Nervous System

1. Introduction. The central nervous system (CNS) is composed of the *brain* and *spinal cord* (Fig. 7–113), enclosed within the bony skull and vertebral column. The brain consists of the cerebrum (largest part), *cerebellum, pons varolii,* and *medulla oblongata.* The *gray matter* of the brain consists of neuron cell bodies; the *white matter* consists of tracts (pathways) of axons. In transverse section, the spinal cord is seen to have an H-shaped configuration of gray matter internally, surrounded by white matter (Fig. 7–114). The brain and spinal cord work together in the perception of sensory stimuli, in integration and correlation of stimuli with memory, and in neural actions resulting in coordinated motor responses to stimuli.

The CNS is enclosed within three tissue membranes, the *meninges.* The *pia mater* is the innermost, vascular membrane, which is closely attached to the brain and spinal cord. The *arachnoid mater* is a thin layer outside the pia mater and attached to it by web-like fibers. The *subarachnoid space* is between the pia and arachnoid mater and is filled with cerebrospinal fluid (CSF). The brain and spinal cord float in CSF, which acts as a shock absorber.

Cerebral artery hemorrhage will leak blood into the CSF. *Lumbar puncture* is performed (between L3 and L4 or L4 and L5) to remove small quantities of CSF for testing and to introduce contrast medium during myelography. The *dura mater* is a double-layered fibrous membrane outside the arachnoid mater. The *subdural space* is located between the arachnoid and dura mater; it does not contain CSF. The *epidural space* is located between the two layers of dura mater.

The cylindrical spinal cord is a continuation of the medulla oblongata, extending through the foramen magnum and spinal canal to its termination at the *conus medullaris* (about the level of L1). The lumbar and sacral nerves have long roots that extend from the spinal cord as the *cauda equina* (horse's tail).

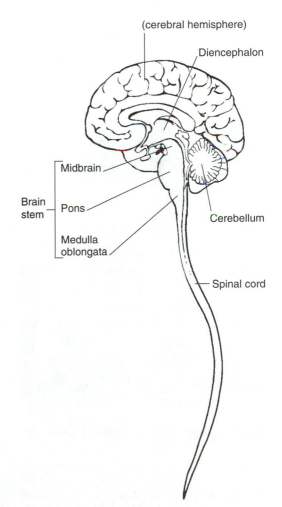

Figure 7–113. The CNS: brain and spinal cord.

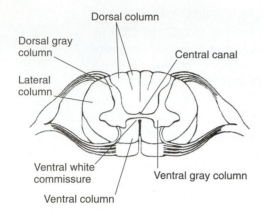

Figure 7–114. Cross-section of the spinal cord.

2. Procedures.
Routine radiographic examination of the bony components of the CNS includes studies of the skull and vertebral column and, occasionally, tomography of these structures. Computerized tomography (CT) and magnetic resonance imaging (MRI) procedures have replaced many plain radiographic procedures in the diagnosis and management of traumatic injuries and pathologic processes of the brain and spinal cord.

3. Myelogram.
Nevertheless, *myelography* remains a valuable diagnostic tool to demonstrate the site and extent of *spinal cord tumors* and *herniated intervertebral discs*. Rupture of an intervertebral disc can be caused by trauma or degeneration. The *nucleus pulposus* protrudes posteriorly through a tear in the *annulus fibrosus* and impinges on nerve roots (Fig. 7–115). More than 90% of disc ruptures occur at the L4–L5 and L5–S1 interspaces. Narrowing of the affected disc space may often be detected radiographically and the defects caused by the rupture can generally be demonstrated through myelography, CT, or MRI.

Water-soluble nonionic iodinated contrast agents are the most widely used contrast media for myelography. Advantages of water-soluble contrast agents (over non–water-soluble) include better visualization of the nerve roots (see Fig. 7–116) and absorption properties that allow it to be left in the subarachnoid space after the examination (because it is easily absorbed by the body). However, the use of water-soluble contrast agents for myelography does require that radiographs be made accurately and without delay, because it is absorbed fairly quickly.

Foot and shoulder supports must be securely attached to the x-ray table. The patient should receive a complete explanation of the examination and must be instructed about the importance of keeping his or her chin extended when the table is lowered into the Trendelenburg position.

A lumbar puncture is performed (usually at the fourth intervertebral space with the patient in the prone or flexed lateral position), a small quantity of CSF is removed from the subarachnoid space and sent to the laboratory for testing, and an equal amount of contrast agent is injected intrathecally (i.e., into the subarachnoid space of the spinal canal). The position of the contrast column will change according to gravitational forces, and its movement is observed fluoroscopically as the x-ray table is angled to varying degrees of Trendelenburg and Fowler's positions. Fluoroscopic spot films are taken as needed, followed by overhead radiographs. Routine protocol generally includes an AP or PA and a horizontal beam (cross-table) lateral view of the vertebral area examined.

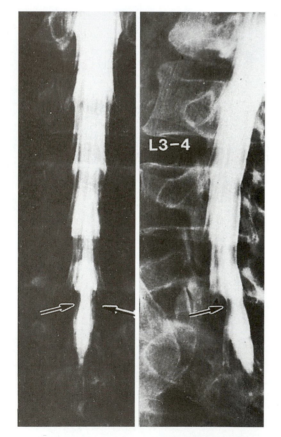

Figure 7–115. Myelograms demonstrating herniated L4–L5 disc. (Reproduced with permission from deGroot, J. *Correlative Neuroanatomy,* 21st ed. East Norwalk, CT: Appleton & Lange, 1991.)

4. Terminology and Pathology.
The following is a list of radiographically significant CNS conditions with which the student radiographer should be familiar.

Degenerative disc disease	Parkinson's disease
Herniated nucleus pulposus	Meningitis
Hydrocephalus	Meningomyelocele
Meningioma	Spondylosis

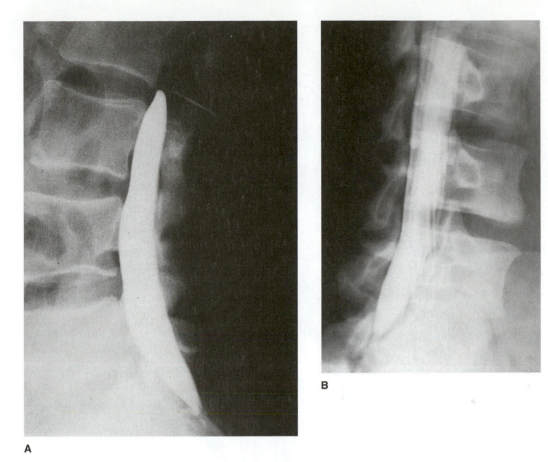

Figure 7–116. **(A)** Non-water-soluble contrast (Pantopaque) myelography. **(B)** Water-soluble contrast myelography; observe improved visualization of nerve roots seen at the level of each pedicle as linear radiolucencies within the small inferolateral extensions of the contrast agent. (**(A)** courtesy of the Stamford Hospital; **(B)** from the American College of Radiology Learning File. Courtesy of the ACR.)

G. CIRCULATORY SYSTEM

1. Introduction. The circulatory system consists of the *heart* and vessels (arteries, capillaries, veins) that distribute blood throughout the body (see Fig. 7–117). The heart is the muscular pump, the *arteries* conduct oxygenated blood throughout the body; the *capillaries* are responsible for diffusion of gases and exchange of nutrients and wastes; and the *veins* collect deoxygenated blood and return it to the heart and lungs.

Contraction of the heart muscle as it pumps blood is called *systole;* relaxation is called *diastole;* these values are measured with a *sphygmomanometer.* Accompanying the contraction and expansion of the heart is contraction and expansion of arterial walls—called *pulse.*

The heart wall is made up of the external *epicardium,* the middle *myocardium,* and the internal *endocardium.* The *pericardium* is the fibroserous sac enclosing the heart and roots of the great vessels. The heart has four chambers. The two upper chambers are the *atria,* and the two lower chambers are the *ventricles.* The apex of the heart is the tip of the left ventricle.

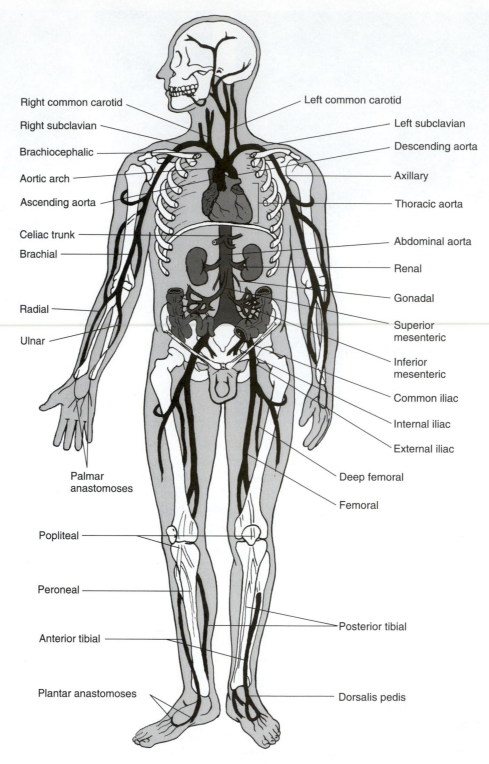

Figure 7–117. The major arteries of the cardiovascular system.

Venous blood is returned to the right atrium of the heart via the *superior* (from the upper part of the body) and *inferior* (from the lower body) *vena cavae* and the *coronary sinus* (from the heart substance; see Fig. 7–118). Upon atrial systole, the blood passes through the *tricuspid valve* into the right ventricle. During ventricular systole, the blood is pumped through the *pulmonary semilunar valve* into the *pulmonary artery* (the only artery to carry deoxygenated blood) to the lungs for oxygenation.

Blood is returned via the *pulmonary veins* (the only veins to carry oxygenated blood) to the left atrium. During atrial systole, blood passes through the *mitral* (bicuspid) *valve* into the left ventricle. During ventricular systole, the oxygenated blood is pumped through the *aortic semilunar valve* into the aorta. When blood pressure is reported, as for example "130 over 85," the top number (130) represents the systolic pressure and the lower number (85) represents the diastolic pressure.

The *aorta* is the trunk artery of the body; it is divided into the ascending aorta, aortic arch (see Fig. 7–119), descending thoracic aorta, and abdominal aorta. Many arteries arise from the aorta to supply destinations throughout the body. The *superior* and *inferior vena cavae* and the *coronary sinus* are the major veins, collecting venous blood from the upper and lower body areas and heart substance re-

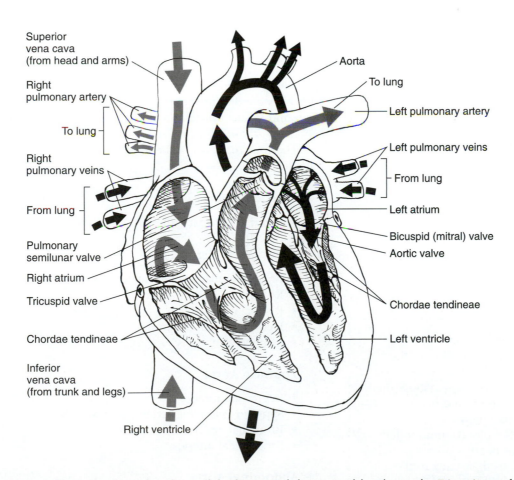

Figure 7–118. The four chambers of the heart and the major blood vessels. Directions of blood flow are indicated.

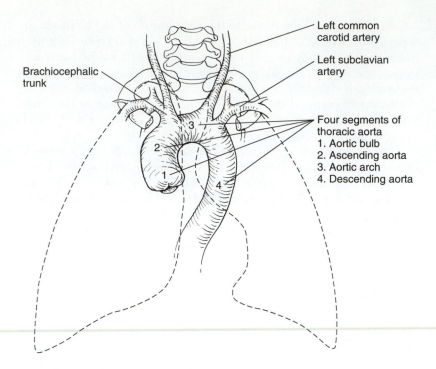

Figure 7–119. Thoracic aorta illustrating major branches of aortic arch.

spectively. The formation of sclerotic plaques (as in *atherosclerosis*) and other conditions that impair the flow of blood can lead to *ischemia* and tissue *infarction*. Atherosclerosis of the coronary arteries can cause *angina pectoris* and *myocardial infarction*.

The *four divisions* of the aorta and *their major branches* are the following.

Ascending aorta

- L and R coronary arteries

Aortic Arch (Fig. 7–119)

- Brachiocephalic (innominate) artery gives rise to:
- R common carotid artery
- R subclavian artery
- L common carotid artery
- L subclavian artery

Thoracic Aorta

- Intercostal arteries
- Superior phrenic arteries
- Bronchial arteries
- Esophageal arteries

Abdominal Aorta

- Inferior phrenic arteries

Pulmonary Circulation
- Unoxygenated blood from the right side of the heart is directed to the lungs for oxygenation, then to the left side of the heart.

Systemic Circulation
- Oxygenated blood from the left side of the heart is pumped to the body tissues then back to the right side of the heart.

- Celiac (axis) artery gives rise to:
  - Common hepatic artery
  - L gastric artery
  - Splenic artery
- Superior mesenteric artery
- Suprarenal arteries
- Renal arteries
- Gonadal arteries (testicular or ovarian)
- Inferior mesenteric artery
- Common iliac arteries give rise to lower extremity arteries:
  - Internal iliac arteries
  - External iliac (hypogastric) arteries

Arteries of the Lower Extremity

- Internal iliac arteries
- External iliac arteries give rise to:
- femoral arteries give rise to:
- popliteal arteries give rise to:
- anterior tibial arteries and posterior tibial arteries give rise to
- dorsalis pedis, peroneal/fibular, medial and lateral plantar arteries

The majority of peripheral and visceral angiographic procedures are performed in a specially equipped angiographic suite by cardiovascular-interventional technologists (Figs. 7–120 and 7–121). Many cardiovascular suites today have equipment available for digital subtraction angiography (DSA). *Subtraction* is a technique that removes unnecessary structures such as bone from superimposition on contrast-filled blood vessels. DSA is subtraction achieved by means of a computer, which can also permit manipulation of contrast and other

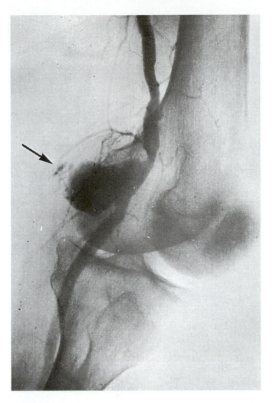

Figure 7–120. Lower-extremity arteriogram demonstrating popliteal aneurysm. (Reproduced with permission from Way, LW, ed. *Current Surgical Diagnosis & Treatment,* 10th ed. East Norwalk, CT: Appleton & Lange, 1994.)

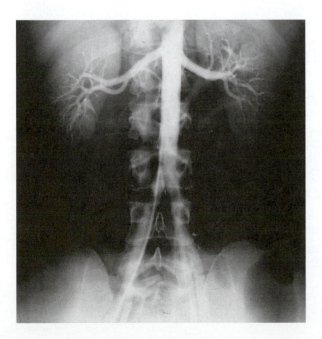

Figure 7–121. The renal arteriogram is one of many types of procedures performed by specially trained teams of health care professionals. (From the American College of Radiology Learning File. Courtesy of the ACR.)

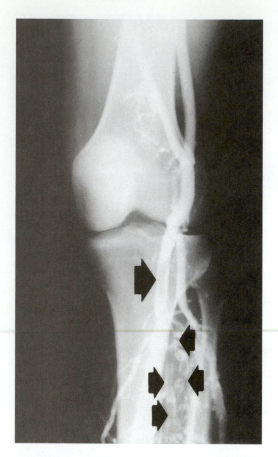

Figure 7–122. AP projection of a lower extremity venogram demonstrating multiple intraluminal filling defects. (Way, LW, ed. *Current Surgical Diagnosis & Treatment,* 10th ed. East Norwalk, CT: Appleton & Lange, 1994.)

image characteristics by the technologist. The student radiographer, while not performing most of these examinations, should be familiar with the names of the most common procedures and the conditions and disorders for which they are performed.

2. Venogram. The one vascular procedure that might still be performed in general radiography is the lower extremity *venogram* (Fig. 7–122). This examination is generally performed to confirm a suspected deep vein thrombosis in an effort to avoid the complications of a pulmonary embolism.

The patient should be examined on a radiographic table that can be tilted to a semierect position of at least 45 degrees. Tourniquest are used to force contrast medium into the deep veins. Sterile technique must be rigorously maintained. An injection of 50 to 100 mL at 1 to 2 mL/sec is usually made through a superficial vein in the foot. Radiographs are made at about 5- to 10-second intervals of the lower leg, thigh, and pelvis.

3. Terminology and Pathology. The following is a list of radiographically significant circulatory conditions with which the student radiographer should be familiar.

Aneurysm	Hypertension
Angina pectoris	Myocardial infarction
Atherosclerosis	Phlebitis
Atrial septal defect	Pulmonary edema
CVA (Cerebrovascular accident)	Pulmonary embolism
Coarctation of aorta	Rheumatic heart disease
Congestive heart failure	Thrombophlebitis
Coronary artery disease	Ventricular septal defect

 Chapter Review Questions

☆ *Congratulations! You have completed your review of a large portion of this chapter. You may go on to the "Registry-type" multiple-choice questions that follow. For greatest success, be sure also to complete the short answer questions found at the end of this chapter.*

1. Which of the following statement(s) regarding myelography is (are) correct?
    1. spinal puncture can be performed in the prone or flexed lateral position
    2. contrast medium distribution is regulated through table angulation
    3. the patient's head must be in acute flexion during Trendelenburg positions
    (A) 1 only
    (B) 1 and 2 only
    (C) 1 and 3 only
    (D) 1, 2, and 3

2. The contraction and expansion of arterial walls in accordance with forceful contraction and relaxation of the heart is called:
   (A) hypertension
   (B) elasticity
   (C) pulse
   (D) pressure

3. The method by which contrast-filled vascular images are removed from superimposition upon bone is called:
   (A) positive masking
   (B) reversal
   (C) subtraction
   (D) registration

4. Indicate the correct sequence of oxygenated blood as it returns from the lungs to the heart:
   (A) pulmonary veins, left atrium, left ventricle, aortic valve
   (B) pulmonary artery, left atrium, left ventricle, aortic valve
   (C) pulmonary veins, right atrium, right ventricle, pulmonary semilunar valve
   (D) pulmonary artery, right atrium, right ventricle, pulmonary semilunar valve

5. In myelography, the contrast medium is generally injected into the:
   (A) cisterna magna
   (B) individual intervertebral discs
   (C) subarachnoid space between the first and second lumbar vertebrae
   (D) subarachnoid space between the third and fourth lumbar vertebrae

6. Lower extremity venography requires an injection of iodinated contrast medium into the:
   (A) superficial veins of the foot
   (B) deep veins of the foot
   (C) femoral vein
   (D) popliteal vein

7. Myelography is a diagnostic examination used to demonstrate:
   1. posterior protrusion of herniated intervertebral disc
   2. anterior protrusion of herniated intervertebral disc
   3. internal disc lesions
   (A) 1 only
   (B) 2 only
   (C) 1 and 2 only
   (D) 1 and 3 only

8. The four major arteries supplying the brain include the:
   1. brachiocephalic artery
   2. common carotid arteries
   3. vertebral arteries
   (A) 1 and 2 only
   (B) 1 and 3 only
   (C) 2 and 3 only
   (D) 1, 2, and 3

9. Which of the following statement(s) is (are) true regarding lower extremity venography?
    1. the patient is often examined in the semi-erect position
    2. tourniquets are used to force contrast medium into the deep veins
    3. all radiographs are AP projections
(A) 1 only
(B) 1 and 2 only
(C) 1 and 3 only
(D) 1, 2, and 3

10. The apex of the heart is formed by the:
(A) left atrium
(B) right atrium
(C) left ventricle
(D) right ventricle

Answers and Explanations

1. (B) Myelography is the radiologic examination of structures within the spinal canal. Opaque contrast medium is usually used. Following injection, the contrast medium is distributed to the vertebral region of interest by gravity; the x-ray table is angled Trendelenburg or visualization of the cervical region and in the Fowler's position for visualization of the thoracic and lumbar regions. While the table is Trendelenburg, care must be taken that the patient's head be kept in acute *extension* in order to compress the cisterna magna and keep contrast medium from traveling into the ventricles of the brain.

2. (C) As the heart contracts and relaxes while functioning to pump blood from the heart, those arteries that are large and those in closest proximity to the heart will feel the effect of the heart's forceful contractions in their walls. The arterial walls pulsate in unison with the heart's contractions. This movement may be detected with the fingers in various parts of the body, and is referred to as the *pulse*.

3. (C) Superimposition of bony details frequently make angiographic demonstration of blood vessels less than optimal. The method used to remove these superimposed bony details is called *subtraction*. *Digital* subtraction can accomplish this through the use of a computer, but *photographic* subtraction may also be performed using films from an angiographic series. *Registration* is the process of matching one series image exactly over another. A reversal film, or *positive mask*, is a reverse of the black and white radiographic tones, obtained using special single emulsion film.

4. (A) Deoxygenated blood is returned by way of the inferior and superior vena cava to the right side of the heart. The blood is emptied into the right atrium, passes through the tricuspid valve, and enters the right ventricle. It is forced through the pulmonary semilunar valve into the pulmonary artery (by contraction of the right ventricle) and passes to the lungs for reoxygenation. From the lungs it is collected by the *pulmonary veins*, which carry the oxygenated blood to the *left atrium*, where it travels through the mitral valve into the *left ventricle*. Upon contraction of the left ventricle, blood passes through the *aortic valve* into the aorta and to all parts of the body.

5. (D) Generally, contrast medium is injected into the subarachnoid space between the 3rd and 4th lumbar vertebrae. Because the spinal cord ends at the level of the 1st or 2nd lumbar vertebrae, this is considered to be a relatively safe injection site. The cisterna magna can be used, but the risk of contrast entering and causing side effects increases.

6. (A) Lower extremity venography requires an injection of contrast medium into the superficial veins of the foot. The skin on top of the patient's foot is very sensitive and every precaution should be taken to minimize the pain involved. Explain the procedure fully and soak the foot in warm water to make the veins more accessible for injection.

7. (A) Rupture of an intervertebral disc can be caused by trauma or degeneration. The nucleus pulposus protrudes *posteriorly* through a tear in the annulus fibrosus and impinges on nerve roots and can be demonstrated by placing positive or negative contrast media into the subarachnoid space. Internal disc lesions can only be demonstrated by injecting contrast into the individual discs (this procedure is termed *discography*). Anterior protrusion of a herniated intervertebral disc does not impinge on the spinal cord, and is not demonstrated in myelography.

8. (C) Major branches of the common carotid arteries (internal carotids) function to supply the anterior brain, while the posterior brain is supplied by the vertebral arteries (branches of the subclavian arteries). The brachiocephalic (innominate) artery is unpaired and is one of three branches of the aortic arch, from which the right common carotid artery is derived. The left common carotid artery comes directly off the aortic arch.

9. (B) To increase the concentration of contrast medium in the deep veins of the leg, a Fowler's position is used with the table angle approximately 45 degrees. Tourniquets can also be used to force the contrast into the deep veins of the leg. Filming may be performed with or without fluoroscopy and may include anteroposterior (AP), lateral, and 30-degree obliques of the lower leg in internal rotation.

10. (C) The heart wall is made up of the external epicardium, the middle myocardium, and the internal endocardium. The pericardium is the fibroserous sac enclosing the heart and roots of the great vessels. The heart has four chambers. The two upper chambers are the atria, and the two lower chambers are the ventricles. The *apex* of the heart is the tip of the left ventricle.

Chapter Exercises

 Congratulations! *You have completed the entire chapter. If you are able to answer the following group of very comprehensive questions, you should feel confident that you have really mastered this section. You can refer back to the indicated pages to check your answers and/or review the subject matter.*

1. Identify the bony structures composing the appendicular skeleton *(pp. 87–94, 100–108)*.

2. Describe the (a) method of positioning, (b) direction and point of entry of the CR, (c) principle structures visualized, and (d) pertinent traumatic or pathologic conditions and any technical adjustments they may necessitate relative to the appendicular skeleton, to include routine and special views of the:

   A. hand and wrist *(pp. 94–97)*

   B. forearm and elbow *(pp. 97, 98)*

   C. humerus and shoulder *(pp. 98, 99)*

   D. clavicle and scapula *(pp. 99, 100)*

   E. foot and ankle *(pp. 109–111)*

   F. lower leg and knee *(pp. 111–113)*

   G. femur and hip *(pp. 113–115)*

   H. pelvis and sacroiliac joints *(pp. 115, 116)*

   I. long bone measurement *(p. 116)*

   J. arthrography *(pp. 116, 117)*

3. Identify the bony structures comprising the axial skeleton *(pp. 123–126, 134–135, 136–143)*.

4. Describe the (a) method of positioning, (b) direction and point of entry of the CR, (c) principle structures visualized, and (d) pertinent traumatic and pathologic conditions and any technical adjustments they may necessitate relative to the axial skeleton, to include routine and special views of the:

   A. cervical spine *(pp. 126–128)*

   B. thoracic spine *(p. 128)*

C. lumbar spine *(pp. 130–132)*

D. sacrum, coccyx *(pp. 132, 133)*

E. scoliosis series *(p. 134)*

F. sternum and ribs *(pp. 135–136)*

G. cranial and facial bones *(pp. 143–148)*

H. mastoids and petrous portions *(pp. 151–153)*

I. paranasal sinuses *(pp. 149–151)*

5. Identify the principle structures comprising the respiratory system and their function(s) *(pp. 157–159)*.

6. Describe the (a) method of positioning, (b) direction and point of entry of the CR, (c) principle structures visualized, and (d) pertinent traumatic and pathologic conditions and any technical adjustments that may be required relative to the routine and special views of the chest (PA, lat, obl, lordotic, decubitus) and airway *(pp. 160, 161)*.

7. Identify the principle structures comprising the biliary system and their function(s) *(p. 166)*.

8. Describe the (a) method of positioning, (b) direction and point of entry of the CR, (c) principle structures visualized, and (d) pertinent traumatic and pathologic conditions and any technical adjustments that may be required relative to the routine and special views of the biliary system, including:

A. OCG *(pp. 167, 169)*

B. OR and T-tube cholangiograms *(p. 169)*

C. ERCP *(p. 169)*

9. Identify the principle structures comprising the digestive system and their function(s) *(pp. 169–173)*.

10. Describe the (a) method of positioning, (b) direction and point of entry of the CR, (c) principle structures visualized, and (d) pertinent traumatic and pathologic conditions and any technical adjustments that may be required relative to the routine and special views of the digestive system, to include:

A. abdomen *(pp. 174, 175, 176)*

B. esophagus *(p. 176)*

C. stomach and small intestine *(pp. 177, 178)*

D. large intestine *(pp. 178–180)*

11. Identify the principle structures comprising the urinary system and their function(s) *(pp. 185–188)*.

12. Describe the (a) method of positioning, (b) direction and point of entry of the CR, (c) principle structures visualized, and (d) pertinent traumatic and pathologic conditions and any technical adjustments that may be required relative to the routine and special views of the urinary system, to include:

    A. KUB *(p. 189)*

    B. retrograde examinations *(pp. 188, 189)*

    C. compression *(p. 187)*

    D. bladder *(p. 190)*

13. Identify the principle structures comprising the female reproductive system and their function(s) *(p. 192)*.

14. Describe the (a) method of positioning, (b) direction and point of entry of the CR, (c) principle structures visualized, and (d) pertinent traumatic and pathologic conditions and any technical adjustments that may be required in hysterosalpingography *(pp. 192, 193)*.

15. Identify the principle structures comprising the CNS and their function(s) *(p. 197)*.

16. Describe the (a) method of positioning, (b) direction and point of entry of the CR, (c) principle structures visualized, and (d) pertinent traumatic and pathologic conditions and any technical adjustments that may be required in myelography *(p. 198)*.

17. Identify the principle structures comprising the circulatory system and their function(s) *(pp. 199–203)*.

18. List the kinds of specialized examinations that might be performed to demonstrate various traumatic and pathologic conditions of the circulatory system *(pp. 203, 204)*.

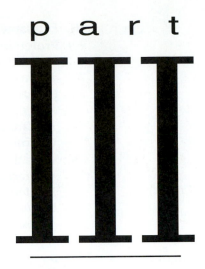

part III

Radiation Protection

Radiation Protection Considerations

I. IONIZING EFFECTS OF X-RAYS

A. ELECTROMAGNETIC RADIATION

A review of electromagnetic radiation and energy is essential to the study of x-rays and other forms of ionizing radiation. *Electromagnetic radiation* can be described as wavelike fluctuations of electric and magnetic fields. There are many kinds of electromagnetic radiation; Figure 8–1 illustrates that visible light, microwaves, and radio

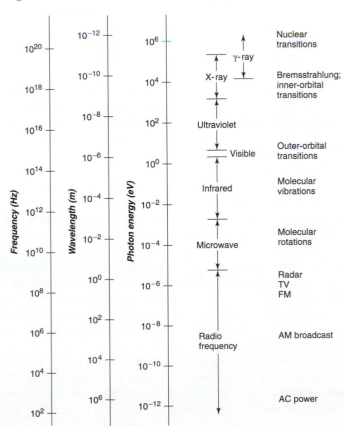

Figure 8–1. The electromagnetic spectrum. Note that frequency and photon energy are directly related and that they are inversely related to wavelength.

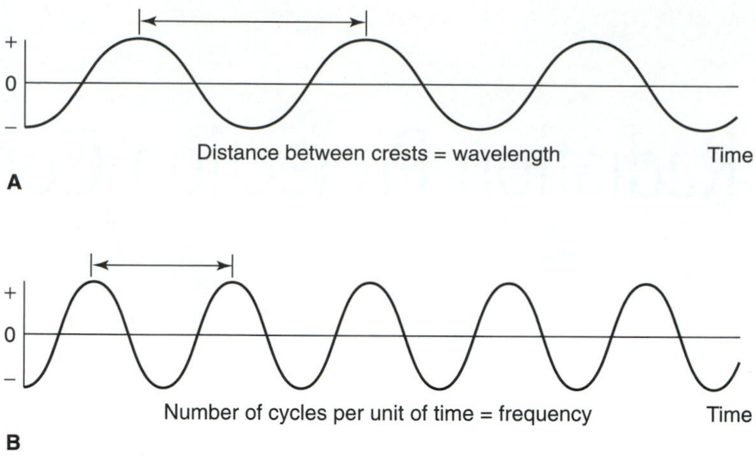

0
+
−
Distance between crests = wavelength   Time

A

0
+
−
Number of cycles per unit of time = frequency   Time

B

Figure 8–2. Wavelength versus frequency. *Wavelength* is described as the distance between successive crests. The shorter the wavelength, the more crests or cycles per unit of time (eg, per second). Therefore, the shorter the wavelength the greater the *frequency* (number of cycles/second). Wavelength and frequency are inversely related.

waves are within the *electromagnetic spectrum*. All the electromagnetic radiations have the same *velocity*, 186,000 miles per second; however, they differ greatly in *wavelength*.

Wavelength refers to the distance between two consecutive wave crests (Fig. 8–2). *Frequency* refers to the number of cycles per second (cps); its unit of measure is the *hertz* (Hz), which is equal to 1 cps.

Frequency and wavelength are closely associated with the relative *energy* of electromagnetic radiations. More energetic radiations have shorter wavelengths and higher frequency. The relationship among frequency, wavelength, and energy is illustrated in the electromagnetic spectrum (see Fig. 8–1).

Some radiations are energetic enough to rearrange atoms in materials through which they pass, and they can therefore be hazardous to living tissue. These radiations are called *ionizing* radiation because they have the energetic potential to break apart electrically neutral atoms, resulting in the production of negative and positive *ions*.

Humans have always been exposed to ionizing radiation. Some ionizing radiations (such as those emitted by uranium) occur naturally in the earth's crust and in its atmosphere (from the sun and cosmic reactions in space). These radiations are present in the structures in which we live and in the food we consume; radioactive gas is present in the air that we breathe, and there are traces of radioactive materials in our bodies themselves. These radiations are referred to as *natural background* (environmental) *radiation*. The levels of natural background radiation vary greatly from one location to another. *The greatest portion of our exposure to background radiation comes from naturally occurring sources such as these.*

In addition to background radiation, we are also exposed to sources of radiation created by humans. *Artificial* or *man-made radiation* includes sources such as medical and dental x-rays, nuclear testing fallout, and radiation associated with nuclear power plants. Figure 8–3 illustrates the approximate quantity of radiation received from natural and artificial sources.

X-ray *photons* are infinitesimal bundles of energy that deposit some of their energy within matter as they travel through it. This deposition of energy and subsequent *ionization* has the potential to cause chemical and biologic damage.

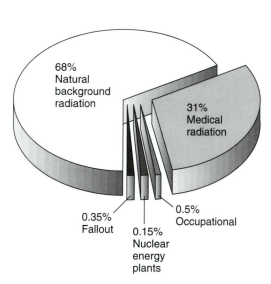

68%
Natural background radiation

31%
Medical radiation

0.35%
Fallout

0.15%
Nuclear energy plants

0.5%
Occupational

Figure 8–3. The population's exposure to various sources of radiation. Natural background radiation (the earth, the sun, building materials) compose the majority of our exposure. Medical irradiation is the largest portion of our exposure to artifical sources of radiation. Occupational radiation, nuclear energy, and a fallout are responsible for only a minute portion of our total exposure.

B. PRODUCTION OF X-RAYS AT THE TUNGSTEN TARGET

Diagnostic x-rays are produced within the x-ray tube as high-speed *electrons* are rapidly decelerated by the tungsten target. The source of electrons is the heated cathode filament; they are driven across to the anode focal spot when high voltage (kVp [kilovoltage peak]) is applied. When the high-speed electrons are suddenly stopped at the focal spot, their kinetic energy is converted to x-ray photon energy. This happens in two ways.

1. Bremsstrahlung (Brems) or "braking" **radiation.** A high-speed electron, accelerated toward a tungsten atom is attracted (and braked, ie: slowed down) by the positively charged nucleus, and therefore is deflected from its course with a resulting loss of energy. This energy loss is given up in the form of an x-ray photon (Fig. 8–4). The electron may not give up all its kinetic energy in one such interaction; it may go on to have several more interactions deeper in the target, each time giving up an x-ray photon having less and less energy. This is one reason the x-ray beam is heterogeneous (ie, has a spectrum of energies). *Brems radiation comprises 70 to 90% of the x-ray beam.*

2. Characteristic radiation. In this case, a high-speed electron encounters the tungsten atom and ejects a K-shell electron (Fig. 8–5A), leaving a vacancy in the K shell (Fig. 8–5B). An electron from the shell above (that is, the L shell) fills the vacancy and in doing so emits a K *characteristic ray* (Fig. 8–5C). The energy of the characteristic ray is equal to the difference in energy between the K and L shell. Characteristic radiation comprises very little of the x-ray beam (10 to 30%).

C. BASIC INTERACTIONS BETWEEN X-RAY PHOTONS AND MATTER

The gradual decrease in exposure rate as radiation passes through tissues is called *attenuation*. Attenuation is principally attributable to the two major types of interactions that occur between x-ray photons and tissue in the diagnostic range.

1. In the *photoelectric effect,* a relatively *low* energy (low kVp) x-ray photon uses all its energy (true/total absorption) to eject an *inner shell* electron, leaving an orbital vacancy. An electron from the shell above drops down to fill the vacancy and, in doing so, gives up energy in the form of a *characteristic ray* (Fig. 8–6).

The photoelectric effect is more likely to occur in absorbers of *high atomic number* (eg, bone, positive contrast media) and contributes significantly to patient dose, as all the photon energy is absorbed by the patient (and for the latter reason, is responsible for the production of short-scale contrast).

2. In *Compton scatter,* a fairly *high* energy (high kVp) x-ray photon ejects an *outer shell* electron (Fig. 8–7). Though the x-ray photon is deflected with somewhat reduced energy (modified scatter), it retains most of its original energy and exits the body as an energetic scattered photon.

Because the scattered photon exits the body, it does not pose a radiation hazard to the patient. It can, however, contribute to *image*

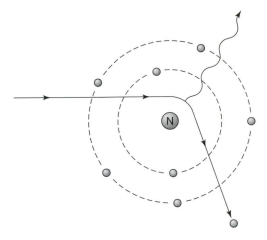

Figure 8–4. Production of Bremsstrahlung (Brems) radiation. A high-speed electron is deflected from its path and the loss of kinetic energy is emitted in the form of an x-ray photon.

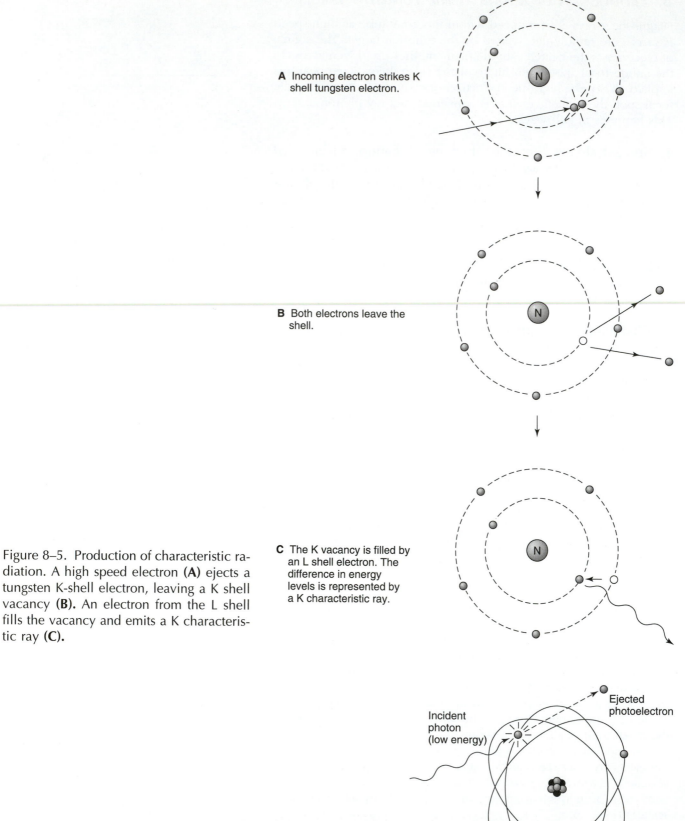

A Incoming electron strikes K shell tungsten electron.

B Both electrons leave the shell.

C The K vacancy is filled by an L shell electron. The difference in energy levels is represented by a K characteristic ray.

Figure 8–5. Production of characteristic radiation. A high speed electron (**A**) ejects a tungsten K-shell electron, leaving a K shell vacancy (**B**). An electron from the L shell fills the vacancy and emits a K characteristic ray (**C**).

Incident photon (low energy)

Ejected photoelectron

Figure 8–6. In the photoelectric effect, the incoming (low energy) photon releases all its energy as it ejects an inner shell electron from orbit.

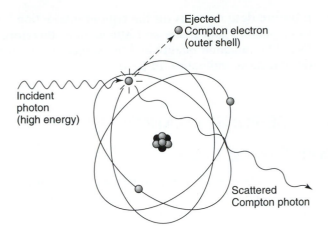

Figure 8–7. In Compton scatter the incoming (high energy) photon uses part of its energy to eject an outer shell electron; in doing so, the photon changes direction (scatters) but retains much of its original energy.

fog and pose a *radiation hazard to personnel* (as in fluoroscopic procedures).

Summary

- The radiations of the electromagnetic spectrum all travel at the same velocity, 186,000 mps, but differ in wavelength.
- Wavelength is the distance between two consecutive wave crests.
- The number of cycles and crests per second is frequency; its unit of measure is the Hz.
- Wavelength and frequency are inversely related.
- Natural background and artificial (man-made) are the two kinds of radiation sources; natural sources account for the largest human exposure to radiation.
- Medical radiation exposure is the largest source of artificial radiation exposure for humans.
- Ionization is caused by high-energy, short-wavelength electromagnetic radiations that break apart electrically neutral atoms.
- Two types of radiation are produced at the anode through energy conversion processes: Brems and characteristic radiation; Brems radiation predominates.
- Characteristics of photoelectric effect:
  - Low energy x-ray photon gives up all its energy ejecting an inner shell electron.
  - Produces a characteristic ray.
  - Major contributor to patient dose.
  - Occurs in absorbers of high atomic number.
  - Produces short-scale contrast.
- Characteristics of Compton scatter:
  - High energy x-ray photon uses a portion of its energy to eject an outer shell electron.
  - Responsible for scattered radiation image fog.
  - Radiation hazard to personnel.

■ **Exposure dose depends on the type of interaction between x-ray photons and tissue and attenuation, therefore, is affected by radiation quality and the subject being irradiated (ie, thickness and nature of part).**

II. DOSE–RESPONSE RELATIONSHIP

A. DOSE–RESPONSE CURVES

The association between a dose of ionizing radiation and the magnitude of the resulting response or effect is referred to as a *dose-response, or dose–effect, relationship.*

Dose–response curves are used to illustrate the relationship between exposure to ionizing radiation and possible resultant biologic effects (Fig. 8–8). The two most frequently used dose–response curves in radiation protection are the *linear, nonthreshold* and the *linear, threshold.* The Committee on Biologic Effects of Ionizing Radiation (BEIR) has evaluated the linear and linear quadratic nonthreshold curves and has pronounced the linear nonthreshold curve (the more conservative of the two) as *the curve of choice for radiation protection standards.*

B. LINEAR, NONTHRESHOLD

The linear nonthreshold curve is used to illustrate responses such as leukemia, cancer, and genetic effects. These are sometimes referred to as *stochastic effects.* Stochastic effects occur randomly and are "all-or-nothing" type effects, that is, they do not occur with degrees of severity. It must be noted that *in a nonthreshold curve there is no safe dose,* that is, no dose below which there will definitely be no biologic response. Theoretically, even one x-ray photon can cause a biologic response. This is the curve of choice to predict effects of low level (eg, medical and occupational) exposure to ionizing radiation.

C. LINEAR, THRESHOLD

A linear, threshold curve illustrates that a certain dose of ionizing radiation must be received before an effect will be manifested, that is, there is a *threshold* dose—a dose *below which no biologic effects are likely to occur.* This is the case in somatic conditions such as skin erythema. These effects are predictable and sometimes referred to as *nonstochastic effects.*

D. LATE (LONG-TERM) EFFECTS

Occupationally exposed individuals are concerned principally with *late* (ie, *long-term,* or *delayed*) effects of radiation such as *genetic effects, leukemia,* and *cancers,* which can occur many years following initial exposure to low levels of ionizing radiation. These long-term/delayed effects are represented by the linear, nonthreshold dose-response curve. History provides us with many examples of the

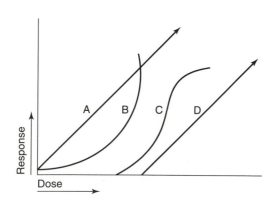

Figure 8–8. Dose-response curves. **(A)** Linear, nonthreshold curve. **(B)** Nonlinear, nonthreshold curve. **(C)** Nonlinear, threshold curve. **(D)** Linear, threshold curve.

delayed effects of ionizing radiation: many of the early radiologists and radiation scientists, A-bomb survivors of Hiroshima and Nagasaki, and ankylosing spondylitis patients in Great Britain in the 1940s developed leukemia and other life-span-shortening diseases as a result of exposure to varying quantities of radiation over a period of time. Some children irradiated in the 1940s for enlarged thymus glands developed thyroid cancer as adults 20 years later. Radium watch-dial painters in the 1920s developed a variety of bone cancers following a latent period of 20 to 30 years. These are all delayed effects of radiation and are represented by the linear, nonthreshold dose–response curve.

Cataractogenesis is another late effect of exposure to ionizing radiation, but is represented by the linear, threshold dose-response curve. An acute dose of about 200 *rad* is required to cause radiogenic cataracts. A far greater occupational or otherwise fractionated dose of approximately 1000 rad is required to induce cataracts.

Summary

- **Ionization of living tissue can cause chemical and biologic damage to somatic and/or genetic cells.**
- **A nonthreshold dose–response curve indicates that there is no safe dose of radiation below which there will be no effects.**
- **The linear nonthreshold dose–response curve illustrates stochastic responses (cancer, genetic effects) and is the curve of choice for occupational exposure.**
- **Occupationally exposed workers are concerned with late effects of radiation such as carcinogenesis, cataractogenesis, and life span shortening.**

III. BIOLOGIC EFFECTS OF RADIATION

Before beginning our review of somatic and genetic effects of radiation, a brief review of *radiobiology* is in order. Radiobiology is the study of the effects of ionizing radiation on biologic material at the cellular level.

A. *LAW OF BERGONIÉ AND TRIBONDEAU*

In 1906, two scientists, Bergonié and Tribondeau, proposed that certain cellular qualities made tissues more or less radiosensitive. The Law of Bergonié and Tribondeau states that the following cells are particularly radiosensitive:

1. Young, immature cells
2. Stem (undifferentiated, or precursor) cells
3. Highly mitotic cells

Thus, very young cells, stem cells, and cells having the most reproductive activity are highly *radiosensitive*. An example of highly radiosensitive tissue is that of the rapidly developing embryo and fetus.

B. QUALITY FACTOR

Ionization causes the removal of electrons from some atoms and the addition of electrons to other atoms. Thus the stage is set for biologic effects; as a result of the ionization, appropriate chemical bonds cannot be maintained.

Similar absorbed doses of *different kinds* of radiation can cause different biologic effects. A *quality factor (QF)* is a number assigned to different types of ionizing radiations so that their effect(s) may be better determined. The QF accounts for differences in biologic effect between different kinds of radiation. For example, to equate the *rad* with the *rem,* the following formula is used.

$$\text{rad} \times \text{QF} = \text{rem}$$

C. LINEAR ENERGY TRANSFER VERSUS BIOLOGIC DAMAGE

Radiation deposits energy as it passes through tissue. The rate at which this occurs is described as *linear energy transfer (LET).* LET is another means of expressing radiation quality and determining QF; it expresses the ability of radiation to do damage. *Diagnostic x-rays are considered low LET radiation.* The more penetrating the radiation, the lower the LET and QF. As the LET of radiation increases, the radiation's ability to produce biological damage also increases. This is described quantitatively by *relative biologic effectiveness (RBE).* LET and RBE are directly related.

Energy transferred to tissue can cause molecular damage. Any manifestation of that damage will depend on the extent of molecular disruption and the type of tissue affected.

D. MOLECULAR EFFECTS OF RADIATION

The interactions that serve to form the radiologic image, the *photoelectric effect* and *Compton scatter,* are ionization processes producing photoelectrons and recoil electrons that traverse tissue and subsequently ionize molecules. This action can lead to molecular damage in the form of *impaired function* or *cell death.*

1. Direct Effect. The two major types of effects that occur are the *direct effect* and the *indirect effect.* The direct effect usually occurs with high LET radiations and when ionization occurs at the deoxyribonucleic acid (DNA) molecule.

2. Indirect Effect. The indirect effect, which occurs most frequently, happens when ionization takes place away from the DNA molecule. However, the energy from the interaction is transferred to the molecule via a *free radical* (formed by radiolysis of cellular water).

Possible damage to the DNA molecule is diverse. A single-strand break on the DNA molecule is *repairable.* A double-strand break, widely spaced, may repair with difficulty or may result in *cell death.* A double-strand break on the same "rung" of the DNA ladder results in *irreparable* damage or *cell death.* Damage to the nitrogenous bases results in alteration of base sequence, causing a cell *mutation.* Any subsequent divisions result in daughter cells with incorrect genetic information.

E. CELLULAR RADIOSENSITIVITY

These types of molecular damage can occur to any of the *somatic* cells or to genetic cells. For example, high levels of radiation exposure to the bone marrow (where blood cells are produced) can cause a decrease in the number of circulating blood cells. *Lymphocytes,* a type of white blood cell that play an important role in the immune system, are particularly radiosensitive. If lymphocytes suffer radiation damage, the body loses its ability to fight infection and becomes more susceptible to disease.

Epithelial tissue, which lines the respiratory system and intestines, is also a highly radiosensitive tissue. In contrast, muscle and nervous tissue are comparatively insensitive to radiation. Because nerve cells in the adult do not undergo mitosis, they comprise the most *radioresistant* somatic tissue. However, nervous tissue *in the fetus* (particularly the second to eighth week) is highly mitotic and hence, highly *radiosensitive.*

The *genetic cells* of the gonads are considered especially radiosensitive tissues. Exposure to ionizing radiation can cause temporary or permanent sterility or mutations in succeeding generations. In particular, the reproductive cells of the fetus and young children are exceptionally radiosensitive. Other factors that determine tissue response to irradiation include the following.

1. *Fractionation or protraction:* The longer the period of time over which a dose of radiation is delivered, the less its effect. (The greatest effect of irradiation will be observed if a *large quantity* of radiation is delivered in a *short time* to the *whole body.*)
2. *Oxygen:* The greater the oxygen content of tissues, the greater their radiosensitivity.
3. *Age:* Fetal tissue is most radiosensitive. As the individual ages, tissue sensitivity decreases. Radiosensitivity increases again in old age, but only slightly.

It is well established that sufficient quantities of ionizing radiation can cause a number of serious *somatic* and/or *genetic* effects. What is not clear, however, are the long-term effects of low-level (diagnostic and occupational) x-radiation.

Health care professionals involved in prescribing and delivering radiologic examinations have an obligation to keep nonproductive radiation exposure to all individuals as low as possible. Possible abusive overuse of radiologic (and other diagnostic) examinations is currently being scrutinized by many health care facilities as part of a continuous quality improvement program. Some formerly routine examinations are now considered excessive and unnecessary, for example, routine chest x-ray on admission to the hospital, are no longer performed unless the patient is admitted to the pulmonary medicine or surgical service; preemployment chest and/or lumbar spine examinations are also considered to have little benefit.

In states having no *licensure* requirements for radiographers, physicians and hospitals often assume the responsibility of hiring only credentialed radiographers. Participation in *quality assurance* ensures that imaging equipment is functioning optimally.

Radiographers must consider patient dose when selecting exposure factors. One component of a radiographer's professionalism, as stated in the seventh principle of the *ARRT Code of Ethics,* is to consistently employ every means possible to decrease radiation exposure to the population.

Radiographers must follow the *ALARA* principle (keeping exposure As Low As Reasonably Achievable) as they carry out their tasks. The radiologic facility must undergo appropriate radiation surveys. Staff must be properly oriented and regular inservice reviews of radiation safety must take place. Proper radiation monitoring and review of monthly radiation reports is essential.

Summary

- **The Law of Bergonié and Tribondeau states that the most radiosensitive cells are young, stem, and highly mitotic cells.**
- **LET is another means of expressing quality and determining QF.**
- **Identical absorbed doses of different kinds of radiation will cause different biologic effects, hence the need for a QF.**
- **Diagnostic x-radiation is low-energy, low-LET radiation.**
- **Radiation effect on cells is named according to the interaction site, namely, direct effect, indirect effect, radiolysis of water.**
- **The most radiosensitive cell is the lymphocyte.**
- **As radiation professionals, we are obligated to keep radiation exposure to our patients and ourselves ALARA.**

IV. GENETIC EFFECTS

A. PREGNANCY

There are a number of situations that require the radiographer's special attention. Irradiation during *pregnancy,* especially in early pregnancy, must be avoided. The fetus is particularly radiosensitive during the first trimester, during much of which time pregnancy may not even be suspected. Especially high-risk examinations include pelvis, hip, femur, lumbar spine, cystograms and urograms, upper gastrointestinal (GI) series, barium enema examinations, and gallbladder (GB) series.

During the first trimester, specifically the second to eighth week of pregnancy (ie, during major organogenesis), if the radiation dose is sufficient, fetal anomalies can be produced. *Skeletal anomalies* can appear if irradiation occurs in the early part of this time period, and *neurologic anomalies* can be formed in the latter part; *mental retardation* and childhood *malignant diseases,* such as cancers or leukemia, can also result from irradiation during the first trimester. Fetal irradiation during the second and third trimester is not likely to produce anomalies, but rather, with sufficient dose, some type of childhood malignant disease. Fetal irradiation during the first 2 weeks of gestation can result in *spontaneous abortion.*

It must be emphasized, however, that the likelihood of producing fetal anomalies at doses below 20 rad is exceedingly small and that most general diagnostic examinations are likely to deliver fetal doses of less than 1 to 2 rad.

B. FEMALES

1. LMP (Last Menstrual Period). In consideration of the potential risk, female patients of child-bearing age should be questioned regarding their *last menstrual period (LMP)* and the possibility of their being pregnant.

2. Ten-day Rule. In addition to supporting the ALARA concept, many institutions also use the *10-day rule* as a guide for scheduling elective abdominal x-ray examinations on women of reproductive age, that is, the exam is scheduled during the first 10 days following the onset of the menstrual period because that is the time when the presence of a recently fertilized ovum is least likely.

Facilities offering radiologic services should make inquiries of their female patients regarding LMP and advise them of the risk associated with radiation exposure during pregnancy. In many institutions, this information is part of a consent form that the patient signs prior to the radiologic examination. Most facilities will also post signs in waiting rooms, dressing rooms, and radiographic rooms cautioning the pregnant patient to advise the radiographer of her condition so that proper precautions may be taken.

Concern is occasionally expressed regarding dose received during diagnostic *mammography*. Yet the risk associated with the x-ray dose received is minimal compared to the benefits of early detection of breast cancer. The use of dedicated mammography equipment with screen–film technique performed by credentialed radiographers delivers the lowest skin and glandular dose of any mammographic method available.

C. MALES

Because of the location of the gonads and *shielding* restrictions thus imposed in the female patient, the female gonads (ovaries) receive more radiation exposure than the male gonads (testes) undergoing similar examinations. The ovaries lie within the abdominal cavity and frequently cannot be effectively shielded during abdominal, pelvic, and lumbar spine radiography. Therefore, they receive far more organ dose than the testes (which are located outside the abdominal cavity) during diagnostic examinations of the abdominal region (eg, lumbar spine, upper and lower GI, intravenous, or retrograde pyelography).

It is important to note that the ovarian stem cells, the oogonia, reproduce only during fetal life. During child-bearing years there are only 400 to 500 mature ova accessible for fertilization; that is, one ovum per menstrual cycle for each of the fertile years. The male germ cells, spermatogonia, are being produced continuously and longevity of fertility is quite different than in the female.

D. CHILDREN

The female oogonia of fetal life and early childhood and male spermatogonia are especially radiosensitive because of their immature stage of development. Consequently, particular care should be taken to adequately shield the reproductive organs of pediatric patients. All too often a radiographer will conscientiously shield adult patients of reproductive age, but fail to consider children whose reproductive cells are particularly radiosensitive and whose reproductive lives are ahead of them.

Very sizable doses of radiation to children are also thought to be associated with increased incidence of leukemia and other radiation-induced malignancies. Examples of high-risk examinations might include pelvic and abdominal radiography and examinations requiring periodic follow-ups, such as scoliosis series. It is advisable to shield the hematopoietic bones of children to reduce radiation dose to blood-forming cells.

E. GENETICALLY SIGNIFICANT DOSE (GSD)

Each member of the world's population bears a particular genetic dose of radiation. Its sources include environmental exposure, radiation received for medical and dental purposes, and occupational exposure. The quantity of exposure to each individual depends on that individual's geographic location (environmental radiation and elevation of terrain), overall general health, the accessibility of health care, and the occupational worker's adherence to radiation protection guidelines. Generally speaking, the genetic dose to an *individual* is very small. Some individuals may receive no genetic dose in a given year, some individuals are past their reproductive years, some individuals will not or cannot bear children. Even if some individuals receive larger quantities of radiation exposure, its impact is "diluted" by the total number of population. This concept is referred to as *genetically significant dose (GSD),* defined as the average annual gonadal dose to the population of child-bearing age, and estimated to be 20 mrem.

It is appropriate to mention *repeat radiographs* at this time. Poor radiographs resulting from technical error (eg, incorrect positioning, improper selection of technical factors) or equipment malfunction must be repeated, thereby subjecting the patient to twice the necessary exposure dose. An exceedingly important feature with significant impact on patient dose is appropriate *collimation.* An important part of radiation protection, then, is care and attention to detail to avoid technical errors requiring repeat radiographs. Another component is a quality assurance program (through an ongoing preventative maintenance program and appropriate inservice education) that assures proper equipment function and compliance with established standards.

V. SOMATIC EFFECTS

Somatic effects of radiation are those that affect the irradiated body itself. Somatic effects are described as being *early* or *late,* depending on the length of time between irradiation and manifestation of effects.

Early somatic effects are manifested within minutes, hours, days, or weeks of irradiation and only occur following a very large dose of ionizing radiation. It must be emphasized that doses received from diagnostic radiologic procedures are not sufficient to produce these early effects. An exceedingly *high dose of radiation delivered to the whole body in a short period of time* is required to produce early somatic effects.

A. CARCINOGENESIS

Late somatic effects are those that can occur years after initial exposure, and are caused by low, chronic exposures. Occupationally exposed personnel are concerned with the late effects of radiation exposure. Some somatic effects like *carcinogenesis* have been mentioned earlier: the bone *malignancies* developed by the radium watchdial painters, the thyroid cancers of the individuals irradiated as children for thymus enlargement, the leukemia eventually developed by patients whose pain from ankylosing spondylitis was relieved by irradiation, and the skin cancers developed by early radiology pioneers working so closely with the "unknown ray." These malignancies are examples of somatic effects of radiation.

B. EMBRYOLOGIC EFFECTS

Embryologic effects are those experienced by the body of the developing embryo or fetus. Spontaneous abortion, skeletal or neurologic anomalies (mental retardation and microcephaly), and leukemia are examples of embryologic somatic effects.

C. CATARACTOGENESIS

Another example of somatic effects of radiation is *cataract* formation to the lenses of eyes of those individuals accidentally exposed to sufficient quantities of radiation (eg, early cyclotron experimenters).

D. LIFE SPAN SHORTENING

The lives of many of the early radiation workers were several years shorter than the lives of the general population. Statistics revealed that radiologists, for example, had a shorter life span than physicians of other specialties. *Life span shortening,* then, *was* another somatic effect of radiation. Certainly, these effects should *never be experienced today.* So much has been learned about the biologic effects of radiation since its discovery and a part of what we have learned has, sadly, been as a result of the experiences of the radiology pioneers.

Summary
- **Delivery of ionizing radiation during early pregnancy is particularly hazardous.**
- **There are five responses of concern to irradiation in utero: spontaneous abortion, congenital anomalies, mental retardation, microcephaly, and childhood malignancies.**
- **Female patients of childbearing age should be questioned regarding LMP and possible pregnancy.**
- **The 10-day rule may be employed to schedule elective radiography for female patients.**
- **Gonadal shielding is easier in the male patient because the reproductive organs are located externally.**
- **Genetic effects refer to damage to reproductive cells, affecting the reproductive capacity of the individual, or creating mutations that will be passed on to future generations.**
- **The genetic dose of radiation borne by each member of the reproductive population is called the genetically significant dose.**

- Somatic effects include those manifesting themselves in the exposed individual and can be described as early or late effects.
    - Early somatic effects can occur only after a very large single exposure of radiation to the whole body.
    - Late somatic effects include carcinogenesis, cataracto-genesis, embryologic effect, and life-span shortening.
- Occupationally exposed personnel are concerned with the late effects of radiation exposure.

Chapter Exercises

 Congratulations! *You have completed this chapter. If you are able to answer the following group of very comprehensive questions, you should feel confident that you have really mastered this section. You are then ready to go on to "Registry-type" questions that follow. For greatest success, do not go to the multiple choice questions without first completing the short answer questions below.*

1. List various kinds of electromagnetic radiation *(p. 213)*.

2. Identify the way in which all electromagnetic radiations are similar and in what respect they differ *(p. 214)*.

3. Define the terms *wavelength* and *frequency* *(p. 214)*.

4. Explain how wavelength and energy and how frequency and energy are related *(p. 214)*.

5. Describe what is meant by the term *ionizing* radiation and how it differs from other electromagnetic radiations *(p. 214)*.

6. Give examples of natural and artificial (man-made) background radiations and identify the percentage each contributes to the population's annual radiation dose *(p. 214)*.

7. What are the two ways in which x-ray photons are produced at the tungsten anode? Describe each. Which occurs more often *(p. 215)*?

8. Describe the photoelectric effect and Compton scatter. The following should be included in your description *(pp. 215–217)*:

    A. energy required for production of each

    B. electron shell involved

    C. any electron shell vacancy or occupancy changes

    D. type of absorber (atomic number) most likely involved

    E. retention or loss of energy of incoming photon

    F. interaction associated with a recoil electron

    G. effect on radiographic contrast

    H. impact on patient dose

9. Describe the difference between threshold and nonthreshold dose–response curves *(p. 218)*.

10. Differentiate between stochastic and nonstochastic effects *(p. 218)*.

11. Name the type of dose–response curve that identifies *no* safe dose *(p. 218)*.

12. Explain why occupationally exposed individuals are mainly concerned with the late, or long-term, effects of radiation exposure *(pp. 218–219)*.

13. List possible long-term effects of radiation exposure *(p. 219)*.

14. List the three types of cells described by Bergonié and Tribondeau in 1906 as being the most radiosensitive *(p. 219)*.

15. What is described as the rate at which radiation deposits energy in tissue *(p. 220)*?

16. Why is a QF assigned to different types of radiation *(p. 220)*?

17. How may the terms *rad* and *rem* be equated *(p. 220)*?

18. How are LET and RBE related *(p. 220)*?

19. With respect to the molecular effects of radiation, describe the difference between the direct and indirect effect; identify the one that occurs more frequently in the diagnostic range *(p. 220)*.

20. What type(s) of DNA damage is/are repairable; which can result in cell death; mutation *(p. 220)*?

21. Identify each of the following as either radiosensitive or radioresistant: muscle, nerve (fetal and adult), and epithelial tissue; lymphocytes; and reproductive cells *(p. 221)*.

22. How does each of the following affect the response of tissue to irradiation: tissue age, oxygen content, fractionation/protraction of radiation delivery *(p. 221)*?

23. Identify the meaning of the acronym ALARA and how it relates to the radiographer *(p. 222)*.

24. What is the most radiosensitive portion of the human gestational period? List four possible results of excessive radiation exposure during this period *(p. 222)*.

25. What can result from excessive radiation exposure during the second and third trimester of pregnancy *(p. 222)*?

26. How much radiation exposure is necessary to produce fetal anomalies? Approximately how much fetal radiation do most diagnostic examinations deliver *(p. 222)*?

27. Explain the value of determining the LMP and/or using the 10-day rule for female patients of child-bearing age *(p. 223)*.

28. Describe the effectiveness of gonadal shielding in the male versus female patient; discuss the importance of shielding children *(p. 223)*.

29. Describe the concept of GSD *(p. 224)*.

30. Why are we concerned with genetic dose? When do genetic effects manifest themselves *(p. 224)?*

31. Distinguish between early and late somatic effects; when does each occur with respect to initial exposure? Can you give historic examples of each *(p. 224)?*

32. What kind of radiation exposure would be required to cause early somatic effects? Give examples of early somatic effects *(p. 224)*.

33. What kind of radiation exposure is characteristic of late somatic effects? Give examples of late somatic effects *(p. 225)*.

A&U Chapter Review Questions

1. How are wavelength and energy related?
   (A) directly
   (B) inversely
   (C) chemically
   (D) empirically

2. A dose of 25 rad to the fetus during the seventh or eighth week of pregnancy is more likely to cause which of the following:
   (A) spontaneous abortion
   (B) skeletal anomalies
   (C) neurologic anomalies
   (D) organogenesis

3. Which of the following accounts for x-ray beam heterogeneity?
   1. incident electrons interacting with several layers of tungsten target atoms
   2. electrons moving to fill different shell vacancies
   3. its nuclear origin
   (A) 1 only
   (B) 1 and 2 only
   (C) 1 and 3 only
   (D) 1, 2, and 3

4. What is the effect on relative biologic effectiveness (RBE) as linear energy transfer (LET) increases?
   (A) as LET increases, RBE increases
   (B) as LET increases, RBE decreases
   (C) as LET increases, RBE stabilizes
   (D) LET has no effect on RBE

5. Long-term effects of radiation include:
   1. formation of cataracts
   2. cancer
   3. genetic effects
   (A) 1 only
   (B) 1 and 2 only
   (C) 2 and 3 only
   (D) 1, 2, and 3

6. Linear energy transfer (LET) is:
   1. a method of expressing radiation quality
   2. a measure of the rate at which radiation energy is transferred to soft tissue
   3. absorption of polyenergetic radiation
   (A) 1 only
   (B) 1 and 2 only
   (C) 1 and 3 only
   (D) 1, 2, and 3

7. In 1906, Bergonié and Tribondeau established a law which states that cells are more radiosensitive if they:
   1. have a low proliferation rate
   2. are stem cells
   3. are young
   (A) 1 only
   (B) 1 and 2 only
   (C) 2 and 3 only
   (D) 1, 2, and 3

8. The type of dose–response curve used to predict genetic effects is the:
   (A) nonlinear nonthreshold
   (B) nonlinear threshold
   (C) linear nonthreshold
   (D) nonlinear nonthreshold

9. The beam of x-ray photons leaving the x-ray tube focus can be described as having what sort of nature?
   (A) homogeneous
   (B) heterogeneous
   (C) homologous
   (D) focused

10. The effects of radiation to biologic material are dependent on several factors. If a quantity of radiation is delivered to a body over a long period of time:
    (A) the effect will be greater than if it were delivered all at one time
    (B) the effect will be less than if it were delivered all at one time
    (C) the effect has no relation to how it is delivered in time
    (D) the effect is solely dependent on the radiation quality

Answers and Explanations

1. (B) Frequency and wavelength are closely associated with the relative energy of electromagnetic radiations. *More energetic radiations have shorter wavelengths and higher frequency,* thus, they are inversely related. The relationship between frequency, wavelength, and energy is illustrated in the electromagnetic spectrum (see Fig. 8–1). Some radiations are energetic enough to rearrange atoms in materials through which they pass, and can therefore be hazardous to living tissue.

2. (C) During the first trimester, specifically the second to eighth week of pregnancy (during major organogenesis), if the radiation dose is at least 20 rad, fetal anomalies can be produced. *Skeletal anomalies* usually appear if irradiation occurs in the early part of this time period, and *neurologic anomalies* are formed in the latter part; mental retardation and childhood malignant diseases, such as cancers or leukemia, can also result from irradiation during the first trimester. Fetal irradiation during the second and third trimester is not likely to produce anomalies, but rather, with sufficient dose, some type of childhood malignant disease. Fetal irradiation during the first 2 weeks of gestation can result in *spontaneous abortion.*

It must be emphasized that the likelihood of producing fetal anomalies at doses below 20 rad is exceedingly small and that most general diagnostic examinations are likely to deliver fetal doses of less than 1 to 2 rad.

3. (B) The x-ray photons produced at the tungsten target comprise a heterogeneous beam, that is, a spectrum of photon energies. This is accounted for by the fact that the incident electrons have different energies. Also, the incident electrons travel through several layers of tungsten target material, lose energy with each interaction, and therefore produce increasingly weaker x-ray photons. During characteristic x-ray production, vacancies may be filled in the K, L, or M shells, differing with each other in binding energies, and therefore, a variety of energy photons are emitted.

4. (A) LET expresses the rate at which photon or particulate energy is transferred to (absorbed by) biologic material (through ionization processes) and is dependent upon the type of radiation and absorber characteristics. RBE describes the degree of response or amount of biologic change we can expect of the irradiated material. As the amount of transferred energy (LET) *increases* (from interactions occurring between radiation and biologic material) the amount of biologic effect or damage will also *increase. LET and biologic effect are directly related.*

5. (D) Occupationally exposed individuals are concerned principally with *late* (ie, *long-term* or *delayed*) effects of radiation, such as *genetic effects, leukemia, cancers,* and *cataractogenesis,* which can occur many years following initial exposure to low levels of ionizing radiation. These long-term, or delayed, effects are represented by the linear, non-threshold dose–response curve, with the exception of cataractogenesis, which is represented by the linear, threshold dose–response curve. An acute dose of about 200 rad would be required to cause radiogenic cataracts. A far greater occupational (ie, fractionated) dose of about 1000 rad would be required to induce cataracts.

6. (B) When biologic material is irradiated, there are a number of modifying factors that determine what kind and how much response will occur in the biologic material. One of these factors is LET, which expresses the rate at which particulate or photon energy is transferred to the absorber. Because different kinds of radiation have different degrees of penetration in different materials, it is also a useful way of expressing the quality of the radiation.

7. (C) The law of Bergonié and Tribondeau states that stem cells (that give rise to a specific type cell, as in hematopoiesis), as well as young cells and tissues, are particularly radiosensitive. It also states that cells with a high rate of proliferation (mitosis) are more sensitive to radiation. This law is historically important in that it was the first to recognize that some tissues have greater radiosensitivity than others, for example, the fetus.

8. (C) The linear-nonthreshold curve is used to illustrate responses such as leukemia, cancer, and genetic effects. These are sometimes referred to as stochastic effects. Stochastic effects occur randomly and are "all-or-nothing" type effects, that is, they do not occur with degrees of severity. Remember that *in a nonthreshold curve there is no safe dose,* that is, no dose below which there will definitely be no biologic response. Theoretically, even one x-ray photon can cause a biologic response. The linear-nonthreshold curve is the curve of choice to predict effects of low level (eg, medical and occupational) exposure to ionizing radiation.

9. (B) Electrons may undergo any one of a few types of interactions as they encounter the target. The emitted photons can therefore have a variety of energies and thus are termed heterogeneous or polyenergetic. It is only at extremely high energies that photon energy becomes more homogeneous; only gamma radiation can be accurately termed homogeneous or monoenergetic.

10. (B) The effects of a quantity of radiation delivered to a body is dependent on a few factors, including the amount of radiation received, the size of the irradiated area, and how the radiation is delivered in time. If the radiation is delivered in portions over a period of time, it is said to be fractionated and has a less harmful effect than if the radiation was delivered all at once. Cells have an opportunity to repair and some recovery occurs between doses.

Patient Protection

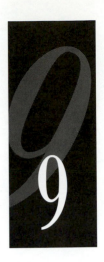

As previously discussed, it is our ethical responsibility to keep radiation exposure to patients (and ourselves) to an absolute minimum. This chapter reviews means of achieving this goal.

Statistics indicate that the number of x-ray examinations performed annually is steadily increasing. Although the benefits of these examinations far outweigh the risks, the concern about the risk of possible long-term effects of x-ray exposure obliges us to practice the *ALARA* (As Low As Reasonably Achievable) principle.

One exceedingly important consideration in reducing patient exposure is *good patient communication.* Explaining the examination and answering the patient's questions will better ensure understanding and cooperation, and reduce the chance for retakes.

Quality control programs are in place to ensure that retakes will not be required as a result of equipment malfunction. Employees receive orientation on new equipment to ensure that it is used to best advantage and to reduce retakes as a result of unfamiliarity with equipment operation. The use of technique charts helps take the guesswork out of selecting exposure factors.

The following topics discuss important factors having impact on patient protection.

I. BEAM RESTRICTION

Beam restriction, or limitation of irradiated field size, is probably the single most important factor in keeping patient dose to a minimum. The primary beam must be confined to the area of interest, thus, only tissues of diagnostic interest should be irradiated.

Another benefit of beam restriction is that, because a smaller quantity of tissue is irradiated, less scattered radiation will be produced. Remember, scattered radiation does not carry useful information; it degrades the radiographic image by adding a layer of fog that impairs image visibility.

There are three basic types of *beam restrictors:* aperture diaphragms, cones, and collimators.

A. APERTURE DIAPHRAGMS

The *aperture diaphragm* is the most elementary of the three types, and is frequently used in dedicated head units and many dedicated chest units. It is simply a flat piece of lead (Pb) having a central opening with a size and shape that determines the size and shape of the x-ray beam. Whereas head units have a variety of aperture diaphragm sizes available for various types of skull exams and required cassette sizes, today's dedicated chest units frequently have a more fixed aperture diaphragm. Regardless of the type, the aperture diaphragm should demonstrate adequate beam restriction by providing an unexposed border around the edge of the radiograph.

B. CONES

Cones are circular, lead-lined devices that slide into place in the tube head or onto the collimator housing. They may be the straight *cylinder* type, with proximal and distal diameters that are identical, or the infrequently used *flare type*, with a distal diameter that is greater than its proximal diameter. Cylinder cones are frequently able to extend, like a telescope, by means of a simple thumbscrew adjustment (Fig. 9–1).

A disadvantage of both the aperture and cone is that they have a fixed opening size, that will provide only one field size at a given distance. To change the size of the field you must change to a different size aperture or cone. Additionally, the cylinder cone can be used only for relatively small field sizes, such as the paranasal sinuses, L5-S1, or other small areas of interest.

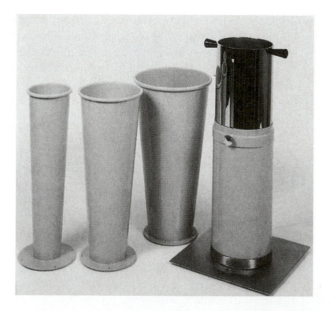

Figure 9–1. Cylinder cones (especially the extendible type) are generally considered more efficient than aperture diaphragms because they restrict the size and shape of the x-ray beam for a greater distance. The closer the distal end of the beam restrictor is to the area of interest, the greater its efficiency. (Courtesy Burkhart Roentgen, Inc.)

C. COLLIMATORS

The *collimator* is, overall, the most efficient beam-restricting device. It is attached to the tube head, and its upper aperture, the first set of shutters, is placed as close as possible to the x-ray tube port window (Fig. 9–2). This is done to control the amount of image degrading "off-focus" radiation leaving the x-ray tube (ie, radiation produced when electrons strike surfaces other than the focal track). The next set of *lead shutters* ("blades" or "leaves") actually consists of two pairs of adjustable shutters—one pair for field length and another pair for field width. It is these shutters that the radiographer adjusts when changing the field size and shape.

D. LIGHT-LOCALIZATION APPARATUS

Another important part of the collimator assembly is the *light localization apparatus*. It consists of a small light bulb (to illuminate the field) and a mirror. For the light field and x-ray field to correspond accurately, *the x-ray tube focal spot and the light bulb must be exactly the same distance from the center of the mirror* (see Fig. 9–2). If the light and x-ray fields do not correspond, image receptor alignment can be "off" enough to require a repeat examination. Collimator accuracy should be regularly checked as part of the quality assurance program. National Council on Radiation Protection and Measurements (NCRP) guidelines state that collimators must be accurate to within 2% of the source-to-image-receptor distance (SID).

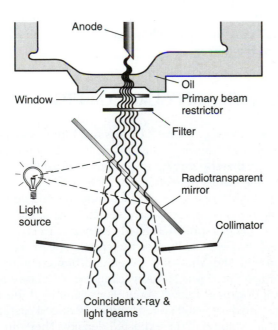

Figure 9–2. X-ray tube, filters, and collimator. The position of the collimator shutters can be seen. Note the position of the first beam restrictor, located at the x-ray tube port window. The oil coolant surrounding the x-ray tube contributes to inherent filtration. Added filtration includes the aluminum filter, the mirror, and collimator. (Reproduced with permission from Wolbarst AB. *Physics of Radiology.* East Norwalk, CT: Appleton & Lange, 1993.)

E. ACCURACY

Cylinder cones are often attached to the tube housing and used in conjunction with collimators. It is important to collimate to the approximate cone diameter size; wide-open collimator shutters can lead to excessive scattered radiation production and can degrade the resulting radiographic image.

As a back-up to the illuminated light field, should the light bulb burn out, there is a calibrated scale on the front of the collimator that indicates the x-ray field size at various source-to-image receptor distances (see Fig. 9–5A on p. 240).

An important feature of nearly all collimators today (radiographic and fluoroscopic) is *positive beam limitation (PBL)*. Sensors located in the Bucky tray or other cassette holder signal the collimator to open or close, according to the cassette size being used in the Bucky tray. A properly calibrated PBL system will provide a small unexposed border on all sides of the finished radiograph, and is required by NCRP guidelines to be accurate to within 2% of the SID.

Summary

- **Beam restriction is the most important way to reduce patient dose.**
- **Beam restrictors reduce the production of scattered radiation.**
- **Types of beam restrictors include aperture diaphragms, cones and cylinders, and collimators (most efficient).**
- **Most x-ray equipment today uses PBL.**
- **A properly calibrated PBL will provide an unexposed border on all sides of the finished radiograph.**
- **For the light and x-ray field to correspond accurately, the focal spot and light bulb must be exactly the same distance from the mirror.**

II. AUTOMATIC EXPOSURE CONTROL

An *automatic exposure control (AEC)* is used to automatically regulate the amount of ionizing radiation delivered to the patient and image recorder, thereby serving to produce consistent and comparable radiographic results time after time. When AEC is installed in the x-ray circuit, it is calibrated to produce radiographic densities as required by the radiologist. AECs have sensors that signal to terminate the exposure once a predetermined, known-correct exposure has been reached. It is essential to use the correct speed screen and film combination with the AEC—the screen and film combination that it has been programmed for. The AEC cannot compensate for a speed system that it does not "know" about. For example, if the system has been programmed for a 400 system and a 200 speed cassette is used, the image will exhibit half the expected density. There are two types of AECs: *ionization chambers* and *phototimers/photomultipliers*.

A. IONIZATION CHAMBER

A parallel plate *ionization chamber* consists of a radiolucent chamber just beneath the tabletop above the cassette and grid (Fig. 9–3). As x-ray photons emerge from the patient, they enter the chamber

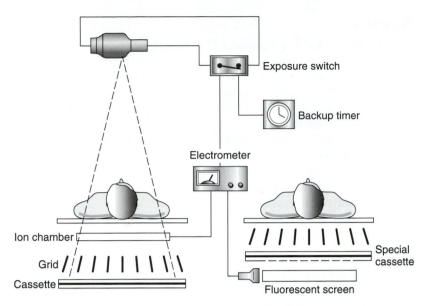

Figure 9–3. Two types of AECs. The ionization chamber is pictured to the left, positioned between the tabletop and cassette. The photomultiplier/phototimer is to the right, located below the cassette. Note that a backup timer, which serves to terminate the exposure in the event of AEC failure, is used in conjunction with both AECs. (Reproduced with permission from Wolbarst AB. *Physics of Radiology.* East Norwalk, CT: Appleton & Lange, 1993.)

and ionize the air within. When a predetermined quantity of ionization has occurred (as determined by the selected exposure factors), the exposure automatically terminates.

B. PHOTOTIMER

In the *phototimer,* a small fluorescent screen is positioned beneath the cassette (see Fig. 9–3). When remnant radiation emerging from the patient exits the cassette, the fluorescent screen emits light. The fluorescent light charges a photomultiplier tube and, once a predetermined charge has been reached, the exposure is terminated.

C. BACKUP TIMER

In either case, the manual timer should be used as *backup timer.* This ensures that, in case of AEC malfunction, the exposure will terminate and *avoid patient overexposure and tube overload.*

D. MINIMUM RESPONSE TIME

Another important feature of the AEC to be familiar with is its *minimum response/reaction time.* This is the length of the *shortest exposure possible* with a particular AEC. If less than the minimum response time is required for a particular exposure, the radiograph will exhibit excessive density.

Exact positioning and centering is particularly critical when using equipment with AECs. The anatomic part of interest must be positioned (centered) accurately with respect to the AEC's sensors; otherwise the result can be over or under exposure.

Summary

- **When used properly, AECs ensure consistency of radiographic density.**
- **There are two types of AECs: ionization chamber type and phototimer/photomultiplier type.**
- **The ionization chamber type is located between the patient and cassette.**
- **The phototimer/photomultiplier type is located beneath the cassette.**
- **Every AEC has a minimum response time.**
- **AECs require accurate positioning and centering to produce predictable results.**
- **The manual timer must be used as backup timer to avoid patient overexposure and tube overload.**

III. EXPOSURE FACTORS

Selection of exposure factors has a significant impact on patient dose. Remember that milliampere-seconds (mAs) is used to regulate the *quantity* of radiation delivered to the patient, and *kVp* (kilovoltage peak) determines the *penetrability* of the x-ray beam. As kilovoltage is increased, more high-energy photons are produced and the overall average energy of the beam is increased. An increase in mAs increases the number of photons produced at the target, but mAs is unrelated to photon energy.

Generally speaking then, in an effort to keep radiation dose to a minimum, it makes sense to use the lowest mAs and the highest kVp that will produce the desired radiographic results. An added benefit is that at high kVp and low mAs values, the heat delivered to the x-ray tube is lower and tube life is extended.

IV. FILTRATION

X-ray photons emanating from the target comprise a *heterogeneous* primary beam. There are many low energy (or "soft") x-rays that, if not removed, would contribute significantly to patient skin dose. These low-energy photons are too weak to penetrate the patient and expose the image receptor; they simply penetrate a small thickness of tissue and are absorbed. Filters, usually made of aluminum, are used in radiography to reduce patient dose by removing this low energy radiation, *resulting in an x-ray beam of higher average energy. Total filtration* is composed of *inherent filtration* plus *added filtration*.

A. INHERENT FILTRATION

Inherent filtration is that which is "built-in," and is composed of materials that are a permanent part of the tube housing, that is, the *glass envelope* of the x-ray tube and the *oil coolant* (0.5 mm aluminum [Al] equivalent).

B. ADDED FILTRATION

Added filtration includes the *collimator structures* and *mirror* (1 mm Al equivalent) and *thin sheets of aluminum* that are added to make the necessary total thickness (see Fig. 9–2).

Filtration Summary

<50 kVp = 0.5 mm Al equivalent
50–70 kVp = 1.5 mm Al equivalent
>70 kVp = 2.5 mm Al equivalent

C. NCRP Guidelines

NCRP guidelines state that equipment operating above 70 kVp must have a minimum total (inherent plus added) filtration of *2.5 mm Al equivalent*. Equipment operating between 50 and 70 kVp must have at least 1.5 mm Al equivalent filtration. X-ray tubes operating below 50 kVp must have at least 0.5 mm Al equivalent filtration. Mammography equipment with a molybdenum target will have 0.025 to 0.03 mm molybdenum (Mo) filtration. For magnification studies, a fractional tungsten (W) target tube, having at least 0.5 mm Al equivalent total filtration, may be used.

Inherent filtration tends to increase as the x-ray tube ages. With use, tungsten evaporates and is deposited on the inner surface of the glass envelope, effectively acting as additional filtration and decreasing tube output.

Summary

- **Low mAs and high kVp factors keep patient dose to a minimum.**
- **Proper calibration of equipment is essential for predictable results.**
- **Proper selection of technical factors and an effective QA system help reduce radiation exposure.**
- **Filtration removes low energy x-rays from primary beam, thereby:**
  - **reducing patient dose**
  - **increasing the average energy of the beam**
- **Filtration is usually expressed in mm of Al equivalent.**
- **Inherent + added filtration = total filtration.**
- **Inherent filtration includes the glass envelope and oil coolant.**
- **Added filtration includes the collimator, mirror, and thin Al sheets.**
- **Equipment operated above 70 kVp must have at least 2.5 mm Al equivalent.**
- **Inherent filtration increases with tube age, thereby decreasing tube output.**

V. SHIELDING

Protective shielding for especially radiosensitive organs (ie, gonads, blood-forming organs) should be provided whenever possible during radiographic and fluoroscopic examinations (Figs. 9–4 and 9–5).

A. Male and Female

Gonadal shielding is far more effective in the male patient because the reproductive organs lie outside the body. Male patients are therefore more easily shielded, and shielding is much less likely to interfere with the diagnostic objectives of the examination. Female reproductive organs are located within the abdominal cavity, where shielding becomes a much-less-feasible option.

B. Guidelines for Use

There are three indications for the effective use of gonadal shields. If the gonads lie in or within 5 cm of a well-collimated field, shield-

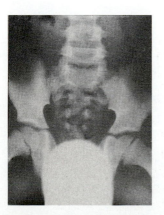

Figure 9–4. Correct placement of shadow shield. (Courtesy of C.B. Radiology Design, Jamestown, NY.)

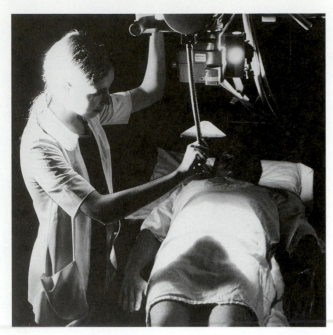

A

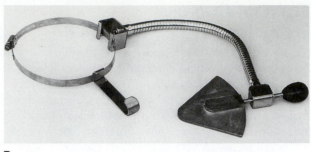

B

Figure 9–5. **(A and B)** A shadow shield is attached to the collimator housing. It has a moveable arm that allows a shield of the desired size and shape to be placed in the radiation field over the gonadal area. It is manually operated and swings away when not in use. (Courtesy of Nuclear Associates.)

ing should be used. A patient with reasonable reproductive potential should be shielded; a generally accepted procedure is to include all patients younger than age 55 years. Gonadal shielding should be used if diagnostic objectives permit, that is, as long as the shield does not obscure important diagnostic information.

C. TYPES OF SHIELDS

There are three types of gonadal shields available: flat, contact shields, shadow shields, and contour (shaped) contact shields.

1. Flat, Contact. The simplest types are flat, *contact shields,* such as pieces of lead-impregnated vinyl that are placed over the patient's gonads. Because they are difficult to secure in place, flat contact shields are useful only for anteroposterior (AP) or posteroanterior (PA) recumbent positions. They cannot be secured adequately for oblique, lateral decubitus, erect, or fluoroscopic procedures.

2. Shadow. *Shadow shields* attach to the x-ray tube head. They consist of a piece of leaded material attached to an arm extending from the tube head (see Fig. 9–5). The leaded material casts a shadow within the illuminated field that corresponds to the shielded area. Although shadow shields are initially more expensive, they are likely to be a one-time expense. Shadow shields can be used for more positions than flat contact shields and may also be used without contaminating a sterile field. They cannot be used for fluoroscopic procedures.

3. Contour (Shaped) Contact Shields.

Contour (shaped) *contact shields* are very effective gonadal shields. They are shaped to enclose the male reproductive organs and are held in place by disposable briefs. They are effective for a variety of positions, including oblique, erect, and fluoroscopic procedures.

4. Breast Shields.

Breast shields should be used for female patients during scoliosis series. Scoliosis series are typically performed at ages when developing breast tissue is particularly radiosensitive. Breast shields are available incorporated in vertebral column compensating filters (Fig. 9–6), and as leaded vinyl vests.

Gonadal Shielding Should Be Used If
- The gonads lie in, or within 5 cm of, a well-collimated field.
- The patient has reasonable reproductive potential.
- Diagnostic objectives permit.

Additional points to remember include the following:

- Lead aprons can be placed under the patient's pillow during GI and BE examinations when the radiographer's assistance is required at the head end of the table during fluoroscopy.
- Half aprons can be used to protect the gonads from *scattered radiation* in chest radiography.
- Lead aprons can also be placed over chest/abdomen during radiography of various body parts to protect radiosensitive organs from exposure to scattered radiation.

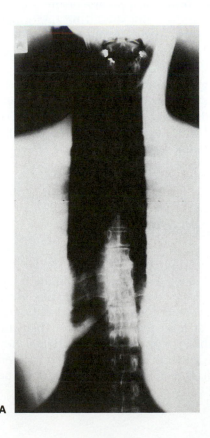
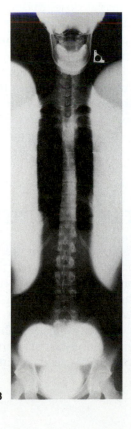

Figure 9–6. Spinal column studies are often required for evaluation of adolescent scoliosis, thus presenting a two-fold problem: radiation exposure to youthful gonadal and breast tissues, and significantly differing tissue densities and thicknesses. Both problems can be resolved with the use of a compensating filter (for uniform density) that incorporates lead shielding for the breasts and gonads. **(A)** Performed without the filter/shield. **(B)** Performed with the filter/shield. Note the improved visualization of the entire vertebral column and appropriate protection of the breasts and gonads. (Courtesy of Nuclear Associates.)

A

B

- Protective shields must be carefully placed; superimposition on diagnostically important anatomic structures can cause retakes and exposure to unnecessary radiation.
- The use of protective shielding during mobile radiography should not be neglected.

Summary

- **Especially radiosensitive organs include the gonads, lenses, and blood-forming organs.**
- **Gonadal shielding should be used:**
  - **if the gonads lie in or within 5 cm of collimated beam**
  - **if the patient has reproductive potential**
  - **if diagnostic objectives permit**
- **Three types of gonadal shields are:**
  - **flat contact**
  - **shadow**
  - **contour contact**
- **Male gonads are more easily and effectively shielded.**
- **Breast shields should be used as needed.**

VI. PATIENT POSITION

Because the primary x-ray beam has a *polyenergetic* (heterogeneous) nature, the entrance or skin dose is significantly greater than the exit dose. This principle may be employed in radiation protection by placing particularly radiosensitive organs away from the primary beam.

To place the gonads further from the primary beam and reduce gonadal dose, abdominal radiography should be performed in the PA position whenever possible. Dose to the lens is significantly decreased when skull radiographs are performed in the PA position.

The same principle applies when performing scoliosis series on young children in an effort to reduce gonadal dose, and to decrease dose to breast tissue in young girls. Dose to breast tissue during scoliosis survey can also be reduced with the use of breast shields. The PA projection does not generally cause a significant adverse effect on recorded detail and is often advocated to decrease dose to the reproductive organs.

VII. FILM AND SCREEN COMBINATION

The higher the speed of the film and screen system, the smaller the dose of radiation required to produce a diagnostic radiograph. As one component of the effort to reduce population dose, rare earth phosphors are used almost exclusively today in general radiography. Rare earth phosphors are at least four times faster than the earlier calcium tungstate phosphors, and the recorded detail they provide is entirely satisfactory. In general, the fastest film and screen combination consistent with diagnostic requirements should be used.

VIII. GRIDS

Grids, both stationary and moving, function to remove a large percentage of scattered (primarily Compton) radiation from the remnant beam before it reaches the image receptor, thereby improving radiographic contrast.

Because scattered radiation often makes a significant contribution to the overall radiographic density, the addition of a grid (or increase in the grid ratio) must be accompanied by an appropriate increase in exposure factors (usually mAs) to maintain adequate density. The improvement in image quality is usually more significant than the increased exposure to the patient (Fig. 9–7). However, the radiographer should avoid using a high-ratio grid with a low kilovoltage; the relatively small amount of scattered radiation produced does not warrant the large increase in mAs required by the high-ratio grid.

It is interesting to note that, to produce a given density, a moving grid generally requires more exposure than a stationary grid of the same ratio. This is because, as the lead strips continually change position moving back and forth, some of the perpendicular rays will unavoidably be "caught" by the lead strips moving into their path.

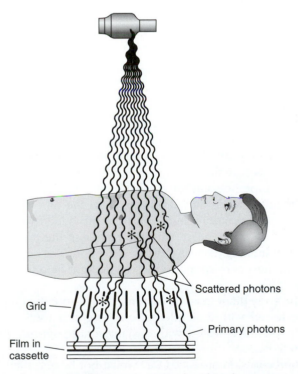

Figure 9–7. Scattered radiation generated within the patient can cause serious degradation of image quality. The improvement in image quality afforded by the use of grids more than makes up for the required increase in patient exposure. (Reproduced with permission from Wolbarst AB. *Physics of Radiology.* East Norwalk, CT: Appleton & Lange, 1993.)

IX. AIR-GAP TECHNIQUE

An *air-gap* technique will function similar to, or in place of, a grid. A distance is introduced between the patient/part and the image recorder. Scattered photons emerging from the patient will continue to diverge and never reach the image recorder.

A "natural" air gap exists in the lateral projection of the cervical spine and a 72-inch SID is used *without* a grid (Fig. 9–8). Because no air gap is introduced in the AP projection of the cervical spine, it is usually radiographed at 40 inches SID *with* the use of a grid.

The SID required in *magnification radiography* is an air-gap and therefore grids are rarely needed when this special imaging technique is performed.

Air-gap technique may also be used in place of a grid in chest radiography. However, to maintain optimum recorded detail and avoid excessive magnification, the SID must be increased considerably, followed by a significant increase in mAs. Air-gap technique is limited in use to radiography of fairly thin parts, as dense tissues would require excessive and impractical radiation exposures.

Additionally, equipment must be properly calibrated to produce consistently predictable results; specifically, the equipment must have *linearity* and *reproducibility*. *Linearity* refers to consistency in exposure with adjacent mA stations and exposure times adjusted to produce the same mAs. *Reproducibility* refers to consistency in exposure output during repeated exposures at a particular setting.

A. NCRP RECOMMENDATIONS FOR PATIENT PROTECTION

Note: Many of the means of patient protection serve to protect the operator as well. (Further recommendations can be found in section II under "NCRP Guidelines.")

- Equipment operating above 70 kVp must have a minimum total (inherent plus added) filtration of 2.5 mm Al equivalent.
- X-ray intensity at a particular mAs and kVp must be consistent within 20% at all combinations of commonly used mA and exposure times.
- X-ray tube housing must keep leakage radiation to less than 100 mR/h when measured 1 m from the tube.
- A device (centering light) must be provided to align the center of the x-ray beam with the center of the image receptor.
- Beam limiting devices must be provided. The collimated x-ray field must correspond to the visible light field to within 2% of the SID.
- The x-ray timer must be accurate. Single-phase equipment can be tested with a simple *spinning-top* test tool. Three phase equipment is tested with a *synchronous spinning top* or an oscilloscope.
- Source-to-skin distance (*SSD*) must not be less than 12 inches for all procedures other than dental radiography.
- The SSD must be at least 12 inches (preferably 15 inches) in stationary (fixed) fluoroscopic equipment.
- When more than one x-ray tube can be energized from a single control panel, there must be an obvious indicator on the control panel and on or near each tube housing that indicates which tube is being operated.

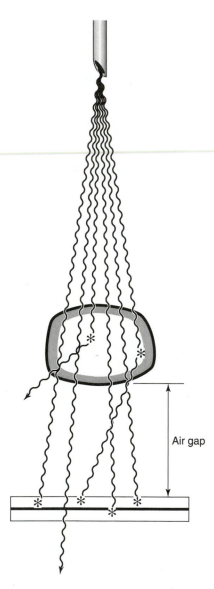

Air gap

Figure 9–8. When an air-gap is used, much of the scattered radiation generated within the patient never reaches the image receptor. An air-gap may occasionally be used in place of a grid. (Reproduced with permission from Wolbarst AB. *Physics of Radiology.* East Norwalk, CT: Appleton & Lange, 1993.)

- The location of the focal spot must be indicated on the outside of the tube housing.
- The film and screen combination selected should be the fastest possible that is consistent with the diagnostic objectives of the examination.
- Radiographic intensifying screens should be cleaned and checked regularly, at least every 6 months.
- X-ray film must be stored in an adequately protected place.
- Radiographic equipment should undergo regular quality assurance (QA) testing.
- The radiographer must be able to see and communicate with the patient at all times.

Summary

- **To reduce exposure to reproductive organs and/or breasts, it is helpful to perform abdominal radiography and scoliosis series in the PA position whenever possible.**
- **The fastest screen and film combination consistent with diagnostic requirements should be used.**
- **Grids improve the radiographic image by reducing the amount of scattered radiation fog, but necessitate an increase in exposure.**
- **An air-gap can have the same effect as a low-ratio grid in decreasing the amount of scattered radiation reaching the image receptor; however, SID, and therefore exposure, must be increased to preserve recorded detail.**
- **There are several important NCRP recommendations governing patient protection with which the radiographer should be familiar.**

Chapter Exercises

 Congratulations! *You have completed your review of this chapter. If you are able to answer the following group of very comprehensive questions, you should feel confident that you have really mastered this section. You are then ready to go on to "Registry-type" questions that follow. For greatest success, do not go to the multiple choice questions without first completing the short answer questions below.*

1. What are some methods of achieving the ALARA goal *(p. 233)?*

2. What is the most important factor in minimizing patient exposure? Give an example of how it affects patient dose *(p. 233).*

3. List the three types of beam restrictors; describe the particular use(s) and efficiency of each *(pp. 233–235).*

4. What effect does beam restriction have on the production of scattered radiation *(p. 233)?*

5. What degree of accuracy must a properly calibrated PBL maintain *(p. 235)?*

6. How is "off focus" radiation minimized *(p. 235)?*

7. Describe the relationship between the focal spot and collimator light bulb with respect to cassette alignment *(p. 235).*

8. Explain the importance of a backup timer *(p. 237).*

9. What is meant by the *minimum response time* of an AEC *(p. 237)?*

10. Why is positioning and centering so critical when using AECs *(p. 237)?*

11. What combination of exposure factors can be used, in general, to keep patient dose to a minimum *(p. 238)?*

12. How does filtration affect patient dose *(p. 238)?*

13. Describe the two types of filtration that comprise total filtration *(p. 238).*

14. What are the NCRP filtration requirements *(p. 239)?*

15. How and why does inherent filtration change as the x-ray tube ages; how does it affect tube output *(p. 239)?*

16. List the three criteria for determining when gonadal shielding should be used *(pp. 239–240)*.

17. Describe the three types of gonadal shielding and indicate the effectiveness of each *(pp. 240–241)*.

18. When might a breast or lens shields be used *(p. 241)*?

19. Explain the value of performing scoliosis series, abdominal, and skull radiography in the PA position *(p. 241)*.

20. How do screen and film combinations impact patient dose *(p. 242)*?

21. The NCRP makes several recommendations that can impact patient dose. Briefly describe the recommendations for each of the following *(pp. 244–245)*:

    A. patient visibility during examination

    B. QA testing

    C. speed and care of intensifying screens

    D. external indication of focal spot

    E. energizing multiple x-ray tubes from one control panel

    F. minimum SSD in fluoroscopy units

    G. x-ray timer testing and accuracy

    H. PBL and accuracy required

    I. beam alignment

    J. leakage radiation

    K. quantity of filtration

    L. linearity and reproducibility

![A&U Review Series] Chapter Review Questions

1. A backup timer for the automatic exposure control serves to:
    1. protect the patient from overexposure
    2. protect the x-ray tube from excessive heat
    3. eventually increase inherent filtration
   (A) 1 only
   (B) 1 and 2 only
   (C) 1 and 3 only
   (D) 1, 2, and 3

2. Which of the following is (are) feature(s) of x-ray equipment designed especially to eliminate unnecessary radiation to the patient?
    1. filtration
    2. minimum SSD of 12 inches
    3. collimation accuracy
   (A) 1 only
   (B) 1 and 2 only
   (C) 1 and 3 only
   (D) 1, 2, and 3

3. The advantages of beam restriction include:
    1. less scattered radiation is produced
    2. less biologic material is irradiated
    3. less total filtration is required
   (A) 1 only
   (B) 1 and 2 only
   (C) 2 and 3 only
   (D) 1, 2, and 3

4. All of the following affect patient dose, *except*:
   (A) inherent filtration
   (B) added filtration
   (C) focal spot size
   (D) source-image distance

5. Which of the following groups of exposure factors will deliver the *least* amount of exposure to the patient?
   (A) 50 mAs, 100 kVp
   (B) 100 mAs, 90 kVp
   (C) 200 mAs, 80 kVp
   (D) 400 mAs, 70 kVp

6. The principle function of filtration is to:
   (A) reduce operator dose
   (B) reduce patient skin dose
   (C) reduce image noise
   (D) reduce scattered radiation

7. Patient dose can be *decreased* by using:
    1. high-speed film and screen combination
    2. high-ratio grids
    3. air-gap technique
   (A) 1 only
   (B) 1 and 2 only
   (C) 1 and 3 only
   (D) 1, 2, and 3

8. Types of gonadal shielding include which of the following?
    1. flat contact
    2. shaped (contour) contact
    3. shadow
   (A) 1 only
   (B) 1 and 2 only
   (C) 2 and 3 only
   (D) 1, 2, and 3

9. How does filtration affect the primary beam?
   (A) filtration increases the average energy of the primary beam
   (B) filtration decreases the average energy of the primary beam
   (C) filtration makes the primary beam more penetrating
   (D) filtration increases the intensity of the primary beam

10. The quality assurance term used to describe consistency in exposure with adjacent mA stations and exposure times adjusted to produce the same mAs is:
    (A) automatic exposure control
    (B) positive beam limitation
    (C) linearity
    (D) reproducibility

Answers and Explanations

1. (B) A parallel plate *ionization chamber* consists of a radiolucent chamber just beneath the tabletop (see Fig. 9–3). As x-ray photons emerge from the patient, they enter the chamber and ionize the air within. When a predetermined quantity of ionization has occurred (as determined by the selected exposure factors), the exposure automatically terminates. In the *phototimer,* a small fluorescent screen is positioned beneath the cassette (see Fig. 9–3). When remnant radiation emerging from the patient exits the cassette, the exposure is terminated. The *manual* timer should be used as *backup timer,* in case the AEC fails to terminate the exposure, *thus protecting the patient from overexposure and the x-ray tube from excessive heat load.* The backup timer is unrelated to filtration.

2. (D) According to NCRP regulations, radiographic and fluoroscopic equipment must have a total Al *filtration* of at least 2.5 mm Al equivalent whenever the equipment is operated at 70 kVp or greater, to reduce excessive exposure to low-energy radiation. *Collimator* and beam alignment must be accurate to within 2%. The *SSD* must not be less than *12 inches* for all procedures other than dental radiography. Distance is the single best protection from radiation. Excessively short SIDs/SSDs cause a significant increase in patient skin dose.

3. (B) With greater beam restriction (ie, smaller field size), less biologic material is irradiated, thereby reducing the possibility of harmful effects. If less tissue is irradiated, less scattered radiation is produced, resulting in improved image contrast. The total filtration is not a function of beam restriction, but rather, is a radiation protection guideline aimed at reducing patient skin dose.

4. (C) *Inherent* filtration is composed of materials that are a permanent part of the tube housing; that is, the glass envelope of the x-ray tube and the oil coolant. *Added* filtration, usually thin sheets of aluminum, is present in order to make a total of 2.5 mm Al equivalent for equipment operated above 70 kVp. Filtration is used to decrease patient dose by removing the weak x-rays having no value but contributing to skin dose. According to the inverse square law of radiation, exposure dose increases as *distance* from the source decreases, and vice versa. The effect of the *focal spot size* is principally on radiographic detail, having no effect on patient dose.

5. (A) mAs regulates the quantity of radiation delivered to the patient. kVp regulates the quality (penetration) of the radiation delivered to the patient. Therefore, higher energy (more penetrating) radiation—which is more likely to *exit* the patient—accompanied by a lower mAs, is the safest combination for the patient.

6. (B) It is our ethical responsibility to minimize radiation dose to our patients. X-rays produced at the target comprise a heterogeneous primary beam. There are many "soft" (low-energy) photons that, if not removed, would only contribute to greater patient dose. They are too weak to penetrate the patient and expose the image receptor; they just penetrate a small thickness of tissue and are absorbed. Filters, usually made of aluminum, are used in *radiography to reduce patient dose by removing this low-energy radiation,* resulting in an x-ray beam of higher average energy. Total filtration is composed of inherent filtration plus added filtration.

7. (A) The *higher the speed* of the film and screen system, the *smaller the dose* of radiation required to produce a diagnostic radiograph. As one component of the effort to reduce population dose, rare earth phosphors are used almost exclusively today in general radiography, as they are at least four times faster than calcium tungstate phosphors.

Grids, both stationary and moving, function to remove a large percentage of scattered (primarily Compton) radiation from the remnant beam before it reaches the image receptor, thereby improving radiographic contrast. Because scattered radiation often makes a significant contribution to the overall radiographic density, the addition of a *grid* (or an increase in the grid ratio) must be accompanied by an appropriate *increase in exposure factors* (usually mAs) in order to maintain adequate density. The improvement in image quality is usually more significant than the increased exposure to the patient (see Fig. 9–7).

Air-gap technique functions similar to, or in place of, a grid. A distance is introduced between the patient and the image receptor. However, to maintain optimum recorded detail and avoid excessive magnification, the SID must be increased considerably, followed by a *significant increase in mAs*.

8. (D) Gonadal shielding should be used whenever appropriate and possible during radiographic and fluoroscopic examinations. *Flat contact* shields (flat sheets of flexible leaded vinyl) are useful for recumbent studies, but when the exam necessitates that oblique, lateral, or erect projections be obtained, they become less efficient. *Shaped contact (contour)* shields are best because they enclose the male reproductive organs, remaining in position in oblique, lateral, and erect positions—but they can be used only for male patients. *Shadow* shields that attach to the tube head are particularly useful for surgical sterile fields.

9. (A) X-rays produced at the target comprise a heterogeneous primary beam. Filtration serves to eliminate the softer, less-penetrating photons leaving an x-ray beam of higher average energy. Filtration is important in patient protection because unfiltered, low-energy photons not energetic enough to reach the image receptor are absorbed by the body and contribute to total patient dose.

10. (C) Equipment must be properly calibrated to produce consistently predictable results; specifically, the equipment must have *linearity* and *reproducibility*. Linearity refers to consistency in exposure with adjacent mA stations (very similar to reciprocity law) and exposure times adjusted to produce the same mAs. *Reproducibility* refers to consistency in exposure output during repeated exposures at a particular setting. Positive beam limitation (PBL) is automatic collimation. The two types of automatic exposure control (AEC) are the photomultiplier and ionization chamber.

Personnel Protection

10

I. GENERAL CONSIDERATIONS

Radiographers must conscientiously avoid unnecessary radiation exposure to themselves as well as strive to keep patient dose to an absolute minimum. The National Council on Radiation Protection and Measurements (NCRP) recommends personal monitoring for individuals who might receive 10% of the occupational dose equivalent limit of 5 rem/y (50 mSv/y). The use of radiation monitoring devices helps us to evaluate the effectiveness of our radiation protection practices. Monthly reports received from dosimeter laboratories are official legal documents that are reviewed, and attempts made to reduce *any* exposure, no matter how small. Radiographers follow the *ALARA* (As Low As Reasonably Achievable) principle as they carry out their tasks. Radiologic facilities undergo appropriate radiation surveys. Staff is oriented and regular inservice education on radiation safety takes place. Proper radiation monitoring and review of monthly radiation reports is essential.

II. OCCUPATIONAL RADIATION SOURCES

A. SCATTERED RADIATION

When primary photons intercept an object and undergo a change in direction, scattered radiation results.

The most significant occupational radiation hazard in diagnostic radiology is scattered radiation from the patient, particularly in fluoroscopy, where use of high kilovoltage results in energetic Compton scatter emerging from the patient. This poses a real occupational hazard to the radiologist and radiographer. *The intensity of scattered radiation 1 m from the patient is approximately 0.1% of the intensity of the primary beam.* That is why, in terms of radiation protection, the patient is considered the most important source of scatter. Other scattering objects include the x-ray table, the *Bucky-slot cover/closer,* and the *control booth* wall.

B. LEAKAGE RADIATION

Leakage radiation is that which is emitted from the x-ray tube housing in directions other than that of the primary beam. Federal regulations (NCRP) state that lead-lined x-ray tubes must limit leakage radiation to less than 100 mR/h at a distance of 1 m from the x-ray tube.

C. NCRP GUIDELINES

NCRP guidelines regulate equipment design, among other things, in an effort to reduce exposure to personnel and patients. Two other guidelines that serve to reduce exposure to personnel are:

- The control panel must somehow indicate when the x-ray tube is energized (ie, "exposure-on" time) by means of an audible or visible sign.
- The x-ray exposure switch must be a *"dead-man" switch* and situated so that it cannot be operated outside the shielded area.

Some patients are unable to maintain the required radiographic position, for example, infants and children. Mechanical immobilizing and restraining devices, thoughtfully and intelligently used, will serve admirably in most cases. Additional help, though rarely required, should ideally be a nonpregnant relative or friend (older than age 18 years) or, as last recourse, another hospital employee. Radiology personnel must *never* be used to hold patients.

NCRP recommendations regarding protection of the *patient and/ or personnel* during *fluoroscopic* procedures include the following:

- During fluoroscopic procedures, the *image intensifier* serves as a protective barrier from the primary beam and must be the equivalent of 2.0 mm Pb.
- The exposure switch must be the "dead-man" type.
- With under-table fluoroscopic tubes, a Bucky-slot closer/cover having at least the equivalent of 0.25 mm Pb must be available to attenuate scattered radiation (which is about at gonad level).
- A cumulative timing device must be available to signal the fluoroscopist (audibly, visibly, or both) when a maximum of 5 minutes of fluoroscopy time has elapsed.
- A leaded screen drape and table-side shield to reduce scattered radiation to the operator must be available having at least 0.25 mm Pb equivalency.
- The tabletop intensity of the fluoroscopic beam must be less than 10 R/min.
- Protective *lead aprons* must be *at least 0.25 mm Pb* equivalent and must be worn by the workers in the fluoroscopy room.
- Protective *lead gloves* must be at least 0.25 mm Pb equivalent. The unshielded hand must not be placed in the unattenuated or useful beam.
- When fluoroscopy is performed with an undertable image intensifier (as in "remote" x-ray units), palpation must be performed mechanically.

Rules for Selecting Someone to Assist the Patient in the Radiographic Room

- A male (older than age 18 years) is preferred; however, a female who is older than age 18 years and not pregnant may also assist.
- The individual must be provided with protective apparel.
- The individual must be as far as possible from the useful beam.
- The individual must not stand in the path of the useful beam.

Summary

- Time, distance, and shielding are the principle guidelines for reducing radiographic exposure; monitoring evaluates their effectiveness.
- The principle scattering object is the patient; others include the x-ray table, Bucky-slot cover, and control booth walls.
- It is important to be familiar with pertinent guidelines established by the NCRP regulating equipment design, performance, and use (NCRP Report no. 102); radiation protection for medical and allied health personnel (NCRP Report no. 105); and recommendations on limits for exposure to ionizing radiation (NCRP no. 116).
- Mechanical restraining devices should be used to immobilize patients when necessary during radiographic examinations.
- Persons occupationally exposed to radiation must never assist (hold) patients during radiographic examinations.
- If someone is required to assist a patient during an examination, it is essential that radiation safety guidelines be adhered to.
- There are several NCRP recommendations regarding protection during fluoroscopic procedures with which the radiographer should be familiar.

III. FUNDAMENTAL METHODS OF PROTECTION

A. CARDINAL RULES

The practice of effective radiation control depends chiefly on common sense. That is, to safeguard yourself from something harmful you generally remove yourself from it as soon as possible, stay as far away from it as possible, and keep a barrier between it and yourself. Hence, the cardinal principles of *time, distance,* and *shielding.*

The greatest amount of occupational exposure is received in fluoroscopy (including special procedures) and mobile radiography. It is here that the radiographer must place special emphasis on the cardinal rules of radiation protection: time, distance, and shielding. Federal government controls also regulate manufacturing standards for the protection of both personnel and patients.

B. INVERSE SQUARE LAW

Reducing the length of time exposed to ionizing radiation, as in reducing fluoroscopy time, results in a reduction of occupational exposure. Increasing the distance from the source of radiation, as illustrated by the *inverse square law,* results in a reduction of occupational exposure. Placing a barrier, like a lead wall or lead apron, between you and the source of radiation results in a reduction of occupational exposure.

Examples:
- If 10 mrem is received in 1 hour of fluoroscopic procedures, how much will be received if the fluoroscopic time is reduced to 30 minutes? (If the fluoroscopic exposure time is cut in half, from 60 to 30 minutes, the exposure dose received would be correspondingly one half of the original, or 5 mrem.)

• If 40 mrem is received at a distance of 40 inches from the x-ray source, what dose will be received at a distance of 80 inches from the source? (According to the inverse square law, if the distance from the radiation source is doubled, exposure dose will be one fourth of the original quantity, or 10 mrem.)

To reduce exposure dose to health care professionals, patients, and the general population, we must minimize the time of exposure to the source of radiation, provide effective shielding from the radiation source and, most importantly, maximize the distance from the source of radiation.

IV. PRIMARY AND SECONDARY BARRIERS

A. NCRP GUIDELINES

Primary barriers protect against direct exposure from the primary, or useful, x-ray beam and have much greater attenuation capability than *secondary barriers,* which only protect from leakage and scattered radiation.

Examples of primary barriers are the lead walls and doors of a radiographic room, that is, any surface that could be struck by the useful beam. Primary protective barriers of typical installations generally consist of walls with 1/16 inch (1.5 mm) lead thickness and 7 feet high.

Secondary radiation is defined as leakage and/or scattered radiation. The x-ray tube housing protects from leakage radiation as stated previously. The patient is the source of most scattered radiation.

Secondary radiation barriers include that portion of the walls above 7 feet in height; this area requires only 1/32 inch lead. The control booth is also a secondary barrier, toward which the primary beam must never be directed (Fig. 10–1). The radiographer must be protected by the control booth shielding during exposures, and the exposure switch

Attenuation Characteristics of Lead Aprons

X-ray attenuation at:

Pb equiv. thickness	75 kVp	100 kVp
0.25 mm	66%	51%
0.50 mm	88%	75%
1.0 mm	99%	94%

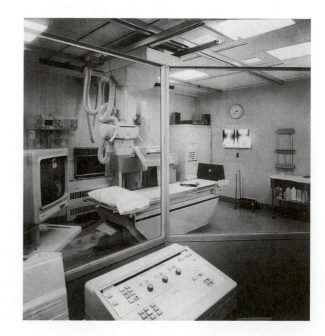

Figure 10–1. The control booth permits the operator to view the patient. The leaded booth and glass protect the operator from exposure to scattered radiation. The control booth is a secondary barrier toward which the primary beam must never be directed. (Courtesy of Nuclear Associates.)

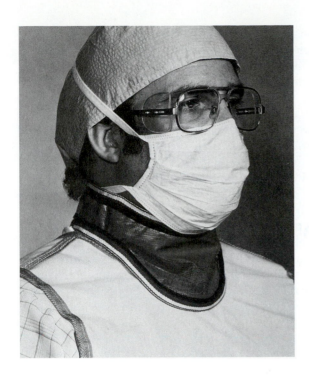

Figure 10–2. Other leaded apparel available for fluoroscopic procedures include thyroid shields and leaded eye wear. (Courtesy of Nuclear Associates.)

or cord must be positioned and attached so that the exposure can only be made *within* the control booth. Leaded glass, usually 1.5 mm Pb equivalent, should be available for patient observation.

B. CARE OF PROTECTIVE APPAREL

During fluoroscopic procedures requiring the radiographer's presence in the radiographic room, the radiographer must wear protective apparel (Fig. 10–2). According to NCRP Report no. 102, lead aprons must provide the equivalent of at least 0.25 mm Pb, and lead gloves at least 0.25 mm Pb equivalent. *Lead aprons and lead gloves are secondary barriers; they will not provide protection from the useful beam!*

Proper care of protective apparel is essential to ensure effectiveness. Lead aprons and gloves should be hung on appropriate racks, not dropped on the floor or folded. Careless handling may result in formation of cracks. Lead aprons and gloves should be imaged annually (either fluoroscopically or radiographically) to check for cracks.

C. PROTECTIVE ACCESSORIES

Another device available for individuals required to remain in the fluoroscopy room is a mobile leaded barrier (Fig. 10–3). Mobile barriers provide full body protection from scattered radiation and are available in a variety of lead equivalents.

V. SPECIAL CONSIDERATIONS

A. PREGNANCY

Deserving special consideration in protection from occupational exposure is the *pregnant radiographer.* As soon as the technologist

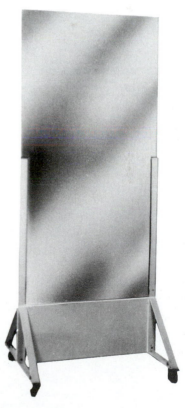

Figure 10–3. Movable leaded barriers provide full body protection for individuals required to remain in the radiographic of fluoroscopic room. Mobile barriers provide protection from secondary radiation and are available in a variety of sizes and lead equivalents. (Courtesy of Nuclear Associates.)

knows she is pregnant, the radiographer *should* notify her supervisor. At that time, her occupational radiation history will be reviewed. She can be supplied with a second (fetal) monitor and any necessary modifications made in her work assignments.

A radiographer who wears his or her radiation monitor on the collar outside the lead apron usually receives less than 100 mrem/y. If a *fetal monitor* were worn under the apron at waist level it would receive 10% of that dose or less than 10 mrem. Because the *gestational dose limit* to the fetus during the gestation period must not exceed *500 mrem,* under typical conditions, when sufficient protection measures are taken, modification of work assignments is not usually necessary. If a fetal, or "baby," monitor is worn, it must be clearly identified and not confused with the radiographer's regular monitor.

However, radiation protection standards should be reviewed during pregnancy and monthly dosimeter reports closely monitored. Many facilities document the counseling received by the pregnant radiographer from the time she advises her supervisor of her pregnancy and makes the signed documents part of the employee's records.

B. MOBILE UNITS

Each *mobile x-ray unit* should have a *lead apron* assigned to it. The radiographer should wear the apron while making the exposure at the furthest distance possible from the x-ray tube. The mobile unit's exposure cord must permit the radiographer to stand at least *6 feet* from the x-ray tube and patient. In *mobile fluoroscopic* units there must be a source to patient skin distance of at least 12 inches.

C. FLUOROSCOPIC UNITS AND PROCEDURES

All *fluoroscopic* equipment must provide at least 12 inches (30 cm), and preferably 15 inches (38 cm), between the x-ray source (focal spot) and the x-ray tabletop (patient), according to NCRP Report no. 102. The *tabletop intensity* of the fluoroscopic beam must not exceed *10 R/min* or 2.1 R/min/mA. Fluoroscopic mA (milliamperes) must not exceed 5, although image intensified fluoroscopy usually operates between 1 and 3 mA. Because the image intensifier functions as a primary barrier, it must have a lead equivalent of at least 2.0 mm.

Beam collimation must be apparent through visualization of unexposed borders on the TV monitor, and *total filtration* must be at least *2.5 mm Al* equivalent. Because occupational exposure to scattered radiation is of considerable importance in fluoroscopy, a *protective curtain* of at least *0.25 mm Pb* equivalent must be placed between the patient and fluoroscopist.

The effect of kVp (kilovoltage peak) and mA adjustment on fluoroscopic images is similar to that on radiographic images. The automatic exposure control automatically varies the exposure required when viewing body tissues of widely differing tissue densities (eg, between the abdomen and chest). *As in radiography, high kVp and low mAs (milliampere-seconds) values are preferred in an effort to reduce dose.*

Summary

- **The cardinal principles of radiation protection are time, distance, and shielding.**

- **Primary barriers protect from the useful (primary) beam; for example, the walls and doors of the radiographic room.**
- **Secondary barriers protect from sources of leakage and scattered radiation; for example, x-ray tube housing, the patient.**
- **Secondary barriers (eg, control panel wall, lead apron) will not afford protection from the primary beam.**
- **There are several NCRP recommendations with which the radiographer should be familiar regarding required thickness and uses of protective shielding (see p. 254).**
- **A pregnant radiographer should advise her supervisor of her condition as soon as possible.**
- **A pregnant radiographer should wear a second monitor at waist level under her lead apron.**
- **Most occupational exposure is received in fluoroscopy, special procedures, and mobile radiography (especially C arm).**

Chapter Exercises

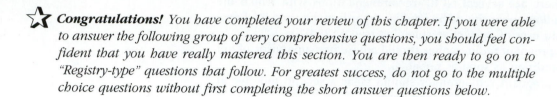 **Congratulations!** *You have completed your review of this chapter. If you were able to answer the following group of very comprehensive questions, you should feel confident that you have really mastered this section. You are then ready to go on to "Registry-type" questions that follow. For greatest success, do not go to the multiple choice questions without first completing the short answer questions below.*

1. What are the three cardinal rules, or principle guidelines, for radiation protection *(p. 255)?*

2. When is personal radiation monitoring required *(p. 253)?*

3. What is the most significant scattering object in fluoroscopy? Why? List other scattering objects *(p. 253).*

4. What are the NCRP rulings on leakage radiation; exposure switches; exposure indicators *(p. 254)?*

5. What resources should be employed to assist and immobilize patients during radioscopic examinations *(p. 254)?*

6. What rules apply if an individual is required in the radiographic room for assistance during a procedure *(p. 254)?*

7. Describe the NCRP rules that are in place for patient and personnel protection during fluoroscopic procedures with respect to *(p. 254):*

    A. image intensifier lead equivalent

    B. exposure switch

    C. Bucky-slot cover

    D. cumulative timer

    E. lead drape or curtain

    F. tabletop intensity maximum

    G. apron and glove lead equivalency

    H. palpation with remote fluoroscopy units

8. Distinguish between and give examples of primary and secondary barriers *(p. 256)*.

9. What is the usual recommended thickness of x-ray room walls; the recommended height *(p. 256)?*

10. What protects from leakage radiation *(p. 256)?*

11. Identify each of the following as primary or secondary barriers: x-ray room walls, control panel, lead aprons, and gloves *(p. 256)*.

12. How should lead aprons and gloves be cared for *(p. 257)?*

13. Describe how a pregnant radiographer might use a second personal monitor *(pp. 257–258)*.

14. What is the gestational fetal dose limit *(p. 258)?*

15. What kinds of counseling and documentation are recommended for the pregnant radiographer *(p. 258)?*

16. What x-ray areas generally have the highest occupational exposure *(p. 258)?*

17. What NCRP rules govern mobile radiography with respect to availability of lead aprons, the exposure cord, the fluoroscope source-to-skin distance (SSD) *(p. 258)?*

18. What NCRP rules govern fluoroscopy equipment with respect to SSD, tabletop intensity, maximum mA, image intensifier lead equivalent, fluoroscopy exposure switch *(p. 258)?*

19. What NCRP rules govern fluoroscopy equipment with respect to collimation, total filtration, protective curtain, Bucky-slot cover, cumulative timer *(p. 258)?*

A&U Chapter Review Questions

1. Which of the following is (are) guidelines used to reduce personnel and/or patient dose in fluoroscopy?
   1. maximum tabletop intensity of 10 R/min
   2. maximum SSD of 12 inches
   3. minimum filtration of 2.5 mm Al equivalent
   (A) 1 only
   (B) 1 and 2 only
   (C) 1 and 3 only
   (D) 1, 2, and 3

2. Which of the following is (are) features of fluoroscopy equipment, designed especially to eliminate unnecessary radiation to patient and personnel?
   1. protective curtain
   2. filtration
   3. collimation
   (A) 1 only
   (B) 1 and 2 only
   (C) 1 and 3 only
   (D) 1, 2, and 3

3. How much protection is provided from a 75 kVp x-ray beam when using a 0.25-mm lead-equivalent apron?
   (A) 51%
   (B) 66%
   (C) 88%
   (D) 99%

4. Radiation dose to personnel is reduced by the following exposure cord guidelines:
   1. exposure cords on fixed equipment must be very short
   2. exposure cords on mobile equipment must be at least 6 feet long
   3. exposure cords on fixed and mobile equipment should be the coiled expandable type
   (A) 1 only
   (B) 1 and 2 only
   (C) 2 and 3 only
   (D) 1, 2, and 3

5. Which of the following groups of exposure factors will deliver the *least* amount of exposure to the patient?
   (A) 100 mAs, 100 kVp
   (B) 200 mAs, 90 kVp
   (C) 400 mAs, 80 kVp
   (D) 800 mAs, 70 kVp

6. Some patients, such as infants and children, are unable to stay in the necessary radiographic position and require assistance. If mechanical restraining devices cannot be used, who of the following is BEST suited to hold these patients?
   (A) floor nurse
   (B) transporter
   (C) friend or relative
   (D) student radiographer

7. Each time an x-ray photon scatters, its intensity at 1 m from the scattering object is what fraction of its original intensity?
   (A) 1/10
   (B) 1/100
   (C) 1/500
   (D) 1/1000

8. If an individual received 45 mR while standing at 4 feet from a source of radiation for 2 minutes, which of the options listed below will *most* effectively reduce his or her radiation exposure?
   (A) standing 6 feet from the source for 2 minutes
   (B) standing 5 feet from the source for 1 minute
   (C) standing 4 feet from the source for 3 minutes
   (D) standing 3 feet from the source for 2 minutes

9. Primary radiation barriers must be at least how high?
   (A) 5 feet
   (B) 6 feet
   (C) 7 feet
   (D) 8 feet

10. The protective control booth from which the radiographer makes the x-ray exposure is a:
   (A) primary barrier
   (B) secondary barrier
   (C) useful beam barrier
   (D) remnant radiation barrier

Answers and Explanations

1. (C) All *fluoroscopic* equipment must provide *at least* 12 inches (30 cm), and preferably 15 inches (38 cm), between the x-ray source (focal spot) and the x-ray tabletop, according to NCRP Report no. 102. The tabletop *intensity* of the fluoroscopic beam must not exceed 10 *R/min* or 2.1 R/min/mA. Fluoroscopic mA must not exceed 5, although image-intensified fluoroscopy usually operates between 1 and 3 mA. The image intensifier functions as a primary barrier and has a lead equivalent of 2.0 mm.

2. (D) The *protective* curtain is usually made of leaded vinyl with at least 0.25 mm Pb equivalent. It must be positioned between the patient and fluoroscopist and greatly reduces exposure of the fluoroscopist to energetic scatter from the patient. Just as overhead radiation barrier equipment, fluoroscopic total *filtration* must be at least 2.5 mm Al equivalent to reduce excessive exposure to low-energy radiation. *Collimator* or beam alignment must be accurate to within 2%.

3. (B) Lead aprons are worn by occupationally exposed individuals during fluoroscopic procedures. Lead aprons are available with various lead equivalents; 0.25, 0.5, and 1.0 mm are the most common. The *1.0-mm* lead-equivalent apron will provide close to 100% protection at most kVp levels, but it is rarely used because it weighs anywhere from 12 to 24 pounds! A *0.25-mm* lead-equivalent apron will attenuate about 97% of a 50-kVp x-ray beam, 66% of a 75-kVp beam, and 51% of a 100-kVp beam. A *0.5-mm* apron will attenuate about 99% of a 50-kVp beam, 88% of a 75-kVp beam, and 75% of a 100-kVp beam.

4. (B) Radiographic and fluoroscopic equipment is designed to help decrease the exposure dose to patient and operator. One of the design features is the exposure cord. Exposure cords on *fixed* equipment must be short enough to prevent the exposure from being made outside the control booth. Exposure cords on *mobile* equipment must be long enough to permit the operator to stand at least 6 feet from the x-ray tube.

5. (A) mAs regulates the *quantity* of radiation delivered to the patient. kVp regulates the *quality* (penetration) of the radiation delivered to the patient. Therefore, higher-energy (more penetrating) radiation—which is more likely to exit the patient—accompanied by lower mAs, is the safest combination for the patient.

6. (C) If mechanical restraint is impossible, a friend or relative accompanying the patient should be requested to hold the patient. If a friend or relative is not available, a nurse or transporter may be asked for help. Protective apparel, such as lead apron and gloves, should be provided to the person(s) holding the patient. *Radiology personnel must NEVER assist in holding patients, and the individual assisting should NEVER be in the path of the primary beam.*

Beam collimation must be apparent through visualization of unexposed borders on the TV monitor, and *total filtration* must be at least 2.5 mm Al equivalent. Because occupational exposure to scattered radiation is of considerable importance in fluoroscopy, a protective curtain of at least 0.25 mm Pb equivalent must be placed between the patient and fluoroscopist.

7. (D) One of the radiation protection guidelines for the occupationally exposed is that the x-ray beam must scatter twice before reaching the operator. Each time the x-ray beam scatters, its intensity at 1 m from the scattering object is approximately 0.1% of the intensity of the primary beam, that is, *one-thousandth* of its original intensity. That is why, in terms of radiation protection, the patient is considered the most important source of scatter. Of course, the operator should be behind a shielded booth while making the exposure, but multiple scatterings further reduce danger of exposure from scatter radiation. Other scattering objects include the x-ray table, the Bucky-slot cover, and the control booth wall.

8. (B) A quick survey of the distractors reveals that options C and D will *increase* exposure dose; thus, they are eliminated as possible correct answers. Both A and B will serve to reduce radiation exposure, as distance is increased and exposure time is decreased in each case. It remains to be seen then, which is the more effective. Using the inverse square law of radiation, it is found that the individual will receive *15 mR at 6 feet in 2 minutes* and *14.4 mR at 5 feet in 1 minute*:

$$\frac{I_1}{I_2} = \frac{D_2^2}{D_1^2}$$

Substituting known values from distractor (A):

$$\frac{45 \text{ mR}}{x} = \frac{6 \text{ ft}^2}{4 \text{ ft}^2}$$

$$\frac{45}{x} = \frac{36}{16}$$

$$36x = 720$$

$$x = 20 \text{ mR at 6 feet for 2 minutes}$$

$$\frac{I_1}{I_2} = \frac{D_2^2}{D_1^2}$$

Substituting known values from distractor (B):

$$\frac{45 \text{ mR}}{x} = \frac{5 \text{ ft}^2}{4 \text{ ft}^2}$$

$$\frac{45}{x} = \frac{25}{16}$$

$$25x = 720$$

$x = 28.8$ mR at 5 feet for 2 minutes, *therefore 14.4 mR in 1 minute*

Note the inverse relationship between distance and dose. As distance from the source of radiation increases, dose rate significantly decreases.

9. (C) Radiation protection guidelines have established that *primary radiation barriers* must be 7 feet high. Primary radiation barriers are walls that the primary beam might be directed toward. They usually contain 1.5 mm lead, but this can vary depending on *use factor* and other factors.

10. (B) *Primary barriers* are those that protect us from the primary or useful beam. They have much greater attenuation capability than secondary barriers, which only protect from leakage and scattered radiation. The radiographic room walls are therefore considered primary barriers because the primary beam is often directed toward them, as in chest radiography. Most control booth barriers, however, are *secondary barriers* and the primary beam is never directed toward them. They are usually constructed of four thicknesses of gypsum board and/or 0.5 to 1 inch of plate glass. Remnant radiation penetrates the patient and forms the latent image on the image receptor.

Radiation Exposure and Monitoring

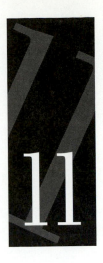

I. UNITS OF MEASURE

W.C. Röntgen's paper, "On A New Kind of Rays," described the ionizing effect of x-rays on air and their effect on photographic emulsions. We still use these principles today to detect and quantify radiation exposure.

The (traditional) radiation units of measure of greatest importance to the radiographer are the roentgen, rad, and rem. The ARRT radiography certification examination identifies SI (International System of Units) units (according to the January 2001 specifications) in parentheses following the traditional unit of measure.

A. THE ROENTGEN

The ARRT examination does not capitalize "roentgen" as a unit of measure, and no "s" is used at the end; for example, 10 roentgen, *not* 10 Roentgens (the same is true for the terms rad and rem). When used to express *rate*, it is abbreviated R/min or R/h. The *roentgen* is a unit of measure of *ionization in air*, and referred to as the *unit of exposure*. Because x-rays ionize air, all the ions of *either* sign (positive or negative) formed in a particular quantity of air are counted and equated to a quantity of radiation expressed in the unit *roentgen*. The roentgen is valid only for *x and gamma radiations* at energies up to 3 MeV (megavolts).

The roentgen SI unit of measure is C/kg (coulomb per kilogram).

B. THE RAD

Rad is an acronym for *radiation absorbed dose*. As radiation passes through matter, a certain amount of energy is deposited in that matter. Absorbed dose refers to the amount of energy deposited per unit mass and is strongly related to chemical change and biologic damage. The amount of energy deposited and, thus, the amount of possible biologic damage is dependent upon the following:

- Type of radiation
- Atomic number of the tissue
- Energy of the radiation

Particulate radiation (alpha, beta, etc.) is highly ionizing. As an *internal* source of radiation, it increases LET (linear energy transfer), and a significant biologic effect can result. As an *external* source of radiation, it is virtually innocuous. As the atomic number of the irradiated tissue increases, more x-ray photons are absorbed by tissues (the photoelectric interaction increases), and LET increases. As the energy of radiation increases, it becomes more penetrating and LET decreases, thereby decreasing the likelihood of biologic effects.

Because the rad does not take into account the biologic effect of various types of radiation, it is not used to express occupational exposure.

The rad SI unit of measure is the Gy (gray).

C. THE REM

Rem is an acronym for *radiation equivalent man*. Rem uses the information collected for the rad, but also uses a quality factor (QF) to predict biologic effects from different types of radiation. Radiations having a high QF have a higher LET and greater potential to produce biologic damage. The rem is described as the unit of *dose equivalency* (DE), and is used to express occupational exposure.

The rem SI unit of measure is the Sv (sievert).

II. MONITORING DEVICES

A. NATIONAL COUNCIL ON RADIATION PROTECTION AND MEASUREMENTS (NCRP) GUIDELINES FOR USE

Radiation monitoring is used to evaluate the effectiveness of the radiation safety policies and practices in place. The Code of Federal Regulations (CFR) states that monitoring be provided for occupationally exposed individuals in a controlled area who are likely to receive more than *one-tenth the dose equivalent limit*.

B. OPTICALLY STIMULATED LUMINESCENCE DOSIMETER

Optically stimulated luminescence (*OSL*) dosimeters are gradually replacing the long-used film badge (Fig. 11–1). The OSL contains a thin layer of *aluminum oxide* (Al_2O_3). Aluminum oxide absorbs and stores the energy associated with exposure to ionizing radiation. When the OSL is returned to the laboratory for processing, the Al_2O_3 chips are stimulated with laser light. This process causes a release of visible light from the Al_2O_3 in proportion to the amount of ionizing radiation absorbed. The quantity of light emitted is equated to a radiation quantity expressed in mrem on the written report returned to the user. The advantages of the OSL include the ability to measure radiation doses as low as 1 mrem (with a precision of ±1 mrem) and to be reanalyzed if necessary. Their tamper-proof plastic package is unaffected by heat, moisture, and pressure.

C. FILM BADGE

A very familiar radiation monitor is the *film badge*. It consists of special radiation dosimetry film packaged like dental film and is enclosed in a special plastic holder. The plastic holder features an open window (through which the user's name appears) and various *filters*, which serve to identify the *type and energy of radiation* (Fig. 11–2).

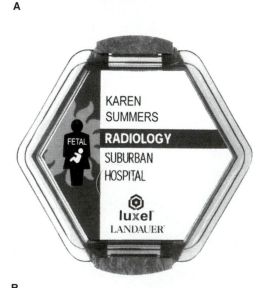

A

B

Figure 11–1. The optically stimulated luminescence dosimeter. (Courtesy of Landauer, Inc., Glenwood, IL.)

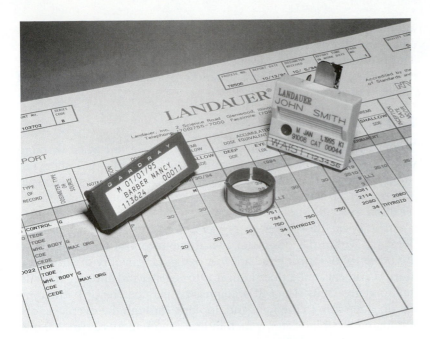

Figure 11–2. The film badge (*left*) contains filters that function to determine the type and energy of radiation received by the wearer. The thermoluminescent dosimeter (*right*) contains thermoluminescent crystals that emit quantities of light proportional to their degree of exposure. The ring badge (*center*) is particularly useful for individuals whose hands are in close proximity to radioactive nuclides or the fluoroscopic x-ray field. A report similar to the one shown is returned monthly, documenting the radiation dose received by each of the personal monitors. (Courtesy of Landauer, Inc., Glenwood, IL.)

Radiation that exposes film behind an aluminum filter is more energetic than radiation that only passes through the open window, and less energetic than radiation penetrating a copper filter. Film badges are used for *1 month,* collected, and sent to a special laboratory for processing. The degree of exposure is carefully evaluated and equated to a dose, usually expressed in *mrem;* the film badge can measure doses as low as 10 mrem. An official written report is sent to the sponsoring institution (see Fig. 11–2).

Film badges have been the most widely used personal radiation monitors, but are gradually being replaced by the OSL.

D. *THERMOLUMINESCENT DOSIMETER*

The thermoluminescent dosimeter (TLD) (see Fig. 11–2) contains crystalline chips of lithium fluoride (LiF). LiF absorbs and stores the energy associated with exposure to ionizing radiation. When the TLD is returned to the laboratory for processing, the LiF chips are heated. This process causes a release of visible light from the chips in proportion to the amount of ionizing radiation absorbed. The quantity of light emitted is equated to a radiation quantity expressed in mrem on the written report returned to the user. The TLD is more sensitive and precise than the film badge because it can measure doses as low as 5 mrem. The TLD is unaffected by heat or humidity and can be worn up to 3 months before processing. However, in the unlikely event that the user had unknowingly received excessive radiation exposure, the user should be made aware of it as soon as possible, and the event should be recent enough to be able to recall. This is often considered the single disadvantage of the TLD. Both the film badge and TLD measure a variety of energies of x, beta, and gamma radiations.

E. POCKET DOSIMETER

The use of a *pocket dosimeter* (Fig. 11–3) is indicated when working with high exposures or large quantities of radiation for a short period of time, so that an immediate reading is available to the user. The pocket dosimeter is sensitive and accurate but has limited application in diagnostic radiography.

The pocket dosimeter, or *pocket isolation chamber,* resembles a penlight. Within the dosimeter is a thimble ionization chamber. In the presence of ionizing radiation, a particular quantity of air will be ionized and cause the fiber indicator to register radiation quantity in milliroentgen (mR). The self-reading type may be "read" by holding the dosimeter up to the light and, looking through the eyepiece, observing the fiber indicator, which indicates a quantity of 0 to 200 mR. The disadvantage of the pocket dosimeter is that it does not provide a permanent legal record of exposure.

Personnel monitors should be worn consistently in the same place and facing forward (ie, with the open window and user's identification visible). The use of a second monitor is occasionally indicated. The *pregnant radiographer* may wear a second, waist level, dosimeter under her lead apron to approximate fetal dose. If the first badge is worn at the collar outside the lead apron it will approximate dose to the head and neck and will provide an overestimation of dose to the shielded organs. Some procedures require the hands to be near the useful beam (eg, some fluoroscopic and vascular procedures). A finger, or ring, monitor will provide information on exposure to the hands.

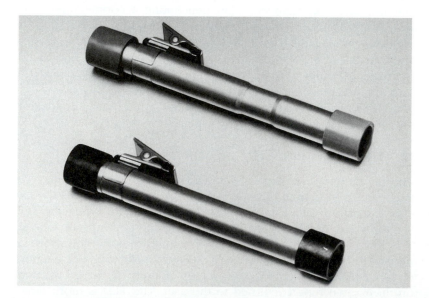

Figure 11–3. The pocket dosimeter contains a small ionization chamber that counts charges in proportion to the exposure received. (Courtesy of Nuclear Associates.)

The radiographer is occupationally exposed to *low energy, low LET* radiation. Monitoring devices are worn only for occupational purposes and never if the individual is exposed for medical or dental reasons.

III. NCRP RECOMMENDATIONS

A part of the professional radiographer's responsibility lies in keeping occupational exposure to a minimum. The use of radiation monitoring devices helps evaluate the effectiveness of radiation protection practices. The periodic reports received from OSL, film badge, or TLD laboratories are official legal documents that must be reviewed, and an attempt should be made to reduce *any* exposure, no matter how small.

NCRP Report no. 105 and the Code of Federal Regulations (10 CFR §20) require that occupationally exposed individuals 18 years of age and older not receive exposures in excess of 5 rem (5000 mrem) annually. A radiography student beginning his or her training before the age of 18 years must not receive an annual dose of more than 0.1 rem (100 mrem).

The lifetime cumulative exposure for the occupationally exposed individual is determined using the formula: 1 rem × age in years. Thus, a 26-year-old radiographer's lifetime occupational exposure must not exceed 26 rem. The pregnant radiographer's *gestational* exposure to the fetus must not exceed 0.5 rem (500 mrem); the *monthly* fetal dose must not exceed 0.05 rem (50 mrem).

These are the recommended maximum dose equivalent limits. The *actual* mean annual exposure to occupationally exposed medical personnel is 100 to 140 mrem, well below the recommended limit! This seems to indicate that we are performing our tasks in a safe, conscientious, and ethical manner.

Summary

- The roentgen (R unit), or unit of exposure, is the unit used to describe quantity of ionization in air.
- The rad describes absorbed dose.
- The rem is the unit of dose equivalency (DE), used to quantify occupational exposure.
- The OSL is the newest, most accurate personal dosimeter. It uses a thin layer of Al_2O_3 to store information.
- Film badges are convenient, low-cost radiation monitors that are processed monthly.
- TLDs use LiF crystals to store exposure information. They are more precise and more expensive than film badges and may be processed quarterly.
- Film badges and TLDs measure exposure to beta, x, and gamma radiation.
- Pocket dosimeters are thimble ionization chambers used to monitor larger quantities of radiation exposure, up to 200 mR.
- Radiographers must strive to keep their occupational dose ALARA.
- NCRP Report no. 91 and the Code of Federal Regulations (10 CFR §20) establish limits for exposure to ionizing radiation with which radiographers should be familiar.

Chapter Exercises

 Congratulations! *You have completed your review of this chapter. If you are able to answer the following group of very comprehensive questions, you should feel confident that you have really mastered this section. You are then ready to go on to "Registry-type" questions that follow. For greatest success, do not go to the multiple choice questions without first completing the short answer questions below.*

1. Discuss the R as a unit of measure, including what it measures, the radiation(s) it measures, and up to what energy *(p. 267)*.

2. What does the acronym *rad* mean? Define rad *(p. 267)*.

3. Name the three things influencing the amount of energy deposited (rad) in tissue *(p. 267)*.

4. Relate particulate radiation to degree of ionization in tissue, to LET, and to possible biologic effects *(p. 268)*.

5. What does the acronym *rem* mean *(p. 268)*?

6. Why can the rem be accurately used to describe occupational DE, whereas the rad cannot *(p. 268)*?

7. Describe the film badge. Include the following in your description *(pp. 268–269)*:

    A. construction

    B. purpose of filters

    C. length of time used

    D. type(s) of radiation detected

    E. how it is "read" and in what unit

    F. any advantages or disadvantages

8. Describe the TLD. Include the following in your description *(pp. 269–270)*:

    A. construction

    B. type of crystals used; their unique characteristics

C. length of time used

D. type(s) of radiation detected

E. how it is "read" and in what unit

F. any advantages or disadvantages

9. Describe the pocket dosimeter. Include the following in your description *(p. 270):*

A. construction

B. indications for use

C. how it is "read," in what unit, and up to what maximum

D. any advantages or disadvantages

10. What is the NCRP recommended dose limit for occupational exposure in individuals younger than 18 years of age? Older than 18 years of age *(p. 271)?*

11. How is lifetime cumulative occupational exposure determined *(p. 271)?*

12. What is the NCRP recommended dose limit for gestational fetal exposure *(p. 271)?*

A&U Chapter Review Questions

1. What is the established fetal dose-limit guideline for pregnant radiographers during the entire gestation period?
   (A) 0.1 rem
   (B) 0.5 rem
   (C) 5.0 rem
   (D) 10.0 rem

2. If a student radiographer who is younger than 18 years of age begins clinical assignments, what is his or her annual dose limit?
   (A) 0.1 rem (1 mSv)
   (B) 0.5 rem (5 mSv)
   (C) 5 rem (50 mSv)
   (D) 10 rem (100 mSv)

3. The NCRP recommends an annual effective occupational dose equivalent limit of:
   (A) 25 mSv (2.5 rem)
   (B) 50 mSv (5 rem)
   (C) 100 mSv (10 rem)
   (D) 200 mSv (20 rem)

4. The dose-limits established for occupationally exposed individuals is valid for:
   (A) alpha, beta, and x-radiations
   (B) x and gamma radiations only
   (C) beta, x, and gamma radiations
   (D) all ionizing radiations

5. The operation of personal radiation monitoring devices depends on which of the following?
   1. ionization
   2. thermoluminescence
   3. resonance
   (A) 1 only
   (B) 1 and 2 only
   (C) 2 and 3 only
   (D) 1, 2, and 3

6. Which of the following is a measure of dose to biologic tissue?
   (A) roentgen (C/kg)
   (B) rad (Gy)
   (C) rem (Sv)
   (D) RBE (relative biologic effectiveness)

7. An optically luminescent dosimetry system would use which of the following crystals?
   (A) silver bromide
   (B) aluminum oxide
   (C) lithium fluoride
   (D) ferrous sulfate

8. During which period of development is the fetus most radiosensitive?
   (A) first trimester
   (B) second trimester
   (C) third trimester
   (D) fourth trimester

9. The unit of measure used to express occupational exposure is the:
   (A) roentgen (C/Kg)
   (B) rad (Gray)
   (C) rem (Sievert)
   (D) RBE

10. The purpose of filters in a film badge is:
   (A) to eliminate harmful rays
   (B) to measure radiation quality
   (C) to prevent exposure from alpha particles
   (D) as a support for film contained within

Answers and Explanations

1. (B) The declared pregnant radiographer poses a special radiation protection consideration, for the safety of the unborn individual must be considered. It must be remembered that the developing fetus is particularly sensitive to radiation exposure. Therefore, established guidelines state that the occupational radiation exposure to the fetus must not exceed 0.5 rem (500 mrem or 5 mSv) during the entire gestation period.

2. (A) Because the established dose limit formula guideline is used for occupationally exposed persons 18 years of age and older, guidelines had to be established in the event a student entered training prior to age 18 years. The guideline states that the occupational dose limit for students younger than age 18 years is 0.1 rem (100 mrem or 1 mSv) in any given year.

3. (B) A 1984 review of radiation exposure data revealed that the average annual dose equivalent for monitored radiation workers was approximately 2.3 mSv (0.23 rem). The fact that this is approximately one-tenth the recommended limit indicates that the limit is adequate for radiation protection purposes. Consequently, the NCRP reiterates its 1971 recommended annual limit of 50 mSv (5 rem). *(NCRP Report No. 105, pp. 14–15.)*

4. (C) The occupational dose-limit is valid for beta, x, and gamma radiations. Because alpha radiation is so rapidly ionizing, traditional personal monitors will not record alpha radiation. Because alpha particles are capable of penetrating only a few cm of air, they are practically harmless as an external source of radiation.

5. (B) Ionization is the fundamental principle of operation of both the film badge and pocket dosimeter. In the film badge, the film's silver halide emulsion is ionized by x-ray photons. The pocket dosimeter contains an ionization chamber, and the number of ionizations taking place may be equated to exposure dose. Resonance refers to motion, and has no application to personal radiation monitoring.

6. (C) Roentgen is the unit of exposure; it measures the quantity of ionization in air. Rad is an acronym for radiation absorbed dose; it measures the energy deposited in any material. Rem is an acronym for radiation equivalent man; it includes the relative biologic effectiveness (RBE) specific to the tissue irradiated, thereby being a valid unit of measure of dose to biologic material.

7. (B) Optically stimulated luminescent dosimeters (OSLs) are personal radiation monitors that use aluminum oxide crystals. These crystals, once exposed to ionizing radiation and then stimulated with a laser, give off light proportional to the amount of radiation received. OSLs are very accurate personal monitors. Thermoluminescent dosimeters (TLDs) use lithium fluoride as the sensitive crystal.

8. (A) The first trimester of the developing fetus is the most radiosensitive. Because the fetus is undergoing major organogenesis, very high doses of radiation at this time can cause congenital anomalies. Radiosensitivity gradually decreases through the rest of the pregnancy.

9. (C) *Roentgen* is the unit of exposure; it measures the quantity of ionizations in air. *Rad* is an acronym for **r**adiation **a**bsorbed **d**ose; it measures the energy deposited in any material. *Rem* is an acronym for **r**adiation **e**quivalent **m**an; it includes the relative biologic effectiveness (RBE) specific to the tissue irradiated, thereby being a valid unit of measure of dose to biologic material.

10. (B) Film badge filters (usually aluminum and copper) serve to help measure radiation quality (energy). Only the most energetic radiation will penetrate the copper; radiation of lower levels will penetrate the aluminum, and the lowest energy radiation will pass readily through the unfiltered area. Thus radiation of different energy levels can be recorded, measured, and reported.

Image Production and Evaluation

Technical Factors

Radiography students occasionally find the area of technical factors, or "technique," to be their first stumbling block. Everything prior to this may have seemed so straightforward and understandable: radiation protection, anatomy, positioning, even physics. Why is it that technique can be so confusing? Perhaps it is because there are so many variables, so many choices to be made, so many factors to consider.

The most obvious variable, and the one in which the least modification is possible, is the *patient.* The importance of careful and accurate patient evaluation cannot be overemphasized. Body habitus, muscle tone, pathology, trauma, and age all require accurate assessment prior to the intelligent selection of technical factors.

Even when using automatic exposure control (AEC) or computerized or digital imaging, the radiographer's accurate evaluation of the patient will result in more efficient use of the technology. Sometimes, AEC selection will require adjustment or modification; sometimes it will be necessary to use manual technique.

After evaluating the patient, various radiographic accessories must be considered: screen and film combinations, grid ratios, and filters, to name a few. Fortunately, these items are fairly standard from one radiographic room to the next within a given department. When it comes to mobile radiography or being able to move from one department to another, however, a good working knowledge of radiographic accessories and their use is required.

What about circumstances that require deviation from the normal source-to-image-receptor distance (SID), or the introduction of an object-to-image-receptor distance (OID)? What if the patient's leg is casted? How does "coning down" (collimating) affect the radiographic image? Why does kVp (kilovoltage peak) affect radiographic density as well as regulate radiographic contrast?

This chapter will structure and show the relationship among these variables, and will provide a clear presentation and complete review of their impact on the radiographic image.

I. FACTORS AFFECTING RECORDED DETAIL AND DISTORTION

The term *recorded detail* refers to the *clarity,* or *resolution,* with which a radiographic image is rendered. If the tiny image details (eg, bony trabeculae, minute calcifications) of a variety of radiographs made under different circumstances were compared, especially with the use of a magnifying glass, it would be noted that the image details appear with varying degrees of clarity. On some of the radiographs, details would be clearly defined, while on other radiographs, the borders of details would have varying degrees of unsharpness, that is they would not be defined as sharply nor with the same degree of resolution. This is the basic concept of recorded detail.

The term *distortion* refers to misrepresentation of the actual *size (magnification)* or *shape (foreshortening* or *elongation)* of the structures imaged, which may be partly or wholly caused by inherent object unsharpness.

The degree of *resolution* transferred to the image receptor is a function of the resolving power of each of the system components and is expressed in *line pairs per millimeter* (lp/mm) (Fig. 12–1). Resolution describes how closely fine details may be associated and still

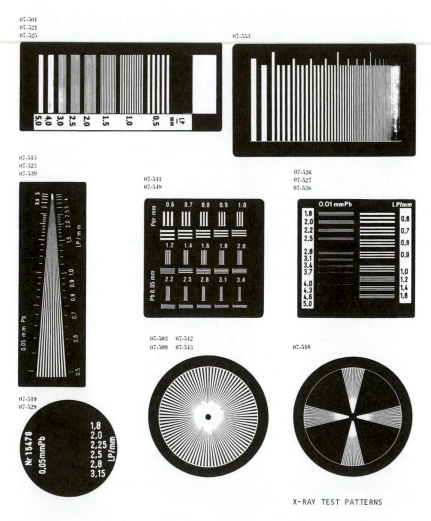

Figure 12–1. *Resolution test pattern.* Resolution is measured with the use of a resolution test pattern and is expressed in *line pairs per millimeter* (lp/mm). The *star pattern* is generally used for focal spot size evaluation, while the *parallel line* type is used for evaluating intensifying screens. (Courtesy of Nuclear Associates.)

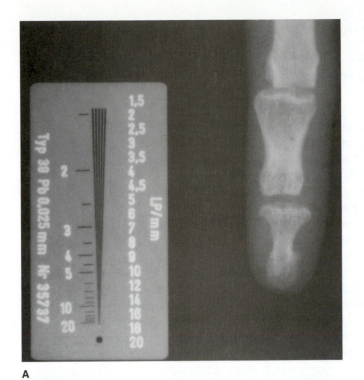

A

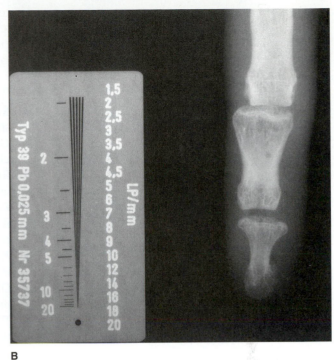

B

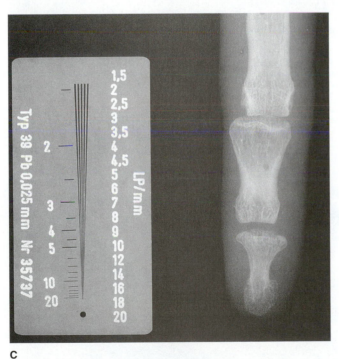

C

Figure 12–2. *Magnified views of the first phalanx and resolution test pattern.* **(A)** Significant blur or unsharpness of image details; resolution is approximately *6 lp/mm.* **(B)** Improved recorded detail; resolution of about *8 lp/mm.* **(C)** Best recorded detail (least blur); resolution of about *12 lp/mm.* (From the American College of Radiology Learning File. Courtesy of the American College of Radiology.)

be recognized as separate details before seeming to blend into each other and appear "as one" (Fig. 12–2).

The term "visibility of detail" refers to *how well the recorded detail can be seen;* for example, excessive density or scattered radiation fog impairs detail visibility because it obscures the details. Density and fog have no effect on how sharply an image detail is rendered; they do, however, determine how easily we are able to recognize those details (ie, *visibility* of detail).

There are a number of technical factors that impact recorded detail. Some of them influence the geometry (size and shape) of the image, and others affect its photographic qualities. Each of the factors having an effect on recorded detail will be discussed further.

Summary

- **Recorded detail refers to the sharpness and abruptness of structural detail borders.**
- **Other terms that refer to *recorded detail* are: resolution, clarity, definition, and sharpness.**
- **Recorded detail is measured with a *resolution test pattern* and expressed in *lp/mm*.**
- **Recorded detail is affected by a number of factors; some influence the geometry of the image, while others affect its photographic qualities.**
- **Anything that affects density or contrast affects *visibility of detail*.**
- **Distortion relates to the size and shape of the *image* compared to the actual size and shape of the *object*.**
- **The terms *magnification, elongation,* and *foreshortening* are used when describing distortion.**

A. DISTANCES

If you place your hand between a flashlight and the wall of a dimly lighted room, the shadow of your hand will vary in size and clarity as it changes position with respect to the flashlight and wall. As your

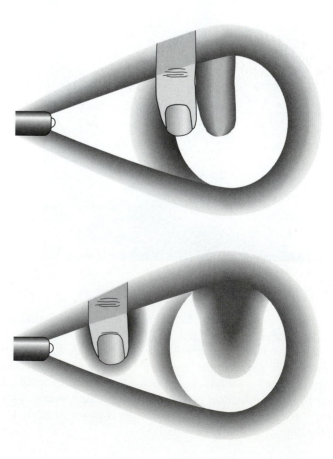

Figure 12–3. *Effect of distance on magnification and detail.* As the finger moves away from the surface (toward the light source), the shadow image becomes magnified and blurry.

hand moves farther from the wall, the shadow becomes larger and less distinct. As your hand is brought closer to the wall (and farther from the flashlight) the shadow becomes more like the actual size of your hand and appears with more clarity (Fig. 12–3).

1. OID. This is the effect object-to-image-receptor distance *(OID)* has on recorded detail. Because (like visible light) the x-ray beam diverges as it leaves its source, an increase in OID will increase *magnification.* X-ray photons strike all parts of the object, continue traveling in a divergent fashion, and "deposit" the (now magnified and unsharp) image on the film or other image receptor (Fig. 12–4). *Geometrically recorded detail improves as OID decreases.*

2. SID. A similar example can be used to show the effect of source-to-image-receptor distance *(SID)* on recorded detail. If your hand is placed a given distance from the wall, any change in the distance between the light source and wall will affect the magnification and clarity of the shadow image. As the flashlight moves closer to your hand, the shadow will become larger and less distinct. As the flashlight is moved farther from the wall, the shadow approaches the actual size of your hand and becomes sharper and more distinct (Fig. 12–5). Similarly, as the distance between the x-ray source and image recorder increases, the x-ray image is less magnified and more distinct (Fig. 12–6). *Geometrically recorded detail improves as SID increases.*

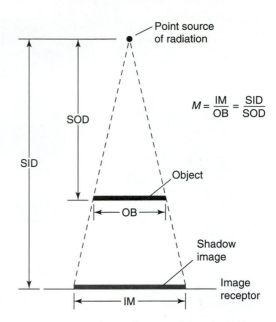

$$M = \frac{IM}{OB} = \frac{SID}{SOD}$$

Figure 12–4. As distance from the object to the image receptor (OID) increases, the projected size of the image increases, that is, magnification increases. (Modified from Wolbarst AB. *Physics of Radiology.* East Norwalk, CT: Appleton & Lange, 1993.)

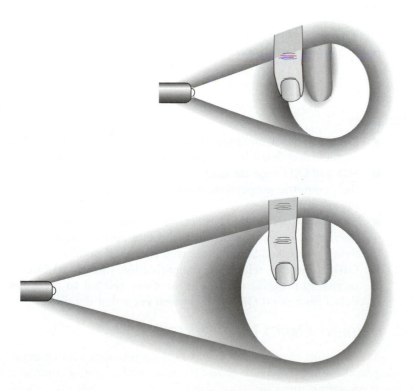

Figure 12–5. *Effect of distance on magnification and detail.* As the flashlight moves closer to the finger, the shadow image becomes magnified and blurry.

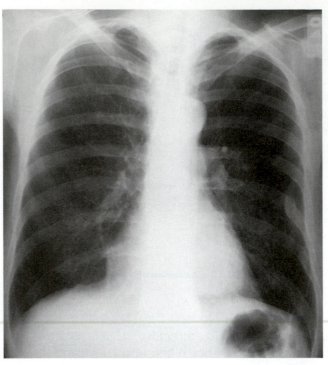

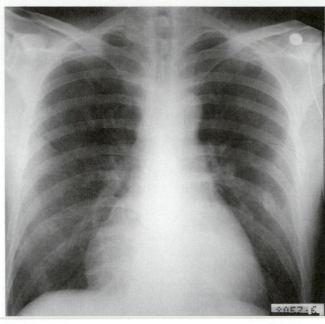

Figure 12–6. **(A)** Posteroanterior (PA) erect chest taken at a distance of 6 feet demonstrates an accurate representation of the heart shadow and various parenchymal and bony structures. **(B)** Anteroposterior (AP) erect at 50 inches of the same patient taken within 24 hours and with no change in patient condition. The heart appears markedly larger (15.5 cm on PA and 20 cm on AP) for two reasons: (1) the heart is farther from the image receptor in the AP projection, and (2) the SID is decreased, thus, the heart is magnified. (From the American College of Radiology Learning File. Courtesy of the American College of Radiology.)

Summary

- **Recorded detail and magnification are inversely related, that is, recorded detail increases as magnification decreases.**
- **SID and OID regulate magnification and therefore influence the geometric properties, and hence recorded detail, of the radiographic image.**
- **SID is inversely related to magnification (increased SID = decreased magnification) and directly related to recorded detail (increased SID = increased recorded detail).**
- **OID is directly related to magnification (increased OID = increased magnification) and inversely related to recorded detail (increased OID = decreased recorded detail).**

B. INHERENT OBJECT UNSHARPNESS

A certain amount of *object unsharpness* is an inherent part of every radiographic image *because of the position and shape of anatomic structures within the body.*

1. Position within the Body. Structures within the three-dimensional human body lie in different planes. For example, the frontal

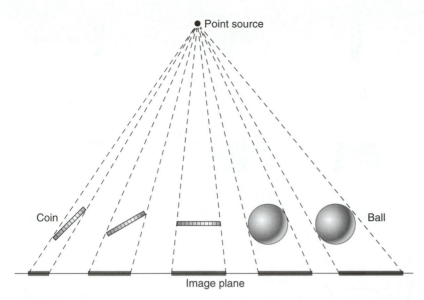

Figure 12–7. The shape of various structures can be radiographically misrepresented (ie, *foreshortened or elongated*) as a result of their position in the body. That misrepresentation can be exaggerated when the part is out of the central axis of the x-ray beam. (From Wolbarst AB. *Physics of Radiology.* East Norwalk, CT: Appleton & Lange, 1993.)

sinuses are more anterior than the sphenoids, the ureters are more anterior than the kidneys, the upper renal poles lie in a plane posterior to the lower renal poles, the fundus of the stomach is more posterior than the body and pylorus, the posterior portions of the sacroiliac joints are more medial than their anterior portions.

2. Structural Shape. Additionally, the three-dimensional shape of solid anatomic structures rarely coincides with the shape of the divergent beam. Consequently, some structures are imaged with more inherent distortion than others and shapes of anatomic structures can be entirely misrepresented. Structures farther from the image receptor will be distorted (ie, *magnified*) more than those closer to the image receptor.

For the shape of anatomic structures to be accurately recorded, the structures must be parallel to the x-ray tube and the image receptor and aligned with the central ray (CR). *The shape of anatomic structures lying at an angle within the body or placed away from the CR will be misrepresented on the image receptor* (Fig. 12–7).

Unless the edges of a three-dimensional *object* conform to the shape of the x-ray beam, blur or unsharpness will occur at the partially attenuating edge of the object. As Figure 12–8 illustrates, this will be accompanied by changes in optical density, according to the thickness of areas traversed by the x-ray beam.

Summary

- **Some geometric unsharpness is intrinsic because of the shape and position of the structure of interest within the body.**

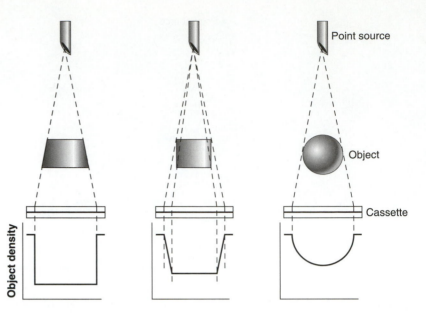

Figure 12–8. Blur or unsharpness results when the *shape* of a three-dimensional object does not coincide with that of the x-ray beam. Blur is accompanied by changes in optical density as a result of differing thicknesses traversed by the x-ray beam. (From Wolbarst AB. *Physics of Radiology.* East Norwalk, CT: Appleton & Lange, 1993.)

■ Structures that do not parallel the x-ray tube and image receptor and/or that lie outside the central axis of the x-ray beam will be foreshortened or elongated.

■ Structures within the body lie at varying distances from the x-ray image receptor, producing varying degrees of magnification.

C. FOCAL SPOT SIZE

Another factor influencing the geometry of the image is focal spot size. If x-ray photons were emitted from a single point source, structures would be recorded and resolved with great clarity. However, because x-ray photons emerge from a measurable focus, image details are represented with unsharp edges. As shown in Figures 12–9 and 12–10, photons emerging from various points on a measurable focal spot are responsible for producing blurred, unsharp edges of anatomic details. The extent or size of the unsharp area is directly related to the focal spot size and OID, and inversely related to the SID; that is, unsharpness increases as focal spot size and OID increase and as the SID decreases.

This border of unsharpness around image details is often referred to as *blur, unsharpness,* or *edge gradient.* The *smaller* the focal spot size, the *better the geometrically recorded detail.*

A distinction is made between the *actual focal spot* and the *effective* (projected or apparent) *focal spot.* The *actual* focal spot is the finite area on the tungsten target that is actually bombarded by electrons from the filament. The *effective* focal spot is the foreshortened size of the focus as it is projected down toward the image receptor; that is, as it would be seen looking up into the emerging x-ray beam. This is called *line focusing* or the *line focus principle* (Fig. 12–11). We generally speak in terms of the effective, or projected, focal spot; manufacturers state effective focal spot size.

The angle of the anode can have a significant effect on recorded detail. Differences in anode angle, all other factors remaining constant, will affect the size of the effective focal spot, as illustrated in

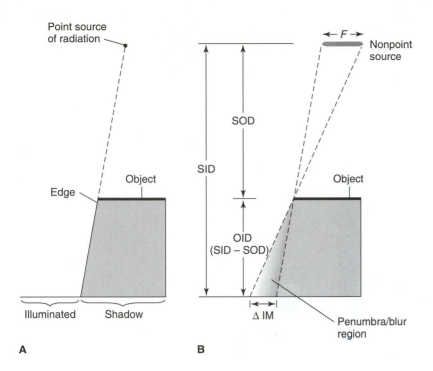

A

B

Figure 12–9. X-ray photons emitted from a point source (**A**) will provide an image having sharply defined borders. X-ray photons emitted from a measurable focal spot (**B**) will produce a zone of blur or unsharpness around each image detail. The degree of blur is directly related to the *size of the focal spot.* (Modified from Wolbarst AB. *Physics of Radiology.* East Norwalk, CT: Appleton & Lange, 1993.)

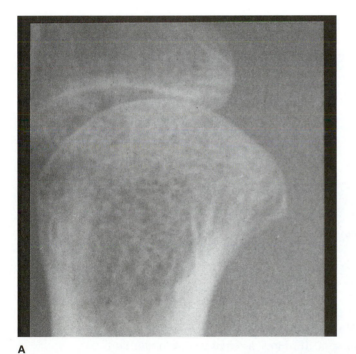

A

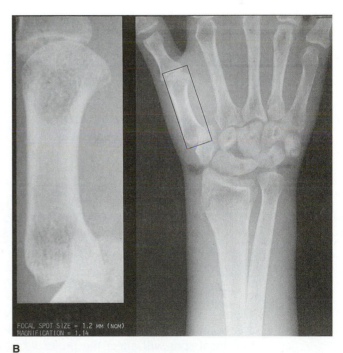

B

Figure 12–10. *Effect of focal spot on recorded detail.* Both images were produced using direct exposure technique to better show the effect of focal spot size on detail, independent of the influence of intensifying screens. (**A**) Magnified image of the first metacarpal, made with a 0.6-mm focal spot. Note the blur or unsharpness associated with bony trabeculae, especially noticeable on the magnified image. (**B**) Image made under identical conditions but using a 1.2-mm focal spot; more severe degradation of recorded detail is demonstrated as a result of blur from the use of a larger focal spot. *Note:* Magnification views must always be made with a 0.3-mm (*fractional*) focal spot, or smaller, to preserve recorded detail. (From the American College of Radiology Learning File. Courtesy of the American College of Radiology.)

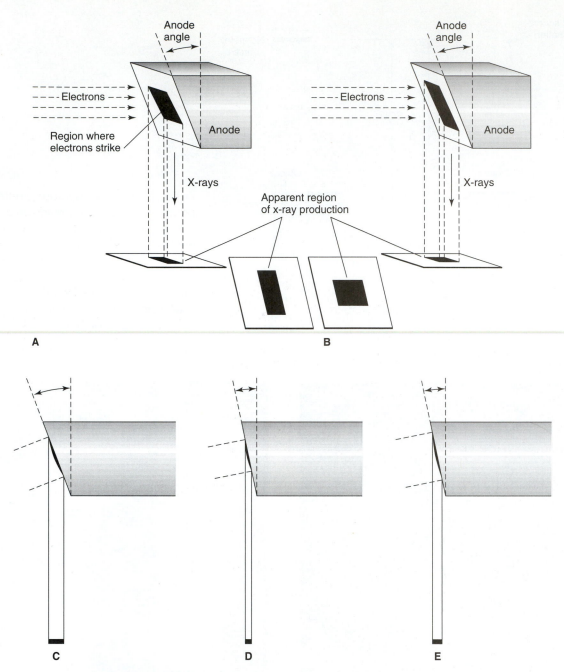

Figure 12–11. **(A)** and **(B)** How the apparent focal spot will differ from the actual focal spot as a result of the *line focus principle*. **(C)** and **(D)** How the *angle/bevel* of the actual focal spot will affect the projected focal spot. **(E)** How a small anode angle combined with a large actual focal spot can result in a small effective focal spot. *The size of the effective focal spot, with its associated blur, actually varies along the length of the image receptor*, being largest at the cathode end of the image receptor and smallest at the anode end (see Figs. 12–12 and 12–13). (**(A)** and **(B)** from Wolbarst AB. *Physics of Radiology.* East Norwalk, CT: Appleton & Lange, 1993.)

Figure 12–11C, D, and E. The *actual* focal spots in Figure 12–11C and D are the same size, but the anode angle in D is half of that in C. Note how much smaller the *effective* or *projected* focal spot is in Figure 12–11D.

Hence, when using a very small anode angle, a larger actual anode area can be bombarded (Fig. 12–11E) while maintaining a small effective focal spot. Thus, a "fractional" (0.3 mm or smaller) effective focal spot can be maintained, recorded detail is improved, and anode heat load tolerance is not compromised. This type of x-ray tube is useful in magnification of small blood vessels.

The size of the effective focal spot, with its associated blur or unsharpness, actually *varies along the length of the image receptor*, being largest at the cathode end of the image receptor and smallest at the anode end (Figs. 12–12 and 12–13).

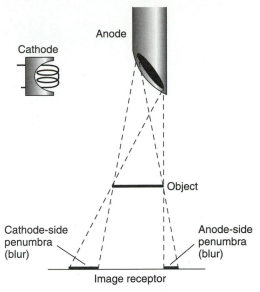

Figure 12–12. Because of the angle of the anode, unsharpness or blur is greatest at the cathode end of the image receptor. (From Wolbarst AB. *Physics of Radiology*. East Norwalk, CT: Appleton & Lange, 1993.)

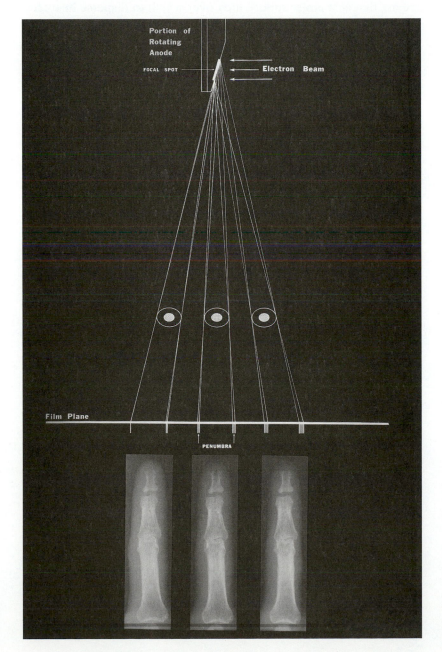

Figure 12–13. *Variation of effective focal spot size along the longitudinal tube axis.* Three images of the third phalanx are shown: one taken at the anode end of the x-ray beam, one at the central portion of the beam, and one at the cathode end. The images clearly illustrate gradual loss of recorded detail toward the cathode end of the x-ray beam. (From the American College of Radiology Learning File. Courtesy of the American College of Radiology.)

If the use of a smaller focal spot size provides us with better recorded detail, why isn't the smallest focal spot available always used? Simply because focal spot size is also associated with the buildup of heat within the x-ray tube. Large quantities of heat delivered to the x-ray tube, especially in a short period of time, can be very damaging to the tube and can shorten its life span.

If the focal spot is small, heat is confined to a tiny area; localized melting of the target material and anode pitting and/or cracking can occur more easily. The larger the focal spot, the greater the surface area available for heat dispersion. The perfect combination would, of course, be a large actual focus that could withstand heat and still provide a small effective focus for optimum recorded detail. This can be achieved by using an x-ray tube with a small target *angle* of approximately 7 to 10 degrees. As previously mentioned, the smaller angle enables a larger "face" to be presented to the electron stream, that is, a larger surface area over which to disperse heat (see Fig. 12–11). The slight target angle causes significant foreshortening of the actual focal spot, creating a very small *effective* focal spot.

A difficulty associated with the use of a small target angle, however, is maintaining a large (14 × 17) field size. The small target angle produces a pronounced *anode heel effect* (Fig. 12–14.) Using a small target angle, a typical radiographic distance of 40 inches SID, and a 14 inch × 17 inch image receptor, there will be approximately 2 inches of unexposed film at the anode end of the radiograph. This can be remedied with an increase in SID, which must be accompanied by an appropriate increase in exposure factors.

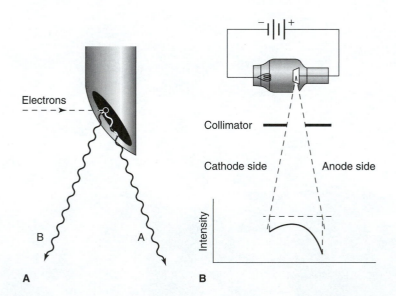

Figure 12–14. *The anode heel effect.* As x-ray photons are produced within the anode, a portion of the divergent beam at its anode end **(A)** is absorbed by the anode's "heel." This represents a decrease in x-ray beam intensity at the anode end of the x-ray beam. The smaller/steeper the target angle/bevel, the more pronounced the heel effect. (From Wolbarst AB. *Physics of Radiology.* East Norwalk, CT: Appleton & Lange, 1993.)

Summary

- Focal spot size affects detail by influencing the degree of blur or unsharpness: increased focal spot size = increased blur = decreased detail.
- Unsharpness or blur is directly related to focal spot size and OID, and inversely related to SID.
- The use of a small focal spot improves recorded detail but generates more heat at the anode.
- The effective or projected focal spot size is always smaller than the actual focal spot according to the line focus principle.
- Effective focal spot size varies along the longitudinal axis of the image receptor, being largest at the cathode end and smallest at the anode end of the x-ray beam.
- Smaller target angles can permit larger actual focal spot sizes while maintaining small effective focal spot sizes—at the expense of accentuating the anode heel effect.
- Use of a small target angle can limit image receptor coverage at traditional and short SIDs.

D. MOTION

Image blur or unsharpness, as a result of motion, can cause severe degradation of recorded detail (Fig. 12–15). The best method of minimizing *voluntary motion* is through good *communication* and suspended respiration. A patient who understands what to expect and what is expected of him or her is better prepared and more likely to cooperate than a patient whose concerns have been inadequately addressed.

Involuntary motion, such as peristaltic activity, muscle spasms, and heart action, cannot be controlled by the patient. The best way to minimize involuntary motion is by using the shortest possible *exposure time*. Motion is often a problem in mobile radiography with machines of limited output (thereby prohibiting the use of short exposure times).

Special positioning devices (such as pediatric immobilizers), positioning sponges, and carefully placed sandbags are frequently used to assist the patient in maintaining the required position.

Equipment motion can cause an effect similar to that caused by patient motion. Bucky motion can cause motion of the part during tabletop examinations; x-ray equipment often has a switch to turn off the Bucky when doing tabletop work. Bumping an improperly balanced tube head just before making the exposure can result in motion blur or unsharpness if the exposure is made while the tube head is still vibrating. Motion blur is probably the greatest enemy of recorded detail and is most obvious when the motion is close to the image receptor (ie, part motion is more damaging to recorded detail than tube motion; Fig. 12–16).

Deliberate motion is occasionally used to blur out unwanted structures so that the area of interest can be seen to better advantage (Fig. 12–17). The "breathing techniques" of lateral thoracic spine and transthoracic shoulder are typical examples. Another is the more specialized procedure of tomography, in which a preselected structure plane will be clearly delineated while structures above and below that plane are blurred.

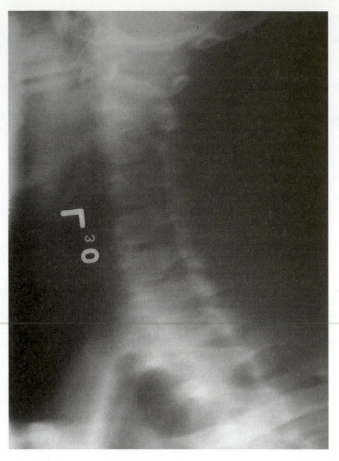

Figure 12–15. Loss of recorded detail as a result of *motion* of the part. (From the American College of Radiology Learning File. Courtesy of the American College of Radiology.)

Summary

- **Motion is the greatest adversary of recorded detail.**
- **Voluntary patient motion can be minimized through good communication.**
- **Involuntary patient motion is best minimized by using the shortest possible exposure time.**
- **Various radiographic accessories are available to help minimize both voluntary and involuntary patient motion.**
- **Equipment motion can also result in loss of recorded detail in the form of image blur.**
- **Special techniques that introduce motion are sometimes employed to see some structures particularly well.**

E. INTENSIFYING SCREENS

In the very early days of radiography, before *intensifying screens* were available, images were produced by exposure of photographic emulsion to x-rays alone. Tremendously lengthy exposures were required for even the smallest parts. These exposures took their toll on the fragile, scarcely understood equipment and, of course, on the unsuspecting victims of excessive radiation exposure. Direct exposure

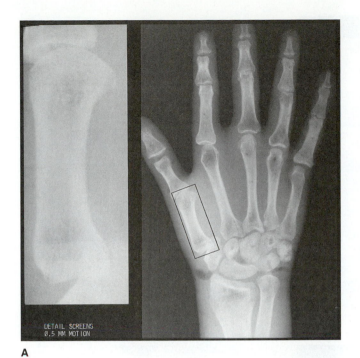

A

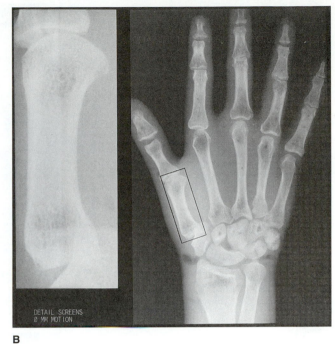

B

C

Figure 12–16. **(A)** Image made using detail (100 speed) screens; 0.5 mm of motion was introduced. Motion blur is noticeable, particularly in the magnified view of the first metacarpal. Compare the recorded detail of image A with that of image **B. (B)** Also made using detail (100 speed) screens, but having no motion. **(C)** Made with fast (400 speed) screens and 0.5 mm motion. Notice how much more obvious detail loss becomes with a faster imaging system. (From the American College of Radiology Learning File. Courtesy of the American College of Radiology.)

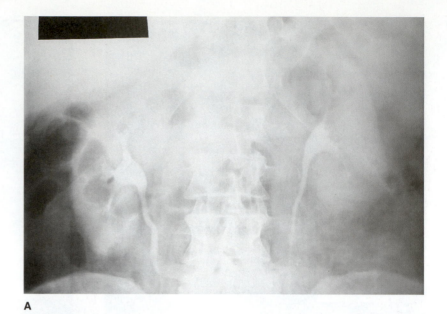

Figure 12–17. **(A)** Plain IVU (intravenous urogram; also termed IVP [intravenous pyelogram] or [EXU excretory urogram]) radiograph with no visible abnormalities. **(B)** An 8-cm tomographic section of the same patient clearly depicting a 7-cm renal cyst overlying the R mid-renal cortex. (From the American College of Radiology Learning File. Courtesy of the American College of Radiology.)

Rare Earth Phosphors

Gadolinium
Lanthanum
Yttrium

technique was frequently used through the 1960s and 1970s for examinations of extremities and other small parts not requiring a grid. Because of the excessive patient dose, direct exposure technique is rarely used today.

In 1896, Thomas Edison developed the *calcium tungstate* intensifying screen that served to reduce the required exposure to a fraction of that needed without screens. Calcium tungstate screens gained wide acceptance during World War I and were used almost exclusively until the advent of *rare earth phosphors* in the early 1970s.

The active ingredient in intensifying screens is the fluorescent *phosphor,* which functions to change x-ray photon energy to fluorescent light energy. More than *98% of the exposure received by the film emulsion is from fluorescent light* emitted by intensifying screen phosphors. For every x-ray photon absorbed by the phosphor, many light photons are emitted. They truly *intensify* the action of x-rays, and thus permit the use of much smaller exposures than those required with direct exposure methods.

In the production of intensifying screens, phosphors are ground to a fine powder and mixed with a transparent binding substance. A somewhat reflective plastic base material is used as a support. The phosphor mixture is spread in a smooth layer onto the plastic base; this is called the *phosphor layer* or *active layer* (Fig. 12–18).

All phosphors are not created equal. Different types of phosphors have different x-ray absorbing and fluorescent light emitting properties. Some types of phosphors are more efficient than others. Some are able to absorb a greater percentage of the x-ray energy. A particular phosphor's ability to absorb x-ray energy and convert it to fluorescent light energy is referred to as its *conversion efficiency.* Phosphors having greater sensitivity (ie, speed) have greater conversion efficiency.

Factors that contribute to the speed of intensifying screens include type of phosphor, phosphor size, active/phosphor layer thickness, and reflective backing.

1. Phosphors. Phosphors with a *high atomic number* have a greater likelihood of interacting with an x-ray photon, and therefore possess greater speed. How well a particular phosphor detects the presence

Relationship Between Screen Speed and Tube Wear (Heat Units)		
Screen Speed	mAs (Milliampere-Seconds)	Heat Units (HU)
100	60	5400
200	30	2700
400	15	1350

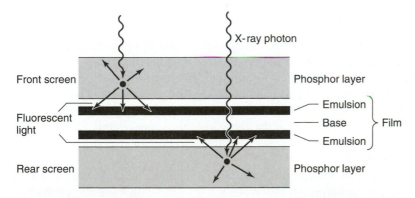

Figure 12–18. *A cross-section of screens and film.* The illustration shows how duplitized x-ray film is sandwiched between two intensifying screens. Phosphors of the adjacent intensifying screens absorb x-ray energy and convert it to fluorescent light, which then exposes the neighboring film emulsion as shown in Figure 12–19. Notice that the rear intensifying screen is thicker. As x-ray photons travel through the cassette front and front screen, they are somewhat attenuated and, as a result, their interaction with the rear screen is somewhat diminished. If the rear screen is made thicker, its speed is increased to compensate for the attenuated x-ray beam. (From Wolbarst AB. *Physics of Radiology.* East Norwalk, CT: Appleton & Lange, 1993.)

Intensifying Screen Speed Increases, and Therefore Recorded Detail Decreases, as

- Phosphor size increases
- Thickness of the active/phosphor layer increases
- Sensitivity of the phosphor increases (ie, calcium tungstate versus rare earth phosphors)
- The degree of screen reflectance increases

Recorded Detail Increases as

- Focal spot size decreases
- SID increases
- OID decreases
- Motion decreases
- (Shape) distortion decreases
- Screen speed decreases

of x-ray photons is referred to as quantum detection efficiency. The phosphor should have a high *conversion efficiency,* that is, it should emit a liberal measure of fluorescent light for each x-ray photon it absorbs. The greater the conversion efficiency, the greater the speed.

Fluorescence should terminate at the same time as the x-ray source; continued fluorescence after termination of exposure is termed *lag* and contributes to an overexposed radiograph. The wavelength, or color, of light emitted must match the particular sensitivity of the film emulsion used. This is known as *spectral matching.* Calcium tungstate emits a blue violet fluorescence and *rare earth phosphors* may fluoresce either green or blue; each must be used with a corresponding green or blue sensitive film emulsion.

Phosphorescence refers to the luminescence from fluoroscopic screen phosphors. Their unique characteristic is the lingering luminescence *after* the termination of x-ray *(afterglow).* This permits the fluoroscopist to continue viewing the part for a short time as the image slowly fades from the monitor. Thus, the fluoroscopist can use intermittent fluoroscopy to reduce patient dose.

Rare earth phosphors possess a much higher conversion efficiency than calcium tungstate, making them the phosphors of choice today. The rare earth phosphors used in radiography are oxysulfides and oxybromides of *lanthanum, gadolinium,* and *yttrium.* The phosphors used in fluoroscopy are *cesium iodide* and *zinc cadmium sulfide.*

2. Phosphor Size.
Screen speed and phosphor size are directly related; that is, *as phosphor size increases*, more surface area is available for x-ray photon capture, resulting in an *increase in screen speed.*

3. Active or Phosphor Layer Thickness.
Screen speed and phosphor layer thickness are directly related; that is, as active layer thickness increases, more x-ray photons are converted to light and, therefore, screen speed increases.

4. Reflective Backing.
Screen speed and the degree of reflectance given the base material are directly related; that is, the greater the reflectance, the greater the number of light photons directed toward the film emulsion and, consequently, the greater the screen speed.

Some manufacturers incorporate a *dye* in the phosphor layer that functions to reduce light diffusion, thus improving resolution. It should be noted however, that the addition of dye does sacrifice a little speed.

Loss of recorded detail may be a result of intensifying screen blur or unsharpness. Fluorescent light emerging from the phosphors diffuses and spreads over a larger area (Fig. 12–19A). It is this diffusion of fluorescent light that causes indistinct, blurry anatomic details. *The degree of diffusion, and hence, the degree of blurriness, is primarily dependent on the factors that regulate intensifying screen speed* (Fig. 12–19B).

Screen speed and screen blurriness are directly related; that is, as intensifying screen speed increases, screen blurriness increases and image resolution/detail decreases.

Radiography departments frequently have more than one speed-intensifying screen available; slower (detail) screens are commonly used for extremity examinations, and faster screens for general radiography.

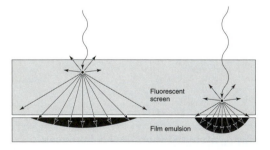

A

Figure 12–19. **(A)** Screen thickness and diffusion of fluorescent light versus recorded detail. As intensifying screen thickness increases, the film is exposed by diffused light from distant phosphors. The phosphors of thinner intensifying screens fluoresce closer to the film; therefore, light is diffused to a lesser degree and recorded detail is maintained. (Modified from Wolbarst AB. *Physics of Radiology,* East Norwalk, CT: Appleton & Lange, 1993.)

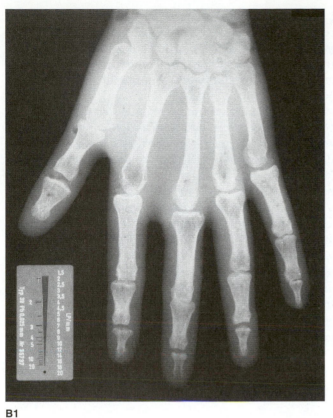

B1

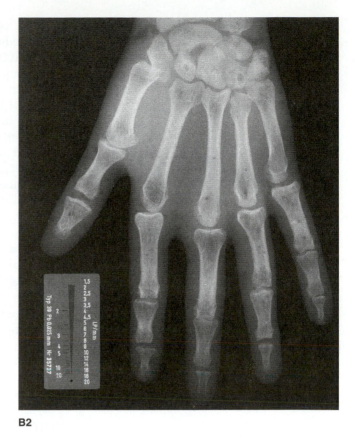

B2

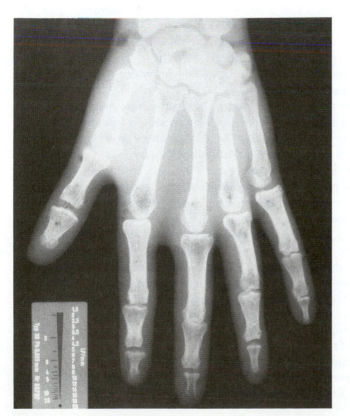

B3

Figure 12–19 (*Continued*). **(B)** Imaging system speed versus required exposure and resolution. Image **1** was made without intensifying screens but required 128 mAs exposure. Image **2** was made using detail (approximately 100 speed) screens and 10 mAs exposure. Image **3** was made with fast (approximately 400) screens and 1.33 mAs exposure. Note the progressive loss of recorded detail accompanying the increase in system speed. (From the American College of Radiology Learning File. Courtesy of the American College of Radiology.)

The use of rare earth phosphors enables the radiographer to greatly reduce patient dose in comparison to exposures required for calcium tungstate screens. The use of rare earth phosphors involves only minimal loss of recorded detail and permits a significant reduction in patient dose; they are, therefore, generally considered the screens of choice.

Another way in which intensifying screens can have a significant impact on recorded detail is through *screen–film contact.* Areas of imperfect screen–film contact result in blurriness that severely degrades recorded detail (Fig. 12–20A). Causes of poor screen–film contact include warped screens, damaged cassette frames, and foreign bodies in the cassette. Elevation of the screen in areas of poor contact allows light to diffuse over a larger area, thus exaggerating screen blur. Larger cassettes are more susceptible to poor screen contact. Proper care of intensifying screens includes *periodic evaluation of screen contact by using a specially designed wire mesh* (Fig. 12–20B).

A related problem associated with screens and resolution is *quantum mottle.* As screen speed and kVp are increased, mAs may be reduced to such a small amount that image *graininess,* or quantum mottle, becomes a problem (Figs. 12–21, 12–22, and 12–23). This graininess becomes apparent and increases as the system speed increases. So few x-ray photons are used (mAs) to produce the image that one can almost count them as the representative black "grains" on the radiographic image!

Summary

- Intensifying screens serve to decrease patient dose and increase tube life.
- As screen speed increases, patient dose decreases and tube life increases.
- Intensifying screen phosphors absorb x-ray photons and emit a large quantity of fluorescent light.
- Fluorescent light is responsible for more than 98% of the image density.
- The color light emitted by the phosphors must be correctly matched with the film emulsion sensitivity (spectral matching).
- Rare earth phosphors have a greater conversion efficiency than do calcium tungstate phosphors.
- The greater the conversion efficiency and speed of screens, the poorer the recorded detail, as a result of greater fluorescent light diffusion at higher screen speeds.
- Screen speed is influenced by the type and size of phosphor used, the thickness of the active/phosphor layer, and the degree of reflectance given the screen base.
- Quantum mottle is more likely to occur when using fast screens with low mAs and high kVp factors.
- Phosphors that continue to fluoresce after the x-ray source has terminated are said to possess "lag" or "afterglow."
- Phosphorescence is associated with fluoroscopic screens.
- Perfect screen–film contact is required to maintain recorded detail.
- Screens may be tested for screen–film contact with the use of a specially designed wire mesh.

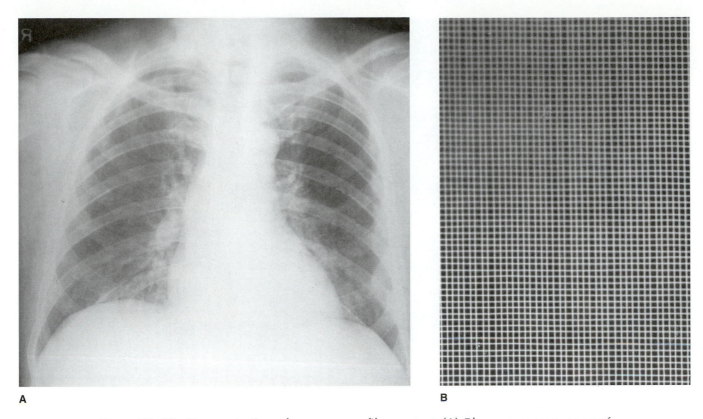

A

B

Figure 12–20. *Demonstration of poor screen–film contact.* **(A)** Blur as a consequence of poor film–screen contact in the apical region of the chest. **(B)** Wire-mesh test of a different cassette illustrates blur caused by poor film to screen contact in the central region of the cassette. (From the American College of Radiology Learning File. Courtesy of the American College of Radiology.)

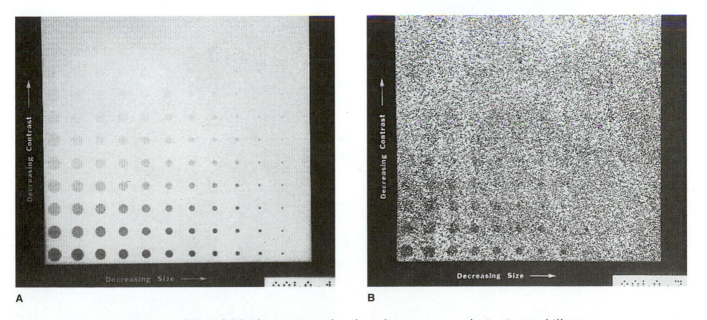

A

B

Figure 12–21. **(A)** and **(B)** The contrast–detail quality assurance device imaged illustrates the effect of x-ray exposure and resulting quantum mottle. Image **(B)** was made using a much lower mAs value (fewer x-ray photons) than image **(A)**; note the striking graininess in **(B).** (From the American College of Radiology Learning File. Courtesy of the American College of Radiology.)

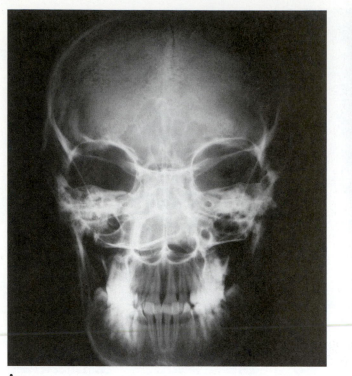
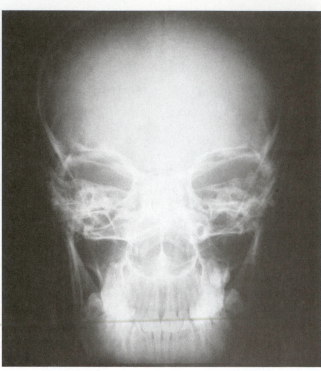

A

B

Figure 12–22. **(A)** and **(B)** The "grainy" appearance of image **(A)** is quantum mottle resulting from a faster screen film combination than image **(B).** (From the American College of Radiology Learning File. Courtesy of the American College of Radiology.)

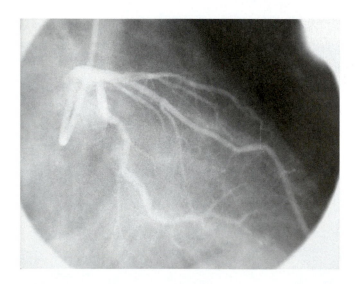
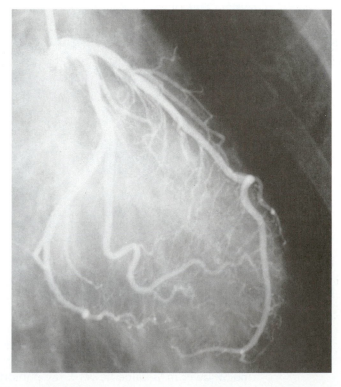

Figure 12–23. Quantum mottle can make visibility of small vessels difficult. (From the American College of Radiology Learning File. Courtesy of the American College of Radiology.)

A&U Chapter Review Questions

⭐ ***Congratulations!*** *You have completed a portion of this chapter. You may go on to the "Registry-type" multiple-choice questions that follow. For greatest success, be sure also to complete the short answer questions found at the end of this chapter.*

1. Which of the following has (have) an effect on recorded detail?
   1. focal spot size
   2. type of rectification
   3. source image distance
   (A) 1 only
   (B) 1 and 2 only
   (C) 1 and 3 only
   (D) 1, 2, and 3

2. A wire mesh is used to test:
   (A) focal spot size
   (B) for screen lag
   (C) film–screen contact
   (D) screen speed

3. Misalignment of the tube–part–image receptor relationship results in:
   (A) shape distortion
   (B) size distortion
   (C) magnification
   (D) blur

4. Which of the following is (are) considered geometric factor(s) controlling recorded detail?
   1. focal spot size
   2. screen speed
   3. object–image receptor distance
   (A) 1 only
   (B) 2 only
   (C) 1 and 3 only
   (D) 1, 2, and 3

5. Although the stated focal spot size is measured directly under the actual focal spot, focal spot size really varies along the length of the x-ray beam. At which portion of the x-ray beam is the effective focal spot the smallest?
   (A) at its outer edge
   (B) along the path of the central ray
   (C) at the cathode end
   (D) at the anode end

6. Which of the following will result in the *best* recorded detail?
   (A) 1.5-mm focal spot
   (B) 1.0-mm focal spot
   (C) 0.6-mm focal spot
   (D) 0.3-mm focal spot

7. All of the following are related to recorded detail, *except*:
   (A) motion
   (B) screen speed
   (C) object–image distance
   (D) grid ratio

8. Foreshortening may be caused by:
   1. the radiographic object being placed at an angle to the image receptor
   2. excessive distance between the object and the image receptor
   3. insufficient distance between the focus and the image receptor
   (A) 1 only
   (B) 2 only
   (C) 1 and 2 only
   (D) 1, 2, and 3

9. When an intensifying screen continues to glow after the x-ray exposure has ended, the screen is said to possess
   (A) fluorescence
   (B) incandescence
   (C) luminescence
   (D) lag

10. Which of the following has an effect on distortion?
    1. source image distance
    2. angulation of the x-ray tube
    3. angulation of the part
    (A) 1 only
    (B) 1 and 2 only
    (C) 2 and 3 only
    (D) 1, 2, and 3

Answers and Explanations

1. (C) Focal spot size affects recorded detail by its effect on blur: the larger the focal spot size the greater the blur produced. Recorded detail is significantly affected by distance changes because of their effect on magnification. As SID increases, magnification decreases and recorded detail increases. The method of rectification has no impact on recorded detail. Single-phase, rectified units produce "pulsed" radiation, whereas three-phase units produce almost constant potential.

2. (C) Intensifying screens can have a considerable impact on recorded detail through *screen–film contact.* Areas of imperfect screen-film contact result in blurriness that severely degrades recorded detail (see Fig. 12–20A). Causes of poor screen–film contact include warped screens, damaged cassette frames, and foreign bodies in the cassette. Larger cassettes are more susceptible to poor screen contact. Proper care of intensifying screens includes *periodic evaluation of screen contact using a specially designed wire mesh* (see Fig. 12–20B). Focal spot testing uses a slit camera or star pattern.

3. (A) Shape distortion (foreshortening, elongation) is caused by improper alignment of the tube, part, and image receptor. Size distortion, or magnification, is caused by too great an object–image distance or too short a source–image distance. Blur is caused principally by use of a large focal spot.

4. (C) The relationship among the focal spot, the anatomic part, and the image receptor determines geometric sharpness. That is, effective focal spot size determines the degree of penumbra, and OID and SID determine the degree of magnification. The OID should be as short as possible and the SID should be as long as practical. The anatomic part should be accurately positioned as closely parallel to the image receptor as possible. Screens also lend a degree of unsharpness to the radiograph, but do not affect the *geometry* of the image (ie, size or shape).

5. (D) X-ray tube targets are constructed according to the *line focus principle;* that is, the focal spot is angled (usually 12 to 17 degrees) to the vertical. As the actual focal spot is projected downward it is foreshortened; thus, the effective focal spot is always smaller than the actual focal spot. As it is projected toward the cathode end of the x-ray beam it becomes larger and approaches its actual size. As it is projected toward the anode end, it gets smaller because of the anode "heel" effect.

6. (D) One factor influencing geometric sharpness is penumbra, or blur. The production of blur is inversely proportional to recorded detail. As focal spot size increases, blur increases, and recorded detail decreases.

7. (D) Motion is said to be the greatest enemy of recorded detail because it completely obliterates image sharpness. Screen speed can reduce recorded detail according to the degree of light diffusion from the phosphors. Object–image distance causes magnification and blurriness of recorded detail. Grid ratio is related to scatter radiation clean-up; it is unrelated to detail.

8. (A) Size distortion (magnification) is inversely proportional to SID and directly proportional to OID. Decreasing the SID and increasing the OID serve to increase size distortion. Aligning the tube, anatomic part, and image receptor so as to be parallel reduces shape distortion. Angulation of the long axis of the part with respect to the image receptor results in foreshortening of the object. Tube angulation causes elongation of the part.

9. (D) When intensifying screen phosphors absorb x-ray photons, the x-ray photon energy is converted to visible light energy. The light emitted by the phosphors is termed luminescence. There are two types of luminescence: fluorescence and phosphorescence. Fluorescence is luminescent light that ceases to be emitted *as soon* as the x-ray photon stimulation ceases. Phosphorescence, on the other hand, is when the phosphors continue to glow *after* x-ray photon stimulation ceases; another term for this is lag.

10. (D) Distortion can be described as being either size or shape. Size distortion is magnification, caused by either insufficient SID or excessive OID. Shape distortion results from misalignment of the x-ray tube, part, and image receptor. Tube angulation can cause elongation of the part. Angulation of the part with respect to the image receptor will foreshorten the image. Focal spot size is unrelated to distortion, but strongly related to production of penumbral unsharpness.

II. FACTORS AFFECTING RADIOGRAPHIC/ OPTICAL DENSITY

Radiographic, or optical, density is defined as the overall amount of blackening on a radiographic image or a particular portion of the image. It provides a degree of background blackening for the anatomic image. Excessive optical density can obscure image details; insufficient optical density can mask pathology. Optical density is a *quantitative* factor; that is, it describes an *amount* of image blackening. Thus, optical density is regulated by the *exposure rate* or *number* of photons reaching the film emulsion image receptor.

Optical density is generally thought of as being optimal, excessive, or insufficient, when in fact it can be precisely measured and quantified. Optical density can be described as the relationship between the amount of light incident upon the radiograph (ie, from the illuminator) compared to the amount of light transmitted through the radiograph. This relationship is expressed in the following equation:

$$OD = \log_{10} \frac{I_o}{I_t}$$

OD is optical density expressed as a logarithm, demonstrating the relationship between the amount of light transmitted through the film (I_t) compared to the amount of light incident upon (I_o) the film. The diagnostically useful range of optical density is 0.25 to 2.5 (Fig. 12–24).

A characteristic curve, like the one shown in Figure 12–25, can be used to illustrate the relationship between the x-ray exposure given the film and the resulting radiographic density.

The study of film emulsion response to exposure is called *sensitometry*. The characteristic curve is discussed further in Section IV: Film, Screen, and Grid Options.

A. MAS

Milliampere-seconds *(mAs)* is the *product* of milliamperes (mA) and exposure time (seconds). Technical factors are usually expressed in terms of mAs rather than mA and time. This is because there are any number of possible combinations of mA and time that will produce the desired mAs. For example,

> It is known that 10 mAs is required to produce a given radiographic density. Therefore, each of the following combinations should produce the required (and identical) results: 100 mA and 0.1 second, 200 mA and 0.05 second, 300 mA and 0.03 second, 400 mA and 0.025 second, and so on.

Any combinations of mA and time that will produce a given mAs (ie, a particular quantity of x-ray photons) will produce identical optical density. This is known as the *reciprocity law*.

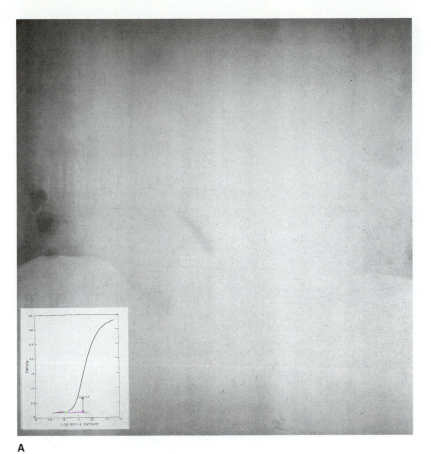

A

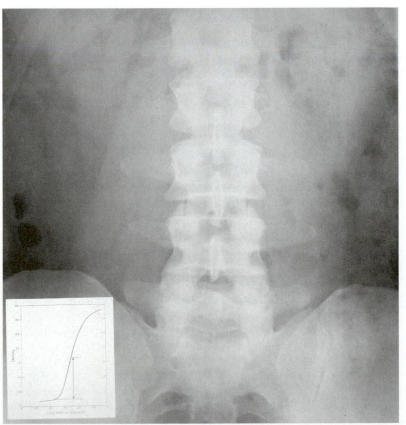

B

Figure 12–24. (A), (B), and (C) *The diagnostically useful range of optical densities is approximately 0.25 to 2.5.* Note the range of densities visualized on each of these radiographs as identified by the accompanying characteristic curve on each film. (From the American College of Radiology Learning File. Courtesy of the American College of Radiology.)

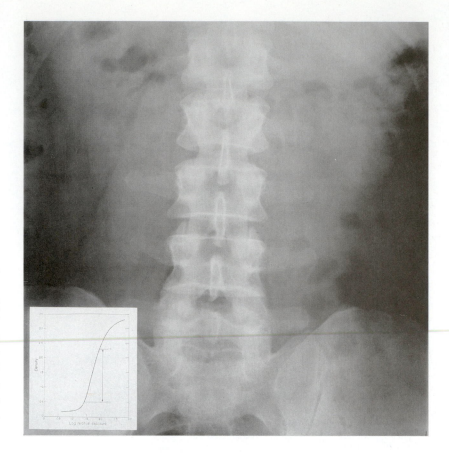

Figure 12–24 (*Continued*). (**C**) The range of densities visualized lie between 0.5 and 2.5, as indicated by the accompanying characteristic curve. Notice the number and visibility of details imaged here as compared with those imaged in (**A**) (density range approximately 0.25 to 0.70) and (**B**) (density range approximately 0.25 to 1.5). (From the American College of Radiology Learning File. Courtesy of the American College of Radiology.)

Radiographic density is a quantitative factor because it describes the amount of image blackening. Milliampere-seconds is also a quantitative factor because it regulates x-ray beam *intensity, exposure rate, quantity,* or *number* of x-ray photons produced (mAs is the single most important technical factor associated with radiographic density and is the factor of choice for regulating radiographic/optical density).

mAs is directly proportional to the intensity (exposure rate, number, quantity) of x-ray photons produced, and the resulting radiographic density. If the mAs is doubled, twice the exposure rate and twice the density occurs. If the mAs is cut in half, the exposure rate and resulting density are cut in half (Fig. 12–26).

It is not surprising then, that to produce just a *perceptible* change in radiographic density, an mAs change of at least 30% is required. For example,

> A particular radiograph was produced using 12 mAs and 78 kVp. The finished image exhibited somewhat insufficient background density. What factors would be required to produce a radiograph having satisfactory radiographic density?

Because the radiographic density requires improvement, the mAs is the technical factor requiring manipulation. The above information implies that background density is only somewhat lacking, therefore a 30% increase in mAs would most likely remedy the situation. Because 30% of 12 mAs is 3.6, a new mAs of 16 should provide ade-

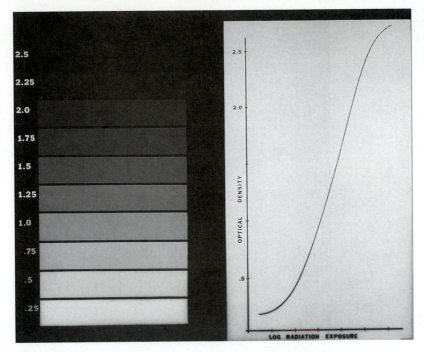

Figure 12–25. *Characteristic curve.* Notice that the intervals of *exposure* appear in increments of 0.3. This is because doubling the exposure (ie, mAs) results in an increase in log relative exposure of 0.3. For example, 100% of the incident light is transmitted through a film having an optical density of zero (0), 50% of the light is transmitted through a film having an optical density of 0.3, 25% of the light through a film with density of 0.6, and so on. (From the American College of Radiology Learning File. Courtesy of the American College of Radiology.)

quate radiographic/optical density. If the radiograph were significantly lacking in density, it would have been appropriate to double the mAs.

Summary

- mAs is the product of mA and exposure time.
- Any combination of mA and time that will produce a given mAs will produce identical radiographic density according to the reciprocity law.
- Radiographic density and mAs are quantitative factors and are directly related.
- Doubling the mAs will double the radiographic density; halving the mAs will cut the density in half.
- At least a 30% change must be made in mAs for there to be a perceptible change in radiographic density.

B. SID

As a child you may have been told to "read your book next to the lamp, where you'll have more light." Perhaps your youthful eyes could see just fine where you were, but in fact your advisor was correct in saying that more light was available closer to the lamp.

As distance from a light source increases, the light diverges and covers a larger area; the quantity of light available per unit area be-

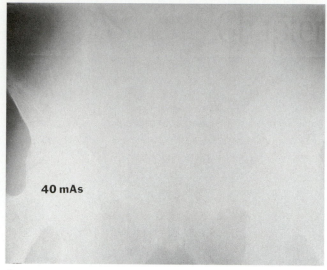

A

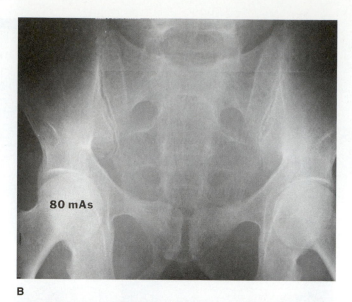

B

Figure 12–26. *Optical density is proportional to mAs.* **(A)** Radiograph made using 40 mAs. **(B)** Radiograph made of the same subject using 80 mAs, all other factors remaining constant; note that doubling the mAs has produced twice the optical density. **(C)** Radiograph made using twice the mAs of **B** (160 mAs), resulting in another doubling of optical density. (From the American College of Radiology Learning File. Courtesy of the American College of Radiology.)

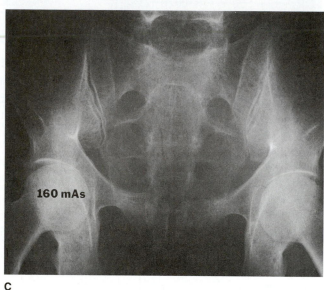

C

comes less and less as distance increases. The intensity (quantity) of light decreases according to the *inverse square law,* that is, the intensity of light at a particular distance from its source is inversely proportional to the square of the distance (Fig. 12–27). For example, if you decreased the distance between your book and the lamp from 6 feet to 3 feet, you would have four times as much light available.

Similarly, source-to-image-receptor distance (SID) has a significant impact on x-ray beam intensity and, hence, radiographic density. *As the distance between the x-ray tube and image receptor increases, exposure rate (and therefore radiographic density) decreases according to the inverse square law.*

Notice that according to the inverse square law the exposure rate is *inversely* proportional to the square of the distance, whereas using the density maintenance formula to determine new mAs because of diminished exposure rate, mAs is *directly* proportional to the distance squared.

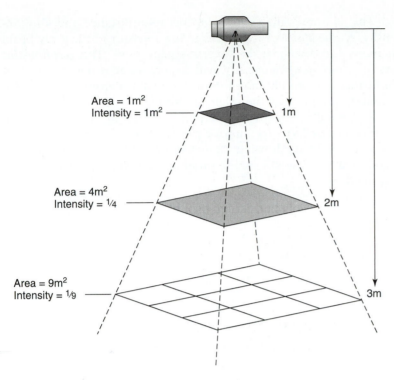

Figure 12–27. *The inverse square law.* Because x-ray beam coverage (area) increases with the square of the distance, the number of x-ray photons per unit area decreases by the same amount. (From Wolbarst AB. *Physics of Radiology.* East Norwalk, CT: Appleton & Lange, 1993.)

The two equations that will be used are:

$$\frac{I_1}{I_2} = \frac{D_2^2}{D_1^2} \qquad \text{Inverse Square Law}$$

and

$$\frac{mAs_1}{mAs_2} = \frac{D_1^2}{D_2^2} \qquad \text{Density Maintenance Formula}$$

In the Inverse Square Law equation, I represents intensity (a quantitative term referring to exposure rate) and D represents distance (SID). The original intensity is represented by I_1, the original distance squared is represented by D_1^2, and the new distance squared by D_2^2. I_2 represents the new intensity (ie, the new exposure rate). Note that the relationship is an *inversely proportional* one. That is, the formula is set up as "old over new = new over old".

Notice that the opposite is true in the Density Maintenance Formula; the relationship is *directly* proportional ("old over new = old over new").

A radiograph made using a particular group of technical factors at 52 inches SID resulted in an exposure rate of 85 mR/min. Another radiograph of the same part will be made at 44 inches SID. What is the exposure rate at the new distance?

$$\frac{85}{x} = \frac{1936\ (44^2)}{2704\ (52^2)}$$

$$1936x = 229{,}840$$

$$x = 118.7 \text{ mR/min at 44 inches SID}$$

Use the Inverse Square Law to Determine

What the new exposure rate is at the new distance, by using the (inverse relationship) equation:

$$\frac{I_1}{I_2} = \frac{D_2^2}{D_1^2}$$

This illustrates the relationship between distance and x-ray intensity. As the *distance* is *decreased*, the *intensity* of the x-ray beam *increases* (according to the inverse square law). The *resulting increase in radiographic density*, will require an adjustment of technical factors, specifically mAs (according to the density maintenance formula), to reproduce the original density.

A particular radiograph was performed at 40 inches SID using 12 mAs and 82 kVp. To improve recorded detail, it is necessary to repeat the radiograph using 72 inches SID. What new mAs will be required at the new distance in order to maintain the original radiographic density?

Using the distance maintenance formula and substituting known factors:

$$\frac{mAs_1}{mAs_2} = \frac{D_1^2}{D_2^2}$$

$$\frac{12}{x} = \frac{1600 \ (40^2)}{5184 \ (72^2)}$$

$$1600x = 62{,}208$$

$$x = 38.9 \text{ mAs at 72 inches SID}$$

At 72 inches SID, 38.9 mAs will be required to produce the same density that was produced at 40 inches SID using 12 mAs.

Use the Density Maintenance Formula to Determine

What change in mAs is required to maintain the original radiographic density, by using the (direct relationship) equation:

$$\frac{mAs_1}{mAs_2} = \frac{D_1^2}{D_2^2}$$

Summary

- **Relatively small changes in SID can have a significant effect on radiographic/optical density.**
- **As the SID increases, exposure rate and radiographic density decrease.**
- **With changes in SID, the inverse square law is used to calculate the new exposure rate.**
- **With changes in SID, the density maintenance formula is used to calculate the new mAs.**

C. *kVp*

As kilovoltage is increased, *more* electrons are driven to the anode with greater speed and energy. More high-energy electrons will result in production of *more high-energy x-rays*. Thus, *kVp* affects both quantity and quality (energy) of the x-ray beam. However, although kVp and radiographic density are directly *related,* they are not directly proportional; that is, twice the radiographic density does not result from doubling the kVp. The effect of kVp on quantity is not proportional because an increase in kVp produces an increase in photons of *all energies*.

With respect to the effect of kVp on radiographic density, there is one convenient rule (*the 15% rule)* that can be followed. If it is desired to double the radiographic density, yet impossible to adjust the mAs, a similar effect can be achieved by *increasing the kVp by 15%.* Conversely, the density may be cut in half by decreasing the kVp by 15% (Fig. 12–28).

A radiograph was made using the following technical factors: 400 mA, 0.025 second, and 84 kVp. It is necessary to produce another image with twice the radiographic density. The maximum mA available is 400 and the exposure time cannot be increased due to involuntary motion. What alternate kVp can be employed to produce a radiograph with the desired radiographic density?

If twice the original density is needed, the kVp may be increased 15% to produce the desired effect. Fifteen percent of 84 is 12.6. Therefore, using the same mAs and increasing the kVp to 97 should produce a radiograph with twice the original density. *Note:* Changing the kVp will change the scale of contrast (discussed in Part III).

Summary

■ **Increased kVp produces more high energy x-ray photons.**

■ **An increase in kVp will result in an increase in optical density; a decrease in kVp will result in a decrease in optical density.**

■ **When mAs manipulation is not possible, optical density can be doubled or halved by using the 15% rule.**

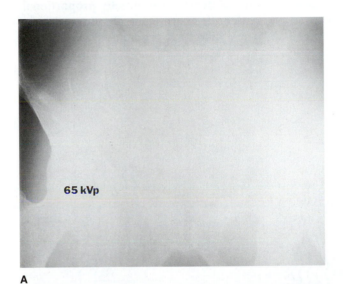

A

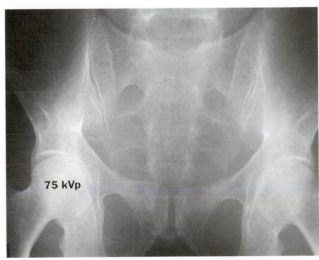

B

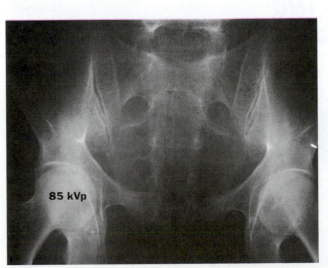

C

Figure 12–28. *Illustration of the 15% rule.* Image **(B)** was made using 15% more kVp than image **(A)** and demonstrates twice the optical density of image **(A)**. Similarly, image **(C)** was made using 15% more kVp than image **(B)** and demonstrates twice the optical density of image **(B)**. (From the American College of Radiology Learning File. Courtesy of the American College of Radiology.)

D. INTENSIFYING SCREENS

Intensifying screens amplify the effect of x-rays on film emulsion by means of fluorescence. For every one x-ray photon interacting with screen phosphors, many light photons are emitted. This effect becomes more pronounced as screen speed increases.

Therefore, with any given group of exposure factors, as *screen speed increases, optical density increases.*

Screen speed and optical density are directly proportional. An increase in intensifying screen speed from 200 to 400 doubles the optical density and enables the optical to cut the mAs in half, thus reducing patient dose (Fig. 12–29) and tube wear (heat units) considerably.

Summary

- **Intensifying screens amplify the action of x-rays through their property of fluorescence.**
- **All other factors remaining constant, an increase in screen speed will result in an increase in optical density.**
- **Screen speed and optical density are directly proportional.**
- **Screen speed and patient dose are inversely proportional.**
- **Screen speed and x-ray tube heat production are inversely related.**

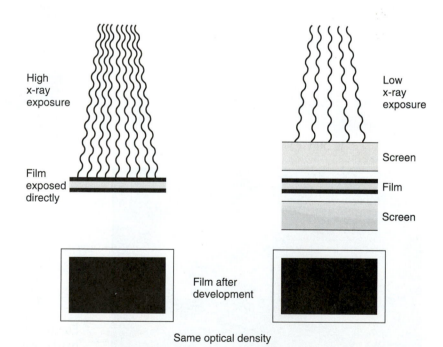

Figure 12–29. Exposure and resulting optical density; *direct exposure versus intensifying screens.* By using intensifying screens, a much smaller patient dose is required to produce the same optical density. (From Wolbarst AB. *Physics of Radiology.* East Norwalk, CT: Appleton & Lange, 1993.)

E. GRIDS

As x-ray photons travel through a part, they either pass all the way through to expose the film/image receptor, or they undergo interaction(s) that may result in their being absorbed by the part or deviated in direction. It is those that change direction (*scattered radiation*) that undermine the image.

Part III discussed the origin of scatter radiation: Compton scatter interactions. Compton scatter can be a personnel radiation hazard, especially in fluoroscopic procedures. With respect to the radiographic image, it is responsible for the scattered radiation that reaches the film/image receptor. *Scattered radiation* adds unwanted, degrading densities to the radiographic image.

The single most important way to reduce the production of scattered radiation is to collimate. Although *collimation,* optimum *kVp,* and *compression* can be used (Fig. 12–30), a large amount of scattered radiation is still generated within the part being radiographed and, because it adds unwanted non information-carrying densities, it can have a severely degrading effect on image quality, as illustrated in the pelvis radiographs shown in Figure 12–31.

A *grid* is a device interposed between the patient and image receptor that functions to absorb a large percentage of scatter radiation before it reaches the image receptor (Fig. 12–32). It is constructed of alternating strips of lead foil and *radiolucent* filler material. X-ray photons traveling in the same direction as the primary beam pass between the lead strips. X-ray photons, having undergone interactions within the body and deviated in various directions, are absorbed by the lead strips; this is referred to as "clean-up" of scattered radiation.

The use of grids is recommended for body parts measuring 11 cm and greater. The major exception to this rule is the chest, which can frequently be examined without a grid because its contents (mostly air) do not generate significant quantities of scatter radiation. Even so, many institutions perform most chest examinations using a grid and high kilovoltage factors.

Without the use of a grid, scatter radiation contributes to more than 50% of the total film emulsion/image receptor exposure. If a grid is introduced, there will be significantly *fewer* photons reaching

Amount of scattered radiation depends upon . . . .

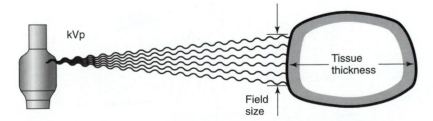

Figure 12–30. *Factors affecting the production of scattered radiation:* kVp level, beam restriction, and thickness and density of tissues. (From Wolbarst AB. *Physics of Radiology.* East Norwalk, CT: Appleton & Lange, 1993.)

Origin of Scattered Radiation and Methods for Controlling Its Production:

- The larger the x-ray field size, the more scatter radiation produced. *Solution:* collimate!
- The higher the kilovoltage, the greater the production of scatter radiation (a result of the higher incidence of Compton scatter interactions). *Solution:* use optimum kVp.
- The thicker and more dense the body tissues, the greater the amount of scatter radiation produced. *Solution:* compression of the part or use of the prone position to decrease the effect of fatty tissue.

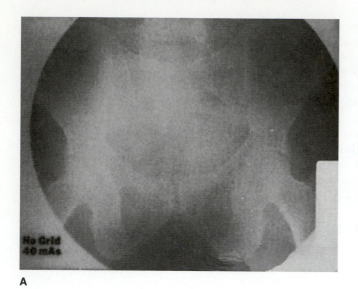

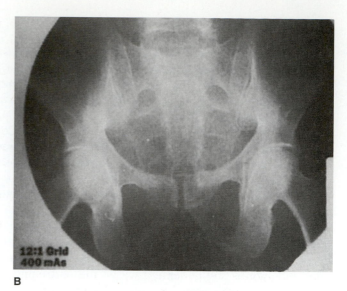

A

B

Figure 12–31. **(A)** Radiograph made at 40 mAs without a grid. Because of the thickness and nature of the part radiographed, a significant amount of scatter radiation was generated and went on to expose the (undiagnostic) film. **(B)** Radiograph made using a 121 grid. Although an exposure increase to 400 mAs was required, scatter radiation was removed before it reached the image receptor and a diagnostic radiograph was obtained. (From the American College of Radiology Learning File. Courtesy of the American College of Radiology.)

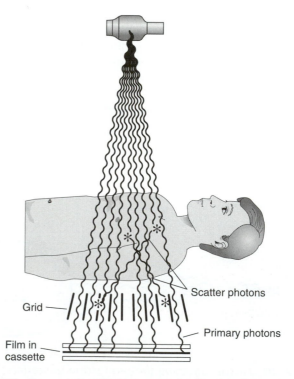

Figure 12–32. Scattered radiation generated in the object is removed (cleaned up) with the use of a grid. (Modified from Wolbarst AB. *Physics of Radiology.* East Norwalk, CT: Appleton & Lange, 1993.)

the image receptor, hence a very significant decrease in radiographic *density*. To maintain adequate density then, the addition of a grid must be accompanied by an appropriately substantial increase in *mAs*.

Before beginning a discussion of the impact of grids on technical factors, a more complete study of them is in order. A grid may be *stationary* or *moving*. Stationary grids are the simplest type and usually consist of alternating *vertical* lead strips (ie, a *parallel* grid) and radiolucent interspace filler material. A grid cassette is an example of a stationary grid. Another example is the "slip-on," or "wafer," grid that may be placed over a regular cassette. *Stationary grids* are useful in mobile radiography and horizontal beam (cross-table lateral) radiography; they are usually low ratio. A disadvantage of stationary grids is visibility of grid lines.

If the grid is in motion during the exposure, as it is in the *moving grid*, the grid lines are effectively blurred out of the radiographic image. The lead strips and interspace material of a moving grid are slightly *angled* so that, at a given distance from the focal spot, the angle of the lead strips will conform with the divergence of the x-ray beam. A grid with lead strips that are angled thus is called a *focused grid*; if an imaginary line is extended up from each lead strip, the point of intersection is called the *convergence line*, and the distance from the convergence line to the surface of the grid is the *focusing distance* (Fig. 12–33). That focusing distance is the ideal SID, although grids usually specify a *focal range* in which they can be safely used.

Another type of grid is the *crossed grid*; it has a second series of lead strips aligned perpendicular to the first. Crossed grids may be parallel or focused, and are extremely efficient in absorbing scat-

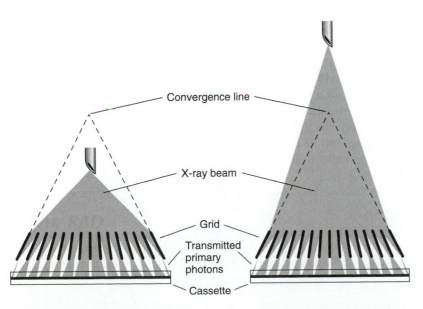

Figure 12–33. Grid cutoff will be apparent if the SID is above or below the specified focal range limits and will be characterized by density loss at the periphery of the image. This is described as an *off-focus error* or *focus-grid distance decentering*. (From Wolbarst AB. *Physics of Radiology.* East Norwalk, CT: Appleton & Lange, 1993.)

tered radiation; however, their use prohibits any x-ray tube angulation and requires that the x-ray tube be exactly centered to the center of the grid. Any misalignment or tube angulation can result in severe *grid cutoff* (absorption of the useful/primary beam). Crossed grids are not used in general radiography; they may have some application in special procedures.

Care must be taken to avoid errors common to the use of focused grids, including angulation errors, off-level errors, off-focus errors, off-center errors, and upside-down grid placement.

- *Angulation errors:* The x-ray tube may be safely angled in the direction of the lead strips; angulation "against" the lead strips causes *grid cut-off;* that is, absorption of the primary beam and resulting loss of density across the image (similar to that exhibited in off-level errors).
- *Off-level errors:* If the planes of the x-ray tube and grid surface are not parallel, grid cutoff will occur. This can happen, for example, when the x-ray tube is tilted or when a grid cassette is placed inaccurately under a patient during mobile radiography. To avoid cutoff, the radiographer must ensure that the grid surface is perpendicular to the central ray.
- *Off-focus errors:* Grid cutoff will occur if the SID is below the lower limits, or above the upper limits, of the specified focal range. This type of error is also referred to as *focus–grid distance decentering.* Off-focus errors are usually characterized by loss of density at the *periphery* of the image.
- *Off-center errors:* If the x-ray beam is not centered to the grid (ie, if it is shifted laterally) grid cutoff will occur. This type of error is referred to as *lateral decentering,* and is characterized by a uniform density loss across the radiographic image (Fig. 12–34).

If the x-ray beam is both *off-center and off-focus below the focusing distance,* the portion of the image below the focus will show *increased* density; if the x-ray beam is *off-center and off-focus above*

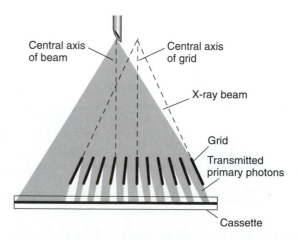

Central axis of beam

Central axis of grid

X-ray beam

Grid

Transmitted primary photons

Cassette

Figure 12–34. A *uniform density loss* across the radiographic image will occur if the x-ray beam is off center laterally. (From Wolbarst AB. *Physics of Radiology.* East Norwalk, CT: Appleton & Lange, 1993.)

the focusing distance, the image below the focus will show *decreased* density.

- *Upside down grid:* A focused grid placed upside down has its lead strips angled exactly opposite the angle of the x-ray beam. So, except for the central area where the lead strips and x-ray beam are vertical, grid cutoff will be severe (Fig. 12–35).

Two of a grid's *physical characteristics* that determine its degree of efficiency in the removal of scattered radiation are:

- *Grid ratio: Grid ratio* is defined as the height of the lead strips compared to the distance between them (Fig. 12–36).

$$\text{Grid ratio} = \frac{\text{height of Pb strip}}{\text{width of interspace material}}$$

For example, a grid having lead strips 1.5 mm tall separated by interspace material 0.15 mm wide has a grid ratio of 10:1.

As the lead strips are made taller, or the distance between them decreases, scattered radiation is more likely to be trapped before

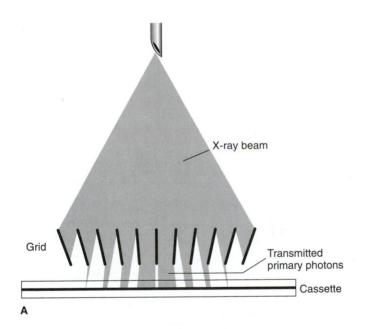

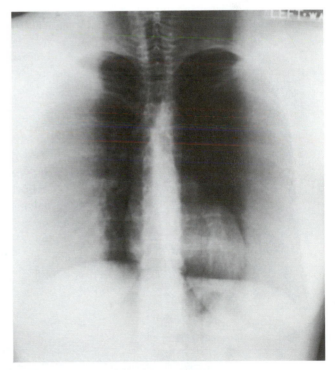

Figure 12–35. **(A)** and **(B)** An *upside-down focused grid* presents its lead strips in the opposite direction to that of the x-ray beam. This results in severe grid cutoff everywhere except in the central portion of the radiographic image. ((A) from Wolbarst AB. *Physics of Radiology.* East Norwalk, CT: Appleton & Lange, 1993; **(B)** from Saia D. *Appleton & Lange's Review for the Radiography Examination.* East Norwalk, CT: Appleton & Lange, 1997.)

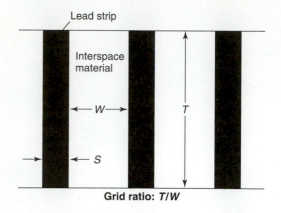

Grid ratio: *T/W*

Figure 12–36. Cross-section of a grid. *Grid ratio* is defined as the height (T) of the lead strips (S) to width of the interspace material (W). Grid ratio = T/W. (Modified from Wolbarst AB. *Physics of Radiology.* East Norwalk, CT: Appleton & Lange, 1993.)

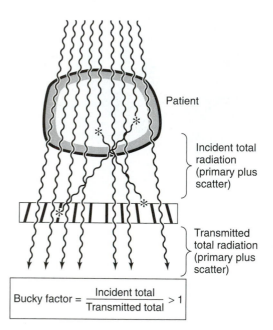

Figure 12–37. The Bucky factor (B) is the *grid conversion factor* and describes the total amount of radiation striking the grid surface compared to the amount of radiation transmitted through the grid. (Modified from Wolbarst AB. *Physics of Radiology.* East Norwalk, CT: Appleton & Lange, 1993.)

reaching the image receptor. A 12:1 ratio grid will absorb more scattered radiation than an 8:1 ratio grid.

- *Number of lead strips per inch:* The number of lead strips per inch may also be referred to as *grid frequency.* The advantage of many lead strips per inch is that there is less *visibility* of the lead strips. As the number of lead foil strips per inch increases, the foil often gets thinner, and therefore less visible. There is, of course, a disadvantage here. If the lead strips get thinner, more energetic scattered radiation can pass through them and reach the *image receptor.* So to maintain the efficiency of a grid having many lead strips per inch, its grid *ratio* is often increased as well; that is, the lead strips are made taller to increase the likelihood of their trapping scattered radiation before it reaches the image receptor.

The radiolucent interspace material is most frequently made of plastic or fiber; some grids use aluminum as the interspace material. Aluminum is more sturdy, gives the radiograph a smoother appearance free of objectionable *grid lines,* and can perhaps have an additional filtering effect on scattered radiation. However, because of this filtering effect, a greater increase in patient dose is required with aluminum interspaced grids. Fiber interspace material, on the other hand, can be affected by moisture and result in warping of the grid.

Other ways of expressing and measuring grid efficiency include:

- *Bucky (grid) factor:* The *Bucky (grid) factor* (B) of a particular grid is the ratio of the total amount of radiation (primary and scattered) incident upon the surface of the grid compared to the amount of radiation transmitted through the grid:

$$B = \frac{\text{incident total}}{\text{transmitted total}}$$

The Bucky factor is the grid conversion factor; that is, that amount by which the mAs must be changed to compensate for the radiation absorbed by the grid (Fig. 12–37). This is discussed in further detail later in this section.

- *Contrast improvement factor:* The ratio of radiographic contrast obtained with a grid compared to the contrast obtained without a grid is referred to as the contrast improvement factor (CIF).

$$CIF = \frac{\text{contrast with grid}}{\text{contrast without grid}}$$

- *Selectivity:* The ratio between the quantity of *primary photons transmitted* through the grid to the quantity of *scattered photons transmitted* is referred to as the selectivity (S) of the grid.

$$S = \frac{\text{primary photon transmission}}{\text{scattered photon transmission}}$$

An undesirable but unavoidable characteristic of grids is that they do absorb some primary photons as well as scattered photons. The higher the ratio grid, the more pronounced this will be. The higher the primary to scattered photon transmission ratio, the more desirable the grid.

- *Lead content:* This is perhaps least familiar to the radiographer because it applies little to the practical use of the grid. The definitions of grid ratio and grid frequency do not take into account the thickness of the lead strip; *lead content* does consider it. Lead content is measured in g/cm^2, and expresses the amount of lead contained within a particular grid.

How must exposure factors be adjusted to maintain appropriate density when changing from nongrid to grid? How can exposure factors be changed to preserve the density level when changing from one ratio grid to another?

In actual practice, the grid conversion factor varies slightly according to kVp range used. The ARRT recognizes that different textbooks cite slightly different grid conversion factors, and has stated that the distractors in calculation problems will not be so close as to cause conflict with the keyed correct answer. The conversion factors listed in the chart to the left can be used to calculate grid conversions in exposure factor problems.

A particular examination was performed tabletop/nongrid at 40 inches SID using 7 mAs and 90 kVp. To reduce the amount of image-degrading scattered radiation, another radiograph will be made using a 12:1 ratio grid. What new mAs factor will be required in order to maintain the original level of optical density?

The grid conversion formula is:

$$\frac{mAs_1}{mAs_2} = \frac{grid\ factor_1}{grid\ factor_2}$$

Substituting known quantities:

$$\frac{7}{x} = \frac{1}{5}$$

$$x = 35 \text{ mAs required with 12:1 grid}$$

A lumbar spine was radiographed laterally at 40 inches SID using 40 mAs and 95 kVp and an 8:1 ratio grid. To improve scattered radiation cleanup, another radiograph will be made using a 12:1 grid. What new mAs factor will be required in order to maintain the original level of optical density?

Using the grid conversion formula shown above, and substituting known quantities:

$$\frac{40}{x} = \frac{4}{5}$$

$$4x = 200$$

$$x = 50 \text{ mAs required with 12:1 grid}$$

An 8:1 grid is satisfactory for radiography up to 90 kVp. A 16:1 grid ratio is frequently advocated for radiography greater than 100 kVp. Routine radiographic equipment generally employs a 10:1 or 12:1 grid.

Grid Conversion Factors for Various Ratio Grids

Grid Ratio	Conversion Factor
No grid	1
5:1	2
6:1	3
8:1	4
10 or 12:1	5
16:1	6

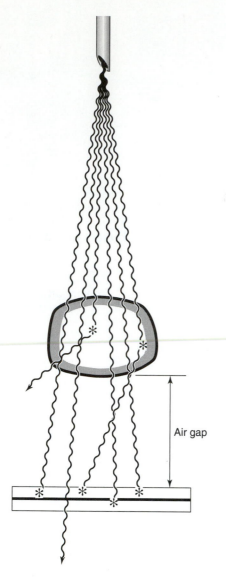

Figure 12–38. Air-gap technique. As scattered radiation emerges from the part, it continues to travel in its divergent fashion, bypassing the image receptor. (From Wolbarst AB. *Physics of Radiology*. East Norwalk, CT: Appleton & Lange, 1993.)

The use of high ratio grids at low kVp levels is discouraged because of the unnecessary patient exposure required.

Remember, to avoid variations in radiographic density, mAs adjustments are essential when changing grid ratios.

A word of caution regarding the use of an *inverted cassette* in place of a grid: the results are unpredictable and this practice is discouraged. Appropriate selection and careful use of a grid provides a far more predictable outcome and a diagnostically superior radiographic image.

An *air gap* introduced between the object and image recorder can have an effect similar to that of a grid. As energetic scattered radiation emerges from the body, it continues to travel in its divergent fashion and, much of the time, will bypass the image recorder (Fig. 12–38). It is usually necessary to increase the SID to reduce magnification caused by increased OID.

Summary

- Scattered radiation is a result of x-ray photon interaction with tissue via Compton scatter processes.
- Scattered radiation adds image-degrading densities to the radiographic image.
- The production of scattered radiation increases with an increase in field size, kVp, and thickness and volume of tissue.
- The single most important way to decrease the production of scattered radiation is to collimate.
- The amount of scattered radiation reaching the image receptor is decreased through the combined use of collimators and grids.
- Grids are made of alternating strips of lead and radiolucent material and are placed between the patient and image receptor to stop scattered radiation.
- Grids may be stationary or moving, parallel or focused.
- Crossed grids are very efficient but require exact centering and prohibit tube angulation.
- Focused grids require that
    - The correct surface be facing the x-ray tube (ie, not upside down)
    - Tube angulation parallels the lead strips
    - The long axis of the x-ray tube and grid surface are parallel
    - The x-ray tube be within the focusing distance/range
    - The x-ray beam not be off center (laterally) with the center of the grid
- If focused grid requirements are not met, the resulting image will demonstrate a loss of density as a consequence of grid cutoff (ie, absorption of the primary beam).
- The most common way of expressing grid efficiency is by grid ratio and number of lead strips per inch.
- Because grids remove many x-ray photons that would have contributed to image density, the addition of a grid requires a significant increase in mAs.
- When implementing a grid or changing grid ratio, a grid-conversion factor must be used to determine appropriate mAs changes to avoid variations in optical density.

F. FILTRATION

As discussed in Chapter 11, the primary beam generally has a total filtration of 2.5 mm Al equivalent for patient protection purposes. In general-purpose radiographic tubes, the glass envelope usually accounts for about 0.5 mm Al equivalent and the collimator provides about 1.0 mm Al equivalent. These are considered *inherent filtration*. The manufacturer adds another 1.0 mm Al *(added filtration)* to meet the minimum requirements of 2.5 mm Al equivalent total filtration for radiographic tubes operated above 70 kVp.

This type of filter serves to remove the diagnostically useless x-ray photons that only contribute to patient (skin) dose. Because this radiation is "soft" (low energy) and would not reach the image receptor anyway, the x-ray tube total filtration *has no real effect on radiographic density*. Filtration serves to increase the overall average energy of the beam; it "hardens" the x-ray beam.

Compensating filters can be used to provide more uniform radiographic density when radiographing structures with widely different x-ray absorbing properties because of thickness or tissue composition. Usually made of aluminum or clear leaded plastic, they slide into tracks in the tube head similar to a cylinder cone, or attach magnetically to the undersurface of the tube housing.

If a foot radiograph demonstrates well-exposed tarsals, the toes will frequently be overexposed (Fig. 12–39A). Conversely, if the exposure is adjusted to improve the image of the toes, the tarsals will be underexposed. Because the foot varies so greatly in thickness and tissue density along its long axis, it is difficult to achieve uniform radiographic density. A simple *wedge*-shaped compensating filter can remedy the situation (Fig. 12–39E and Fig. 12–40B and C). The filter is attached to the tube head so that the thin portion is over the tarsals and the thick portion over the toes. Exposure factors appropriate for tarsals are used, and the thick portion of the filter removes enough of the primary beam to prevent overexposure of the toes. Thus, a foot radiograph having uniform density throughout is achieved (Fig. 12–39A and B). A wedge filter is also useful for femur examinations and decubitus abdomen images (Fig. 12–39C and D).

Another type of compensating filter is the *trough* filter (Fig. 12–40A), so named because its central portion is thin and the portions extending laterally are thicker, thus forming a central trough. A trough filter can be used in chest radiography to permit visualization of the denser mediastinal structures without overexposing the more radiolucent lungs and pulmonary vascular markings.

Another simple, yet effective, application of compensating filtration is the use of a saline bag. The saline bag is placed over the thinner body part and serves to filter out excessive exposure. This technique is effectively employed in the AP projection of the thoracic spine, however its use should be noted on the requisition as its use can cause an artifact.

Summary

- **Ordinary x-ray tube filtration of 2.5 mm Al has no effect on radiographic density.**
- **When anatomic parts vary greatly in thickness or tissue composition, compensating filters may be used to "even out" radiographic densities.**

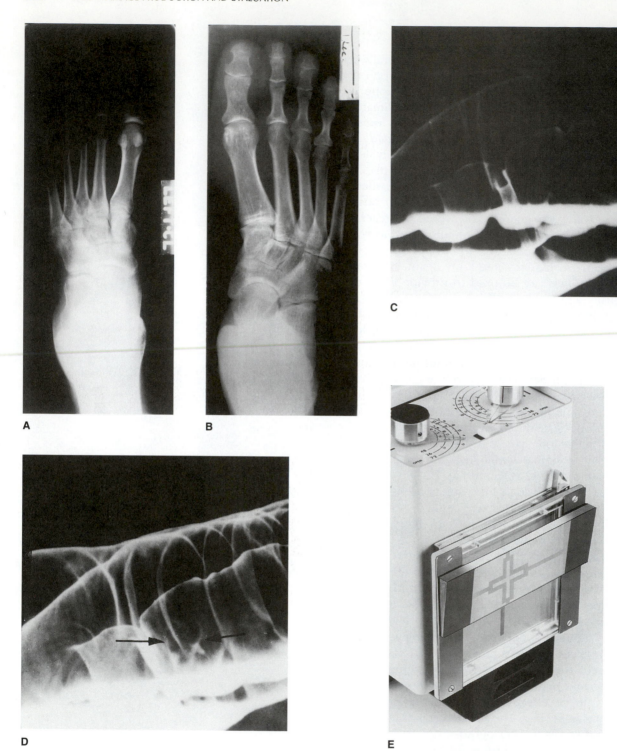

Figure 12–39. **(A)** Typical foot radiograph performed without the use of a *compensating filter;* although the tarsals and metatarsals are well demonstrated, the phalanges are significantly overexposed. **(B)** Image made using a compensating filter whose thicker portion was placed over the phalanges to balance radiographic densities. **(C)** Lateral decubitus image of an air and barium-filled colon. Abdominal tissues often shift to the dependent side in the decubitus position, making the "down" side thicker than the "up" side. Excessive density of the air-filled structures can obliterate pathology. **(D)** Use of a wedge-shaped compensating filter can equalize tissue density differences, thus providing more uniform optical density and improved visualization of any pathology (a polypoid lesion is demonstrated). **(E)** Compensating (wedge) filter magnetically attached to the x-ray tube housing. (Courtesy of Nuclear Associates.)

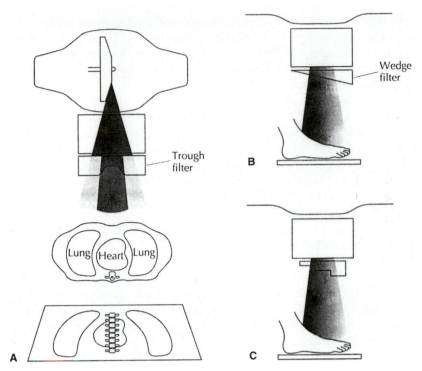

Figure 12–40. **(A)** *Trough filter* in place for chest radiograph. The thicker lateral portions of the trough reduce the intensity of the beam directed toward the lungs, while the thinner central portion does not attenuate the beam directed to the more dense mediastinal structures. **(B)** and **(C)** Two types of *wedge filters* used to "graduate" the x-ray beam intensity, with a greater number of photons directed to the thicker tarsal area and fewer photons toward the thinner areas of metatarsals and phalanges. (Reproduced with permission from Shephard CT. *Radiographic Image Production and Manipulation.* New York: McGraw-Hill, 2003.)

- Compensating filters slide into place by means of tracks on the tube housing.
- Compensating filters are available in various shapes: their thicker portions absorb more of the x-ray beam and are therefore placed over thinner body parts, while their thinner portions (absorbing fewer x-rays) are placed over thicker body parts.

G. STRUCTURAL (NORMAL VERSUS PATHOLOGIC) CONSIDERATIONS

Normal tissue variants and pathologic processes can alter tissue thickness and composition and thereby have a significant effect on radiographic density. The radiographer must be aware of these variants and processes to make an intelligent and accurate selection of technical factors.

In 1916, R. Walter Mills presented a paper at the American Roentgen Ray Society meeting in Chicago (published in *American Journal of Roentgenology*, April 1917) describing "The Relation of Bodily Habitus to Visceral Form, Position, Tonus and Motility." Here he coined

Examples of Additive Pathologic Conditions

- Ascites
- Rheumatoid arthritis
- Paget's disease
- Pneumonia
- Atelectasis
- Congestive heart failure
- Edematous tissue

Examples of Destructive Pathologic Conditions

- Osteoporosis
- Osteomalacia
- Pneumoperitoneum
- Emphysema
- Degenerative arthritis
- Atrophic and necrotic conditions

the terms *hypersthenic, sthenic, hyposthenic,* and *asthenic* (defined in Chapter 6) to describe the various body types. He noted that most physicians came into the field prejudiced by their early anatomic teachings and had fixed conceptions, "which the revelations of the roentgen ray ruthlessly outraged."

Radiographers still use these terms today to describe *body habitus* and its normal variants. Knowledge of each of the body types and its associated tissue characteristics, position and tonus of associated organs, and so on helps us to position more accurately and to select appropriate technical factors. The same body part, such as the stomach, in two different individuals will require very different central ray points of entry if one individual is hypersthenic and the other asthenic. A particular body part, such as the shoulder, may measure the same on two different individuals, yet it may not be appropriate to select identical exposure factors for each if one is a muscular sthenic build and the other a hyposthenic type with little muscle tone.

Other factors that influence radiographic density, and consequently the selection of technical factors, are age, gender, and pathology. Various abnormal pathologic conditions, disease processes, and trauma can affect tissue density and, hence, radiographic density. Normal variants of muscle development result from different lifestyles, occupations, and age, and will affect radiographic density.

Some pathologic conditions are referred to as *destructive*, such as osteoporosis and conditions involving necrosis or atrophy. These conditions can cause an undesirable increase in radiographic density unless they are recognized and appropriate changes made in exposure factors. Other conditions such as ascites, rheumatoid arthritis, and Paget's disease are *additive*, and an increase in exposure factors is required to maintain adequate radiographic density.

Summary

- Variations in tissue density will be noted as radiographic density variations in the x-ray image.
- Normal tissue density differences exist as a result of body habitus, age, gender, and level of activity.
- Abnormal density differences exist as a result of trauma or pathologic conditions.
- The radiographer must be knowledgeable about the conditions affecting normal and abnormal changes in tissue density to make accurate selection of technical factors.

H. GENERATOR TYPE

Three-phase x-ray generation is much more efficient than *single phase* because the voltage never drops to zero. Three-phase equipment has a small voltage ripple, and thus produces more high-energy x-ray photons (Fig. 12–41). Therefore, if two radiographs were made of the same part and using the same factors, one made with a single-phase machine and one with a three-phase machine, the three-phase radiograph would show considerably more radiographic density. Consequently, to reproduce similar radiographic densities when using different generators, exposure factor adjustment is necessary.

If 92 kVp and 60 mAs were used for a particular abdominal exposure using single phase equipment, what mAs would be required

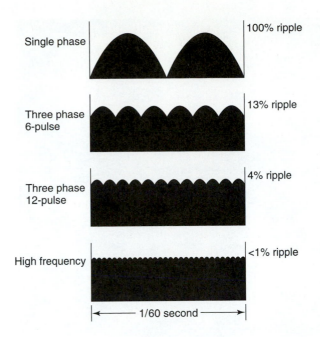

Figure 12–41. *Single-phase (1φ) and three-phase (3φ) wave-forms. Compared to the one useful impulse available per 1/60th second with alternating current, single-phase rectified current has two useful impulses, 3φ 6p rectified has six useful impulses, and 3φ 12p has 12.*

to produce a similar radiographic image using three phase, six pulse equipment?

The correction table in the box in this section indicates that only two-thirds of the original single-phase mAs would be required to produce similar optical density with three-phase equipment.

Thus:

$$2/3 \times 60 = 40 \text{ mAs with } 3\phi \text{ 6p equipment}$$

(note that kVp is irrelevant)

It should be noted that approximately the same quantity of radiation is delivered to *the image receptor* from each x-ray machine (1φ and 3φ) to produce similar radiographic images. The entrance skin exposures (ESEs), however, differ significantly (Fig. 12–42). This is because the single-phase machine produces many more low-energy photons, contributing only to patient skin dose.

When technical factors are modified for single-phase or three-phase changes, it is usually the mAs that is adjusted; however, kVp adjustment is also workable. Changing from single-phase to three-phase requires a 12% decrease in kVp; conversely, changing from three-phase to single-phase requires a 12% increase in kVp.

Conventional 60 Hz full-wave rectified power is converted to a higher frequency of 500 to 25,000 Hz in the most recent generator design—the high-frequency generator. The high-frequency generator is small in size, in addition to producing an almost constant potential waveform.

Summary

- **Three-phase (3φ) equipment produces nearly peak potential voltage whereas single-phase (1φ) voltage drops periodically to zero between voltage peaks.**
- **mAs is usually adjusted to compensate for differences between 1φ and 3φ waveform equipment.**

Correction Factor	
Single Phase	**Three Phase**
x mAs	2/3 × (6p)
x mAs	1/2 × (12p)
x kVp	x − 12%

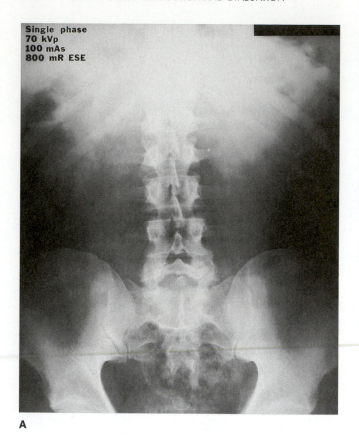

Single phase
70 kVp
100 mAs
800 mR ESE

A

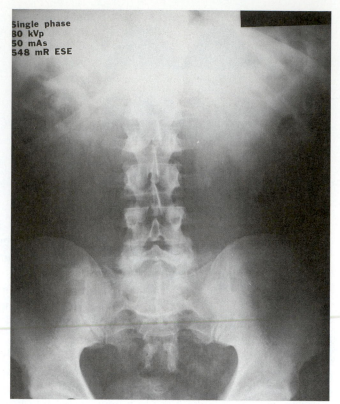

Single phase
80 kVp
50 mAs
548 mR ESE

B

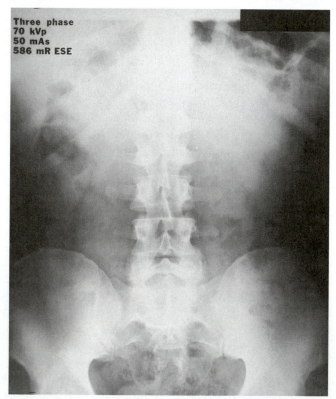

Three phase
70 kVp
50 mAs
586 mR ESE

C

Figure 12–42. Images **(A)** and **(C)** are good examples of 1φ to 3φ conversion and the difference in entrance skin exposure (ESE). Images **(A)** and **(B)** demonstrate the radiation protection factor in increasing from 70 kVp at 100 mAs to 80 kVp at 50 mAs; note the big difference in ESE. (From the American College of Radiology Learning File. Courtesy of the American College of Radiology.)

■ **When changing from 1φ to 3φ 6p, two-thirds less mAs is required; from 1φ to 3φ 12p, one-half the original mAs is required (the reverse is true when changing from 3φ to 1φ).**

I. BEAM RESTRICTION

A change in radiographic density will occur with changes in the size of the irradiated field, all other factors remaining constant. *Beam restriction* (ie, reducing the volume of tissue irradiated) reduces the production of scattered radiation and, consequently, decreases radiographic density. The reverse is also true: as field size increases, radiographic density increases as a result of increased production of scattered radiation fog. *Therefore, as changes are made in the size of the irradiated field, an accompanying change in mAs is required to maintain the same radiographic density.*

J. ANODE HEEL EFFECT

The anode heel effect was discussed earlier with respect to focal spot size and recorded detail. Figures 12–43 and 12–44 illustrate how a portion of the divergent x-ray beam is absorbed by the anode resulting in diminished radiographic density at the anode end of the radiograph.

When using general radiographic tubes at standard distances, the heel effect is only noticeable when radiographing parts of uneven thickness, such as the femur and thoracic spine. In these cases, the heel effect may be used to advantage by placing the thicker body portion under the cathode end of the x-ray beam, thus having the effect of "evening out" tissue densities.

The Anode Heel Effect is Emphasized Under the Following Conditions
• At short SIDs • With large cassettes • With small target-angle x-ray tubes

K. PROCESSING

Radiographic film emulsion is very sensitive to even small changes in chemical processing. A decrease in developer temperature of 2° to 3°F will produce a dramatic decrease in radiographic density (Fig. 12–45) and, conversely, a rise in developer temperature results in a density increase (Fig. 12–46). Figure 12–47 illustrates the impact of developer temperature on the characteristic curve.

Radiographic density is also directly related to length of development and replenishment rate; that is, density increases as development time increases or as replenishment rate increases.

Summary

■ **Changing the size of the irradiated field affects radiographic density as a result of increased or decreased scattered radiation production.**

■ **The anode heel effect is characterized by greater x-ray intensity at the cathode end of the beam.**

■ **The anode heel effect is most pronounced at short SIDs, with large image receptors, and with x-ray tubes having small target angles.**

■ **The anode heel effect can be used to "even out" densities when radiographing parts of uneven thickness.**

■ **Radiographic density increases as developer temperature increases.**

■ **Radiographic density increases as the replenishment rate and/or length of development increase.**

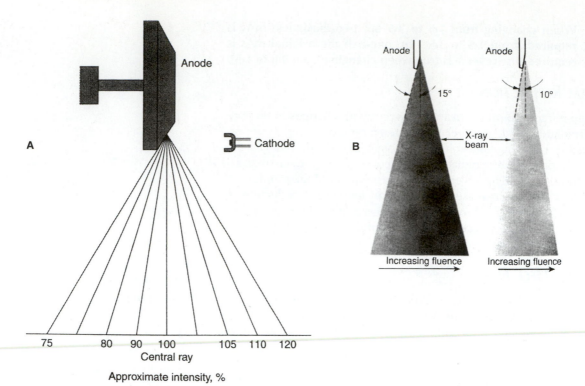

Figure 12–43. **(A)** and **(B)**. *The anode heel effect.* As x-ray photons are produced within the anode, a portion of the divergent beam is absorbed by the anode's "heel." This represents a decrease in x-ray beam intensity at the anode end of the x-ray beam. (Reproduced with permission from Shephard CT. *Radiographic Image Production and Manipulation.* New York: McGraw-Hill, 2003.)

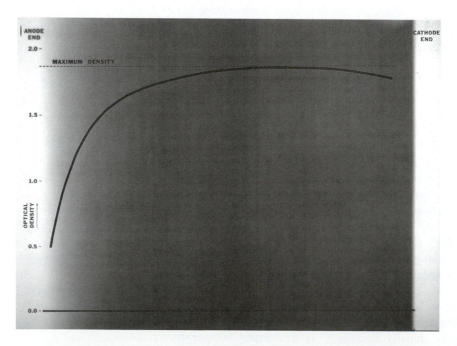

Figure 12–44. *Radiographic illustration of the anode heel effect.* Note the gradual increase in radiographic density toward the cathode end of the beam. (From the American College of Radiology Learning File. Courtesy of the American College of Radiology.)

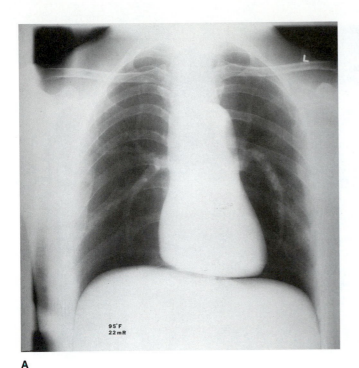

A

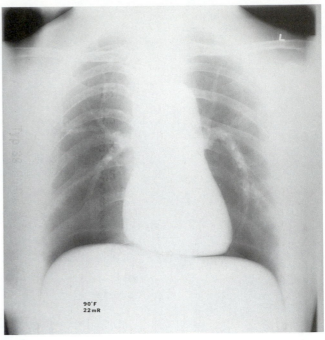

B

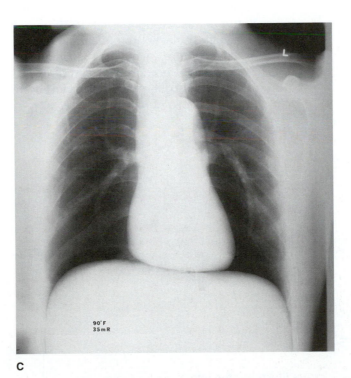

C

Figure 12–45. *Developer temperature* versus image density and patient exposure. **(A)** Radiograph of a chest phantom made using 22 mR and processed at the recommended temperature of 95°F. **(B)** Radiograph exposed and produced under the same conditions except that the developer temperature was 5° lower, at 90°F; note the significant change in radiographic density. **(C)** Radiograph using the same 90°F developer, but with exposure compensated to provide the required density; note the increase in exposure dose to 35 mR. (From the American College of Radiology Learning File. Courtesy of the American College of Radiology.)

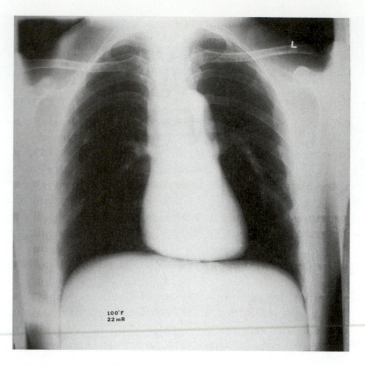

Figure 12–46. This radiograph was exposed under the same conditions as Figure 12–45A, but was processed at a developer temperature 5° above normal (at 100°F), producing a dark radiograph. Although a diagnostic radiograph might be produced by reducing the film exposure, higher-than-recommended processing temperatures are not advised because they can produce inconsistent results. (From the American College of Radiology Learning File. Courtesy of the American College of Radiology.)

Figure 12–47. The characteristic curve illustrates the effect of *developer temperature* changes seen in Figures 12–45 and 12–46. The relative position of the lower temperature (90°F) curve is to the right of the optimal temperature (95°F) curve; to achieve the same density, the exposure must be increased to compensate for decreased development. The 100°F curve illustrates a shift to the left of the optimal curve, illustrating that less exposure is required to compensate for decreased development. (Modified from the American College of Radiology Learning File. Courtesy of the American College of Radiology.)

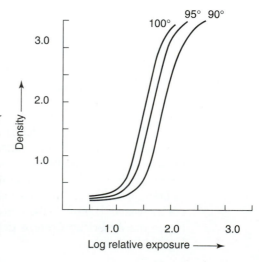

Chapter Review Questions

⭐ ***Congratulations!*** *You have completed a portion of this chapter. You may go on to the "Registry-type" multiple choice questions that follow. For greatest success, be sure also to complete the short answer questions found at the end of this chapter.*

1. Grid ratio is defined as the relationship between the height of the lead strip and the:
   (A) width of the lead strip
   (B) distance between the lead strips
   (C) number of lead strips per inch
   (D) angle of the lead strip

2. Of the following groups of exposure factors, which will produce the greatest radiographic density?
   (A) 200 mA, 0.05 sec, 36 inches SID
   (B) 400 mA, 0.05 sec, 72 inches SID
   (C) 400 mA, 0.10 sec, 72 inches SID
   (D) 200 mA, 0.10 sec, 36 inches SID

3. How is source-image distance related to exposure rate and optical density?
   (A) as SID increases, exposure rate increases and optical density increases
   (B) as SID increases, exposure rate increases and optical density decreases
   (C) as SID increases, exposure rate decreases and optical density increases
   (D) as SID increases, exposure rate decreases and optical density decreases

4. If the radiographer is unable to adjust the mAs, yet needs to double the optical density on a particular image, which of the following would *best* accomplish this?
   (A) increase the kVp by 50%
   (B) increase the kVp by 15%
   (C) decrease the SID by 25%
   (D) increase the grid ratio

5. Exposure factors of 85 kVp and 10 mAs are used for a particular nongrid exposure. What should be the new mAs if a 12:1 grid is added?
   (A) 20 mAs
   (B) 30 mAs
   (C) 40 mAs
   (D) 50 mAs

6. An image lacking sufficient optical density may be attributable to insufficient
      1. SID
      2. developer temperature
      3. kilovoltage
   (A) 2 only
   (B) 1 and 2 only
   (C) 2 and 3 only
   (D) 1, 2, and 3

7. The quantity of x-ray photons delivered to the patient in a given exposure is *primarily* regulated by:
   - (A) mAs
   - (B) kVp
   - (C) SID
   - (D) focal spot size

8. An exposure was made using 200 mA, 0.05 second exposure, and 75 kVp. Each of the following changes will function to double radiographic density, *except*:
   - (A) change to 0.1 second exposure
   - (B) change to 86 kVp
   - (C) change to 20 mAs
   - (D) change to 100 mA

9. An exposure was made at 40 inches SID using 300 mA, 0.12 second exposure and 70 kVp with a 200 film–screen combination and an 8:1 grid. It is desired to repeat the radiograph and, in order to produce improved detail, use 48 inches SID and 100 film–screen combination. Using 0.25 second exposure, and with all other factors remaining constant, what mA will be required to maintain the original radiographic density?
   - (A) 100 mA
   - (B) 200 mA
   - (C) 300 mA
   - (D) 400 mA

10. Compared to a low-ratio grid, a higher-ratio grid could have:
    1. taller lead strips
    2. more distance between the lead strips
    3. thicker lead strips
    - (A) 1 only
    - (B) 1 and 2 only
    - (C) 2 and 3 only
    - (D) 1, 2, and 3

Answers and Explanations

1. (B) A grid consists of alternate strips of lead and interspace material. The lead strips are used to trap scatter radiation before it reaches the image receptor, thus decreasing the effect of scatter radiation fog on the radiograph. Grid ratio is defined as the height of the lead strip to the distance between the strips (or width of the interspace material).

2. (D) Using the formula mA × sec = mAs, determine each mAs. The greatest radiographic density will be produced by the combination of greatest mAs and shortest SID. Groups A and C should produce identical radiographic density, according to the inverse square law, because group C is twice the distance and four times the mAs of group A. Group B has twice the distance of group A, but only twice the mAs; it has, therefore, less density than groups A and C. Group D has the same distance as group A, and twice the mAs, making it the group of technical factors that will produce the greatest radiographic density.

3. (D) According to the inverse square law of radiation, the intensity or exposure rate of radiation from its source is inversely proportional to the square of the distance. Thus, as distance from the source of radiation increases, exposure rate decreases. Because exposure rate and radiographic density are directly proportional, if the exposure rate of a beam directed to an image receptor is decreased, the resultant optical density would be decreased proportionally.

4. (B) Radiographic/optical density is proportional to mAs. However, other methods may be used to adjust optical density. When adjusting mAs is not possible, an increase in kVp by 15% will effectively double the radiographic density. Decreasing the source-image distance (SID) will increase density, but increased patient dose and size distortion make this an impractical approach. Increasing the grid ratio will decrease optical density.

5. (D) To change nongrid to grid exposure, or to adjust exposure when changing from one grid ratio to another, recall the factor for each grid ratio:

no grid = 1 × original mAs

5:1 grid = 2 × original mAs

6:1 grid = 3 × original mAs

8:1 grid = 4 × original mAs

12:1 grid = 5 × original mAs

16:1 grid = 6 × original mAs

Therefore, to change from nongrid to 12:1 grid, multiply the original mAs by a factor of 5. A new mAs of 50 is required.

6. (C) Insufficient kVp can result in underpenetration of an anatomic part and inadequate radiographic density. If developer temperature is too low, the developing agents (especially hydroquinone) may become inactive, resulting in an underdeveloped image with insufficient density. Insufficient SID (ie, SID too low) will result in an image with excessive radiographic density.

7. (A) While mAs is primarily used to regulate x-ray *quantity*, the number of x-ray photons produced in a given exposure, kVp is generally used to regulate x-ray *quality*, the energy or wavelength of x-ray photons produced at the target during a given exposure. Although source–image distance significantly *affects* optical density, it is not used to *regulate* the quantity of photons produced. Focal spot size is unrelated to radiation quantity or quality.

8. (D) Optical density is directly proportional to mAs. If exposure time is doubled from 0.05 (1/20) second to 0.1 (1/10) second, optical density will double. If the mAs is doubled from 10 to 20 mAs, optical density will double. If the kVp is increased by 15%, from 75 to 86 kVp, optical density will double according to the 15% rule. Changing to 100 mA will halve the mAs, effectively halving the optical density.

9. (D) A review of the problem reveals that *three changes* are being made: an increase in SID, a change from 200 speed system to 100 speed system, and an increase in exposure time (to be considered last). Because the original mAs was 36, cutting the speed of the system in half (from 200 to 100) will require a doubling of the mAs, to 72, in order to maintain density. Now we must deal with the distance change. Using the density maintenance formula (remember 72 is now the *old* mAs!) we find that the required new mAs at 48 inches is 103. Because the problem states that we are now using 0.25 second exposure, it is left to determine what mA, used with 0.25 second, will provide 103 mAs.

$$0.25 \, x = 103$$

$$x = 412 \, mA$$

10. (A) As the lead strips are made *taller*, or the *distance between them decreases*, scattered radiation is more likely to be trapped before reaching the image receptor. For example, a 12:1 ratio grid will absorb more scattered radiation than an 8:1 ratio grid. Thickness of the lead strips refers to its lead content, which is unrelated to grid ratio. Lead content is measured in g/cm^2, and expresses the amount of lead contained within a particular grid.

III. FACTORS AFFECTING RADIOGRAPHIC CONTRAST

A. TERMINOLOGY

Radiographic contrast exists whenever two or more different densities are present in a radiographic image. When there is a big difference between shades of densities, radiographic *contrast* is said to be *high*. When there is little difference between densities, radiographic *contrast* is *low*.

Radiographic contrast is the sum of subject contrast and film contrast.

Subject contrast is a result of differential absorption by tissues of varying densities and thicknesses. X-ray photons are attenuated to differing degrees by various body tissues, with less exit radiation emerging from thicker, denser structures, and more exit radiation from thinner or less-dense structures. Hence, subject contrast produces the various density *differences* visible on the radiographic image, and is exhibited as a *scale of grays* having varying tones representative of differential tissue absorption.

Exposure factor selection and various other methods are used to *modify* the effect of differential absorption properties of tissue, thereby enabling the radiographer to produce the desired scale of contrast.

Subject contrast is regulated by the quality (energy, wavelength, penetrability) of x-ray photons.

Film contrast describes the response of the film emulsion to the variety of x-ray intensities emerging from the irradiated part. Film contrast is affected by the manufacturing process (film type, base fog), processing conditions, and fluorescent properties of the intensifying screens. Film contrast characteristics are illustrated by the characteristic (D log E) curve.

A radiograph exhibiting a variety of different shades of gray possesses *long-scale* (low) *contrast;* that is, there is *little difference* among the various shades. One that exhibits only a few shades possesses *short-scale* (high) *contrast.*

The function of contrast is to make image details visible. Most anatomic structures have an infinite number of details that compose the

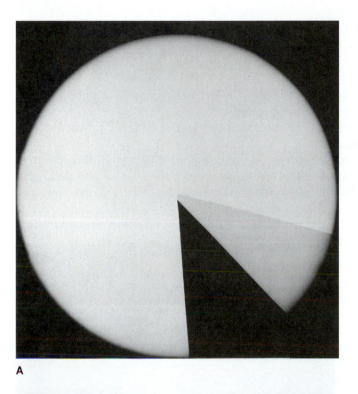

A

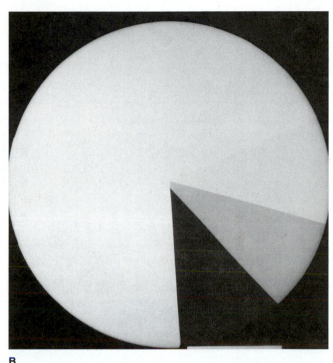

B

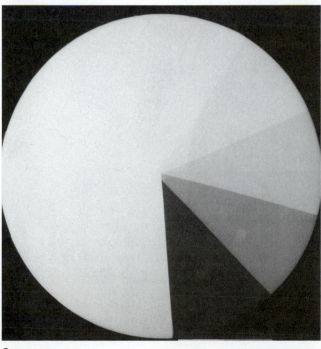

C

Figure 12–48. *Contrast functions to make details visible.* Radiographs were made of a circular phantom having a variety of wedge-shaped thicknesses; a circular "lesion" of greater density is embedded in each wedge. Note that the level of contrast between adjacent areas is strongly related to the degree of visibility of the "lesions." **(A)** Illustrates the highest contrast; only two wedges (thicknesses) are visualized and only one "lesion" is barely visible. **(B)** The contrast scale is a little longer; a third wedge begins to be seen and two "lesions" are visualized. **(C)** Five wedges are visualized (hopefully the printing process shows them!) and at least three "lesions" can be seen clearly. Methods that can be used to adjust the level of contrast between adjacent areas include (1) increasing kVp; (2) using compensating filtration; and (3) using lower contrast (higher latitude) film. (From the American College of Radiology Learning File. Courtesy of the American College of Radiology.)

Contrast Terminology

HIGHER CONTRAST	LOWER CONTRAST
shorter scale contrast	longer scale contrast
↓	↓
IS A PRODUCT OF:	IS A PRODUCT OF:
lower kVp	higher kVp
fewer, widely different tissue densities	many similar tissue densities

image and these structural details often represent a variety of tissue densities having different absorption properties. If the anatomic part is represented radiographically by only a few shades of gray, then many anatomic details are not being visualized at all. If, however, the radiograph displays a wide range of gray tones more anatomic details will be represented and visualized (Fig. 12–48). Hence, long-scale contrast *usually* provides more information (but short-scale, ie, high, contrast may be required for certain examinations or body parts; see Fig. 12–49).

A number of factors affect the production of radiographic contrast and each is discussed individually.

Summary

- **Radiographic contrast refers to the degree of difference between image densities.**
- **Radiographic contrast is the sum of subject contrast and film contrast.**
- **Subject contrast is the result of differential absorption of x-rays by body tissues of various thicknesses and densities.**
- **Film contrast is the result of manufacturing, processing, and intensifying screens.**
- **Subject contrast is regulated by selection of x-ray beam quality.**

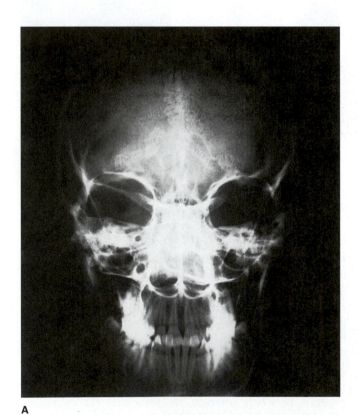

A

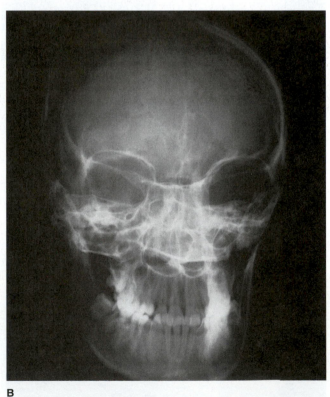

B

Figure 12–49. **(A)** Example of *high, or short-scale, contrast.* **(B)** Example of *low, or long-scale, contrast.* Rotation of the skull is also seen. (From the American College of Radiology Learning File. Courtesy of the American College of Radiology.)

- Radiographic images with several diverse density differences are said to possess long-scale (or low) contrast.
- Radiographic images possessing few density differences, strikingly different from each other, are said to possess short-scale (or high) contrast.

B. KVP

Kilovoltage peak (kVp), which governs x-ray *penetrability,* is the primary exposure factor affecting radiographic contrast. In general, as kVp increases so does the scale of contrast (Fig. 12–50).

In general, parts having *low subject contrast* will produce long-scale radiographic contrast, and if high kVp is used to image these parts, unacceptably low radiographic contrast will result.

Scattered radiation fog reduces the visibility of low contrast objects. When imaging *structures having low subject contrast, use of lower kVp frequently helps to emphasize what little contrast exists in the subject tissues.*

Because kVp determines the penetrating ability of the x-ray photons, *low kVp can be used to emphasize the differences between tissue densities,* for example, in mammography, foreign-body localization, and iodine-containing renal collecting systems (Fig. 12–51).

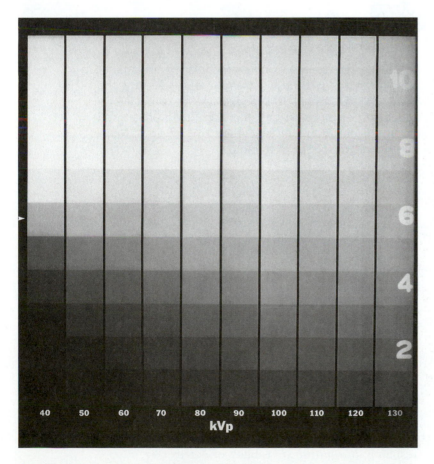

Figure 12–50. *Aluminum step wedge test.* As kVp increases, a greater number of steps (and the subtle differences between them) are discernible. (From the American College of Radiology Learning File. Courtesy of the American College of Radiology.)

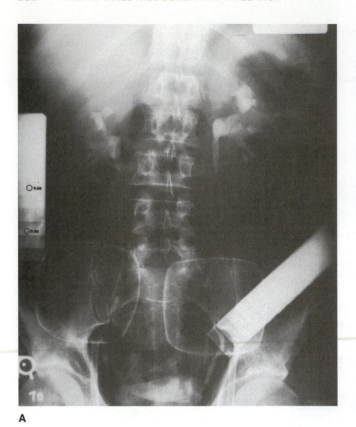
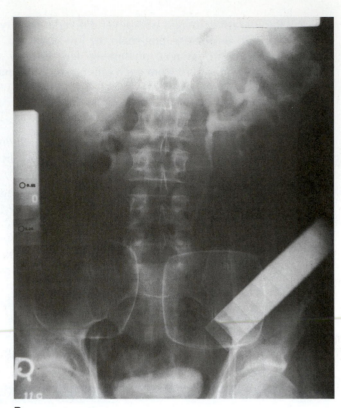

A   B

Figure 12–51. In anatomic regions having *low subject contrast* such as the abdominal viscera, artificial contrast agents are often introduced to demonstrate organs such as the kidneys. **(A)** IVU made using 70 kVp. **(B)** IVU using 110 kVp. The use of too high kVp with iodinated media and the production of more scatter radiation has almost obliterated the contrast-filled collecting systems in image **(B).** (From the American College of Radiology Learning File. Courtesy of the American College of Radiology.)

Higher/Shorter Scale Contrast Results When

- Subject contrast increases
- kVp decreases
- Scattered radiation decreases
- Grid ratio increases
- Exposure latitude decreases

Anatomic parts having *high subject contrast* will produce short-scale radiographic contrast, and if low kVp is used to image these parts, unacceptably high radiographic contrast will result (Fig. 12–52). Visibility of structures within the very light and very dark areas is greatly diminished. *When imaging structures having high subject contrast, the use of higher kVp will promote more uniform penetration of the part,* thus it "evens out" big differences in tissue densities and bringing about visualization of small image details (as in high kVp chest radiography).

C. SCATTERED RADIATION

High kVp may be desirable in terms of patient dose, tube life, and making more details visible, but use of excessively high kVp will result in production of excessive amounts of scatter radiation and fog, resulting in *diminished* visibility of details (Fig. 12–53).

Much of the scatter radiation produced is highly energetic and exits the patient along with useful image forming radiation. Scattered radiation carries no useful information, but adds noise in the form of fog, thereby impairing visibility of detail.

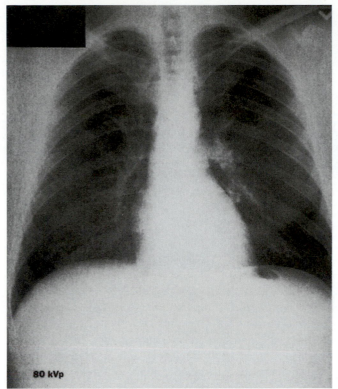
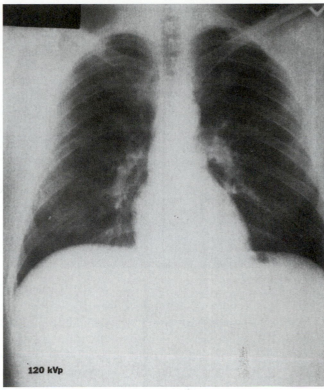

A   **B**

Figure 12–52. Posteroanterior (PA) chest radiographs made using 80 kVp **(A)** and 120 kVp **(B)**. Image **(A)** PA chest radiograph made using 80 kVp demonstrates shorter-scale contrast, and pulmonary vascular markings are not well visualized. **(B)** Chest radiograph made using 120 kVp demonstrates longer-scale contrast, and visualization of pulmonary vascular markings *through* the bony rib details, and requires a smaller patient dose. (From the American College of Radiology Learning File. Courtesy of the American College of Radiology.)

Because scattered radiation can have such a devastating effect on image contrast, it is essential that radiographers are knowledgeable about methods of reducing its production. The three factors that have a significant effect on the *production of scattered radiation* are:

- Beam restriction
- Kilovoltage
- Thickness/volume and density of tissues

Perhaps the most important way to limit the production of scattered radiation is by limiting the size of the irradiated field; that is, through beam restriction (Fig. 12–54). *As the size of the field is reduced, there is less area and tissue volume for scatter radiation to be generated.*

As the volume and/or density of the irradiated tissues increase(s) so does scatter radiation (Fig. 12–55). *Thicker and denser anatomic structures will generate more scattered radiation production.* Compression of certain parts can occasionally be used to minimize the effect of scatter, but close collimation can always be used effectively.

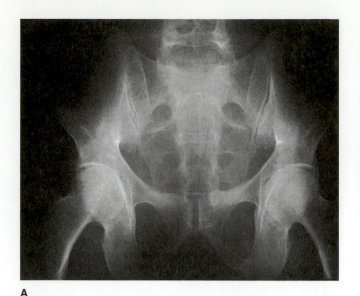

A

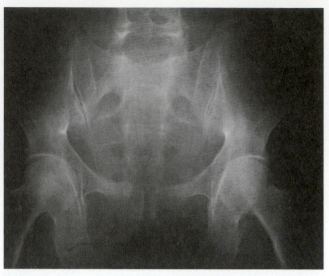

B

Figure 12–53. *Kilovoltage is directly related to the production of scatter radiation.* **(A)** Image made using 80 kVp and 75 mAs. **(B)** Image made using 100 kVp and 18 mAs, all other factors remaining the same. As kVp is increased, the percentage of scattered radiation relative to primary radiation increases. Use of optimum kilovoltage for each anatomic part is helpful in keeping scatter to a minimum. (From the American College of Radiology Learning File. Courtesy of the American College of Radiology.)

Introduction of an OID (*air gap*) can have a noticeable effect on radiographic contrast. An air gap introduced between the object and image recorder can have an effect similar to that of a grid. As energetic scattered radiation emerges from the body, it continues to travel in its divergent fashion and, much of the time, will bypass the image recorder (see Fig. 12–38).

D. STRUCTURAL AND PATHOLOGIC CONDITIONS

Various tissue types and pathologic processes can alter tissue thickness and composition and thereby have a significant effect on radiographic contrast. Anatomic structures having high atomic numbers and pathologic conditions that increase tissue density tend to produce a higher contrast.

The radiographer must be aware of the nature of pathology under investigation to make an intelligent and accurate selection of technical factors.

Summary

- kVp selection determines the energy of x-ray photons and therefore degree of penetration of various tissues, thereby determining the contrast characteristics of the image.
- Images of low subject contrast structures often benefit from the use of lower kVp, while high subject contrast structures can be represented with a longer range of grays by using higher kVp.
- The use of high kVp reduces patient dose and reduces the production of x-ray tube heat, but increases the production of scatter radiation fog.

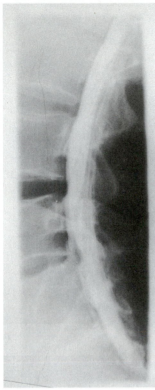

A

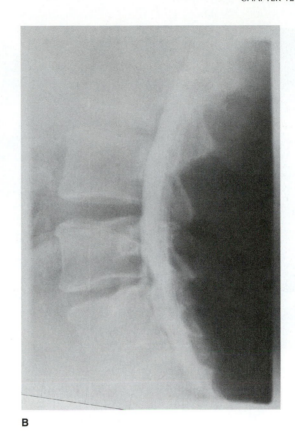

B

Figure 12–54. Note the striking improvement in radiographic quality in image (**A**) as beam restriction is increased in this lateral lumbar myelogram. Although a 50% increase in exposure was required to maintain appropriate density in image (**A**) (to compensate for less scattered radiation reaching the image receptor), radiation protection is maintained because the volume of irradiated tissue is decreased. (From the American College of Radiology Learning File. Courtesy of the American College of Radiology.)

■ **Radiation that has scattered carries no useful information, but rather, adds noise that impairs visibility of image details. The production of scattered radiation can be minimized by using optimum kVp techniques and by restricting the size of the x-ray beam as much as possible.**

■ **As the thickness and density of tissues increase, so does the production of scattered radiation; tissue thickness can sometimes be minimized with compression.**

■ **As normal tissues undergo pathologic change, their penetrability frequently also changes in ways characteristic of the disease process.**

E. GRIDS

An image produced with a grid usually differs considerably from an image produced without a grid. Since thicker, denser parts can generate significant amounts of scattered radiation, a grid should be used whenever a part measures 11 cm or greater in thickness. A possible exception to this rule is the chest, although much chest radiography performed today employs high kVp and grids.

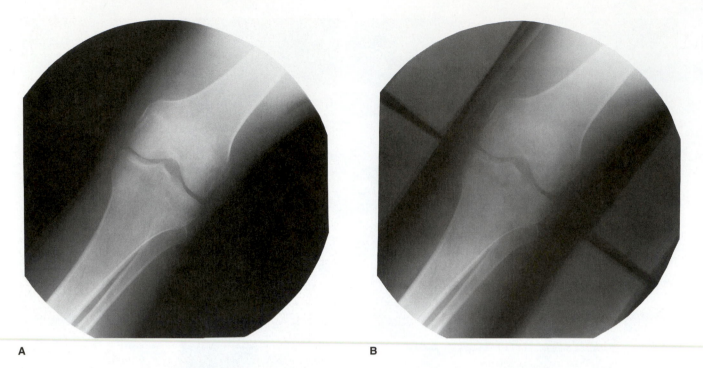

A   **B**

Figure 12–55. The *volume of irradiated tissue is directly related to the quantity of scatter radiation generated.* **(A)** Anteroposterior (AP) of knee. **(B)** AP with paraffin absorbers *around* the knee. The loss of contrast exhibited in **(B)** is caused by increased *volume* of irradiated material within the beam, resulting in increased scattered-radiation fog. Note that the part need not be *thicker* to generate significant scatter, just that the total irradiated *volume* be greater. (From the American College of Radiology Learning File. Courtesy of the American College of Radiology.)

Although collimation, optimum kVp, and compression may be used, a large amount of scattered radiation can still be generated within the part being radiographed and can have a severely degrading effect on image contrast. Without the use of a grid, scattered radiation can contribute 50 to 90% of the total image exposure. The function of a grid, then, is to remove scattered radiation exiting the patient *before* it reaches the image receptor thereby improving contrast (Fig. 12–56).

As discussed earlier in this part, two of a grid's physical characteristics that determine its degree of efficiency in the removal of scattered radiation are *grid ratio* (the height of the lead strips compared to the distance between them) and number of *lead strips per inch.* Other familiar ways of expressing and measuring grid efficiency include the *Bucky factor* (grid conversion factor), *contrast improvement factor,* and *selectivity.*

The *Bucky factor (B)* is the ratio of the total amount of radiation (primary and scattered) incident upon the surface of the grid to the amount of radiation transmitted through the grid.

$$B = \frac{\text{total incident}}{\text{total transmitted}}$$

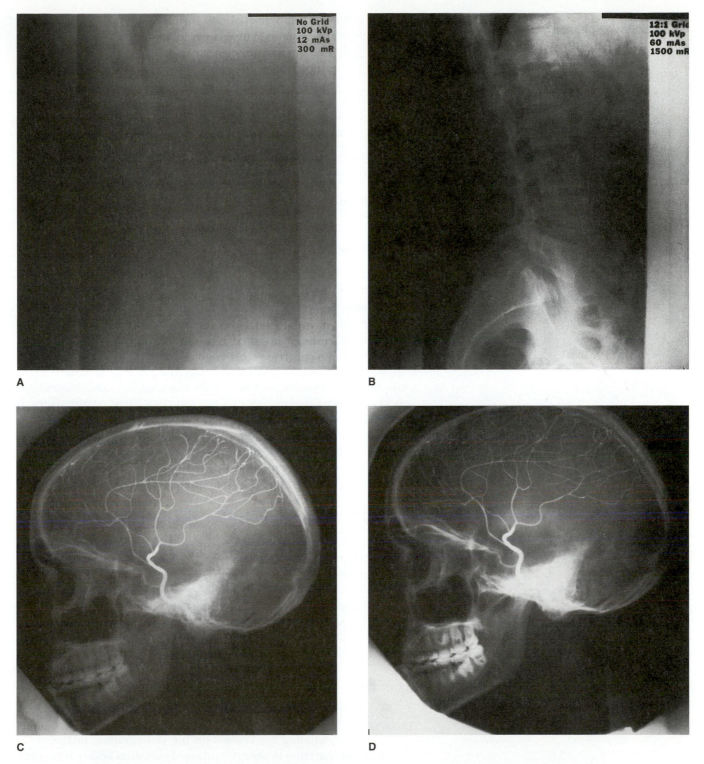

Figure 12–56. *Effect of grids on image contrast* and radiographic quality. **(A)** Made using 100 kVp and 12 mAs without a grid; scatter radiation fog obliterates recorded detail almost entirely. **(B)** Made with 100 kVp, 60 mAs, and using a 12:1 grid, all other factors remaining constant; scatter radiation is "cleaned up" and image details are more readily perceptible. **(C)** Made without a grid using 70 kVp and 4 mAs. **(D)** Made with a 12:1 grid using 70 kVp and 20 mAs. Note the improved contrast and detail visibility. (From the American College of Radiology Learning File. Courtesy of the American College of Radiology.)

As Grid Ratio Increases

- Scatter radiation clean-up increases
- Contrast scale decreases (higher contrast produced)
- Exposure factors (usually mAs) must increase

The *contrast improvement factor (CIF)* is the ratio of radiographic contrast obtained with a grid to that obtained without a grid.

$$CIF = \frac{\text{contrast with grid}}{\text{contrast without grid}}$$

Selectivity (S) is the ratio between the quantity of primary photons transmitted through the grid and the quantity of scattered photons transmitted.

$$S = \frac{\text{primary photon transmission}}{\text{scattered photon transmission}}$$

As previously discussed, the introduction of an *air gap can have an effect similar to that obtained through the addition of a grid.*

F. FILTRATION

The primary beam usually has a total filtration of 2.5 mm Al equivalent. Inherent filtration includes 0.5 mm Al from the glass envelope and 1.0 mm Al from the collimator. The manufacturer adds another 1.0 mm Al to meet the minimum requirements of 2.5 mm Al equivalent total filtration for radiographic tubes operated above 70 kVp.

Filtration serves to increase the overall average energy of the beam; it "hardens" the x-ray beam. The 2.5 mm Al equivalent functions to remove the diagnostically worthless x-ray photons that contribute to patient dose. Since these photons do not have sufficient energy to reach the image receptor, the usual required filtration in the x-ray tube *has no significant effect on radiographic contrast* (Fig. 12–57).

The addition or removal of *compensating* filters (as discussed in section II-F) will impact the radiographic contrast unless exposure factors are adjusted to compensate for the change.

G. INTENSIFYING SCREENS

Radiographic images produced with intensifying screens possess higher contrast than those produced by direct exposure. In general, when comparing radiographs produced using different speed intensifying screens, *the higher the screen speed, the higher the contrast;* that is, 400 speed screens will produce somewhat higher contrast than 200 and 100 speed screens, and 200 screens will produce higher contrast than 100 screens, and so on. Contrast differences among various speed screens, however, are slight.

Summary

- X-rays scattering within a part and having enough energy to exit the body and reach the image receptor produce scattered radiation fog (noise) on the radiographic image.
- Grids function to absorb scattered radiation before it reaches the image receptor.
- Scattered radiation cleanup increases as grid ratio increases.
- The higher the grid ratio, the higher (shorter scale) the resulting contrast.
- X-ray tube filtration ordinarily has little effect on contrast; it functions primarily for patient protection.
- Compensating filters added or removed from the x-ray beam will affect contrast unless exposure adjustment is made.

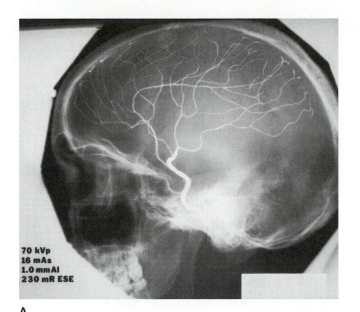
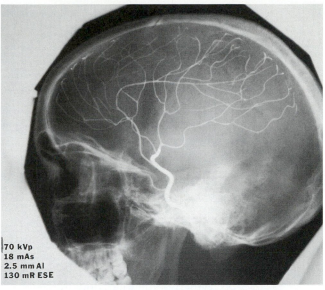

A **B**

Figure 12–57. **(A)** and **(B)**. *The effect of filtration on image contrast.* The contrast displayed in **(A)** and **(B)** is very similar. An increase in filtration, however, results in a lower ESE (entrance skin exposure) and greater tube load (mAs). As filtration is increased above 2.5 mm Al, minimal dose reduction occurs and tube loading is significantly increased. (From the American College of Radiology Learning File. Courtesy of the American College of Radiology.)

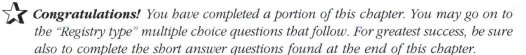 Chapter Review Questions

☆ ***Congratulations!*** *You have completed a portion of this chapter. You may go on to the "Registry type" multiple choice questions that follow. For greatest success, be sure also to complete the short answer questions found at the end of this chapter.*

1. What are the effects of scattered radiation on the radiographic image?
   1. it produces fog
   2. it increases contrast
   3. it increases grid cutoff
   (A) 1 only
   (B) 2 only
   (C) 1 and 2 only
   (D) 1, 2, and 3

2. In comparison to 60 kVp, 80 kVp will:
   1. permit greater exposure latitude
   2. produce longer scale contrast
   3. produce more scatter radiation
   (A) 1 only
   (B) 2 only
   (C) 1 and 2 only
   (D) 1, 2, and 3

3. An increase in the kilovoltage applied to the x-ray tube increases the:
   1. x-ray wavelength
   2. exposure rate
   3. patient absorption
   (A) 1 only
   (B) 2 only
   (C) 2 and 3 only
   (D) 1, 2, and 3

4. All of the following are related to radiographic contrast *except*:
   (A) photon energy
   (B) grid ratio
   (C) object image distance
   (D) focal spot size

5. Which of the following groups of exposure factors will produce the longest scale of contrast?
   (A) 200 mA, 1/20 sec, 70 kVp, 12:1 grid
   (B) 500 mA, 0.02 sec, 80 kVp, 16:1 grid
   (C) 300 mA, 0.03 sec, 90 kVp, 8:1 grid
   (D) 600 mA, 0.015 sec, 70 kVp, 8:1 grid

6. Which of the following anatomic parts exhibits the highest subject contrast?
   (A) elbow
   (B) kidney
   (C) esophagus
   (D) lumbar spine

7. A radiograph that exhibits many shades of gray from white to black may be described as having:
   (A) long-scale contrast
   (B) short-scale contrast
   (C) more density
   (D) good recorded detail

8. The advantages of high kilovoltage chest radiography include
   1. greater exposure latitude
   2. longer scale contrast
   3. reduced patient dose
   (A) 1 only
   (B) 1 and 2 only
   (C) 1 and 3 only
   (D) 1, 2, and 3

9. Which of the following exposure factors is used to regulate radiographic contrast?
   (A) mA
   (B) exposure time
   (C) mAs
   (D) kVp

10. Which of the following contribute(s) to the radiographic contrast present on the finished radiograph?
    1. tissue density
    2. pathology
    3. muscle development
    (A) 1 and 2 only
    (B) 1 and 3 only
    (C) 2 and 3 only
    (D) 1, 2, and 3

Answers and Explanations

1. (A) Scattered radiation is produced as x-ray photons travel through matter, interact with atoms, and are scattered (change direction). If these scattered rays are energetic enough to exit the body, they will strike the image receptor from all different angles. They therefore do not carry useful information and merely produce a flat, gray (low contrast) fog over the image. Grid cutoff increases contrast and is caused by improper relationship between the x-ray tube and grid.

2. (D) The higher the kVp range, the greater the exposure latitude (margin of error in exposure). Higher kVp is more penetrating and produces more grays on the radiograph, lengthening the scale of contrast. As kVp increases, the percentage of scatter radiation also increases.

3. (B) As the kilovoltage is increased, a *greater number* of electrons are driven across to the anode with *greater force*. Therefore as energy conversion takes place at the anode, *more high-energy* (short wavelength) photons are produced. However, because they are higher-energy photons, there will be *less* patient absorption.

4. (D) As photon energy increases, more penetration and greater production of scattered radiation occurs, producing a longer scale of contrast. As grid ratio increases, more scattered radiation is absorbed, producing a higher contrast. As OID (object-to-image-receptor distance) increases, the distance between the part and image receptor acts as a grid and consequently less scatter radiation reaches the image receptor, producing a higher contrast. Focal spot size is related only to recorded detail.

5. (C) Of the given factors, kilovoltage and grid ratio will have a significant effect on radiographic contrast. The mAs values are almost identical. Because an increased kilovoltage and low-ratio grid combination would allow the greatest amount of scattered radiation to reach the image receptor, thereby producing more gray tones, C is the best answer. D also uses a low ratio grid, but the kV is too low to produce as much gray as C.

6. (A) The greatest subject contrast is found in body parts made of a few widely differing tissue densities. The elbow has but bone, some muscle, and soft tissues constituting high subject contrast. The abdomen, containing the kidneys, stomach, small and large intestines, and other viscera, is a heavy body part composed of many similar tissue densities, and thus, normally has very-low subject contrast.

7. (A) Radiographic contrast is described as the difference between the densities present on a radiograph. A radiograph possessing many shades of gray between black and white is said to exhibit long-scale, or low, contrast. A radiograph possessing only a few widely different shades of gray between black and white is said to exhibit short-scale, or high, contrast.

8. (D) The chest is composed of widely differing tissue densities (bone and air). In an effort to "even out" these tissue densities and better visualize pulmonary vascular markings, high kV is generally used. This produces more uniform penetration and results in a longer scale of contrast with visualization of the pulmonary vascular markings as well as bone (which is better penetrated) and air densities. The increased kV also affords the advantage of greater exposure latitude (an error of a few kV will make little if any difference). The fact that the kV is increased means that the mAs is accordingly reduced and thus, patient dose is reduced as well.

9. (D) Kilovoltage regulates the energy, and therefore penetration, of the photons produced at the target. The greater the photon energy, the less the total absorption by dense tissues and the more that tissue densities will be "evened out," that is, showing a longer scale of grays. Time and mA are the quantitative exposure factors controlling radiographic density.

10. (D) The radiographic subject, that is, the patient, is composed of many different tissue types of varying densities, resulting in varying degrees of photon attenuation and absorption. This *differential absorption* contributes to the various shades of gray (ie, scale of radiographic contrast) on the finished radiograph. Normal tissue density may be significantly altered in the presence of pathology. For example, destructive bone disease can cause a dramatic decrease in tissue density. Abnormal accumulation of fluid (as in ascites) will cause a significant increase in tissue density. Muscle atrophy, or highly developed muscles, will similarly decrease or increase tissue density.

IV. FILM, SCREEN, AND GRID OPTIONS

X-ray film may be described as being made of *silver bromide grains suspended in a gelatin emulsion and coated on a plastic base material*. X-ray film is an important means of recording and storing the radiographic image and so a brief overview of the process of x-ray film production is in order here.

First, gelatin is extracted from cattle hooves and hides and rendered into a very pure, uncontaminated state. Nitric acid is combined with pure silver to form *silver nitrate*. Then, *in total darkness, silver nitrate is added to potassium bromide to form silver bromide*. Silver bromide is then combined with the gelatin mixture to form the emulsion, which is coated onto one (single emulsion film) or both sides (*duplitized*) of the film base.

The base material is a durable *polyester* plastic that will not tear, and with a dimensional stability that will be unaffected as it travels through the processor roller system and various chemical temperatures. Film base is not absolutely clear; it has a measurable density, referred to as *base fog* or *base density*. Base fog or density is the sum of environmental exposure received during production and storage as well as the density resulting from the base material tint and dye. An additional, approximately equal, amount of fog results from processing. The total *base plus fog* should not exceed 0.2 density as measured by a densitometer.

A *protective coat* of hard, clear gelatin is placed over the emulsion to help prevent damage in the form of scratches.

A. FILM CONTRAST AND LATITUDE

Each type of x-ray *film emulsion* is manufactured with certain characteristics required for its particular use (eg, latitude film, mammography film), each having its own particular response to exposure (ie, *film latitude*). Some film emulsion is manufactured especially to produce high contrast, for example, film used in mammography and vascular procedures. Others are produced to provide a long range of grays; this type of emulsion possesses more film *latitude*, that is, it is more "forgiving" of errors in technical factors (Fig. 12–58). The study of film emulsion response to exposure is called *sensitometry* and is illustrated by the characteristic Hurter and Driffield (H&D) curve.

The characteristic curve (Fig. 12–59) illustrates the degree of film density as a result of exposure. Density is represented by the vertical axis, log exposure by the horizontal axis. The *characteristic curve* has three portions: the *toe* (D_{min}), *straight-line portion,* and *shoulder* (D_{max}). Exposures made in the toe and shoulder portions of the curve will be excessively under or overexposed. The useful diagnostic range of densities lies between 0.25 and 2.5, corresponding to the *straight line portion* (average gradient) of the curve and is generally regarded

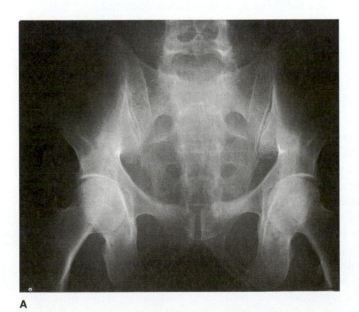
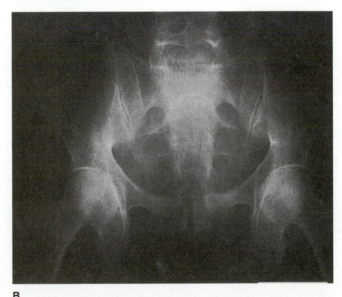

A   B

Figure 12–58. **(A)** Made using 80 kVp, 75 mAs, and regular film. **(B)** Made under identical conditions and using the same factors, but with latitude (ie, low-contrast) film. (From the American College of Radiology Learning File. Courtesy of the American College of Radiology.)

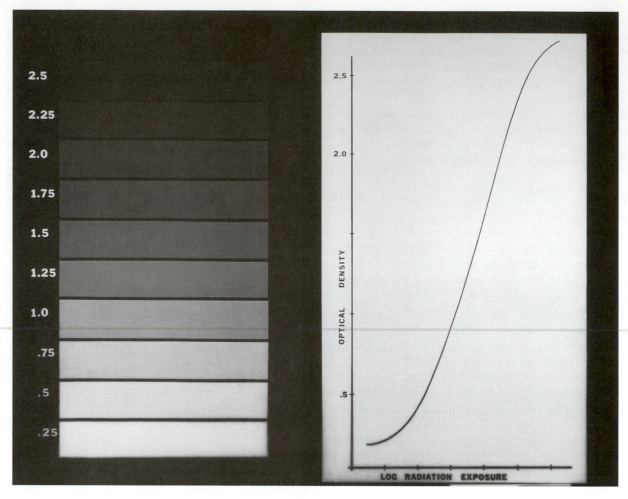

Figure 12–59. *Characteristic curve.* Notice that the toe portion of the curve does not begin at zero; this represents the slight exposure due to base fog. Total base plus fog should not exceed 0.2 density. (From the American College of Radiology Learning File. Courtesy of the American College of Radiology.)

as the *region of correct exposure.* Exposures made outside of this region do not record diagnostically useful information.

The highest point on the characteristic curve is where maximum density occurs, and is referred to as D_{max}. Just beyond D_{max}, the curve begins to descend again, representing a decrease in density. This is the *solarization point,* where additional exposure will actually cause a reversal of the image.

Have you noticed that an unexposed and processed duplicating film emerges from the processor black? If regular x-ray film were used for film duplication, a black and white reversed image would result. This is because, using regular film, the print box light will pass through the whiter areas causing exposure and darkening, while little light will pass through the darker areas, causing little or no exposure on the x-ray film: hence, a reversed image. Duplicating film emulsion, however, has been chemically brought up to the solarization point so that further exposure will cause a reversal, thus remedying the problem of reversed images with regular film.

A glance at a film's characteristic curve will tell you about its *speed, latitude, and contrast.* A curve having a steep slope (*average gradient*) is likely to be fast, having little latitude and producing high contrast. A fast film responds readily to fluorescent light or x-rays, and has the advantage of permitting a decrease in exposure factors, and ultimately, patient dose. When two or more curves are being compared, the curve farthest to the left represents the fastest emulsion.

The average gradient of a characteristic curve gives a good indication of that film's *contrast.* A steep characteristic curve (average gradient) is representative of high contrast, shorter scale, contrast. *Latitude* refers to the *range* of exposure that will provide densities within the diagnostically useful range; fast film generally offers less latitude (Fig. 12–60). Film and screen protocols are generally established at the radiographer's workplace; however, the radiographer should be knowledgeable enough to use the types available to best advantage.

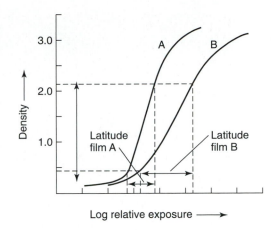

Figure 12–60. *Film latitude.* Note the differences in film latitude within the useful density range. Latitude and contrast are inversely related. **(A)** High-contrast, low-latitude film. **(B)** Low-contrast, high-latitude film.

B. EXPOSURE LATITUDE

While *film latitude* is related to emulsion characteristics, *exposure latitude* is related to the technical factors selected. Exposure latitude is the leeway, or margin of error, one has with a given group of exposure factors; the degree of exposure latitude is generally determined by the kilovoltage. At higher kilovoltages, a difference of a few kVp will make little, if any, difference radiographically (recall the 15% rule). At low kilovoltages, however, an error of just a few kVp can make a very noticeable difference in the radiographic image. While the radiographer has little control over film latitude, he or she has much control of exposure latitude.

Summary

- **X-ray film emulsion consists of silver bromide grains suspended in gelatin.**
- **Film base is a tough polyester plastic.**
- **Base plus fog is a result of environmental factors, base tint, and processing.**
- **Base plus fog should not exceed 0.2 density.**
- **Various kinds of film emulsion are available from the manufacturer; emulsion characteristics differ according to their use and the desired radiographic requirements.**
- **Film emulsions are made to be slow speed or high speed, low contrast or high contrast.**
- **Sensitometry is the study of film emulsion response to exposure.**
- **Characteristic curves are used to illustrate and compare film emulsion response to exposure.**
- **The typical characteristic curve has a toe (D_{min}), straight-line portion (average gradient), and shoulder (D_{max}).**
- **Diagnostically useful densities are within 0.25 to 2.5 on the vertical axis.**
- **A characteristic curve with a steep slope usually represents higher contrast emulsion; a characteristic curve with a gentle slope usually represents lower contrast emulsion.**
- **Exposure latitude is related to kVp level: as kVp increases, exposure latitude increases, and vice versa.**

C. ANATOMIC FACTORS

Consideration of patient habitus, tissue density, and pathology is important in the appropriate selection of radiographic accessories. For example, routine protocol may call for knee and shoulder examinations to be performed using the table or upright Bucky. However, children, the elderly, and patients with degenerative conditions may not require the use of a grid. Small, thin parts and parts undergoing degenerative changes (such as in osteoporosis) can frequently be performed tabletop (ie, using intensifying screens without a grid), thereby significantly reducing patient dose.

Many radiology departments have two screen types available. Slower speed screens (eg, 100 speed) are generally used for extremities and other structures where better detail is desired. Faster screens (eg, 400 speed) are usually used for general radiography of larger, thicker, denser structures to reduce exposure while still maintaining reasonably good image detail.

The usual use of intensifying screens may be modified to suit the particular circumstances of the examination. With all other factors remaining the same, the use of faster screens results in less exposure dose to the patient. Faster screens permit the use of shorter exposure times, and therefore may be used for extremities of children and other examinations where motion may be a problem; they can also be helpful when the affected extremity is unusually large or casted. Slower screens may be used when improved detail of a small area is desired, keeping in mind that exposure dose will be increased.

mAs Conversions for Screen Speed Changes

Screen Speed	mAs Conversion Factor
100	2
200	1
400	1/2 (.50)
800	1/4 (.25)

Relationship Between Grid Ratio and mAs

Grid Ratio	mAs Conversion Factor
No grid	1
5:1	2
6:1	3
8:1	4
10/12:1	5
16:1	6

D. CONVERSION FACTORS: INTENSIFYING SCREENS AND GRIDS

There are many variables associated with the practice of radiography. It is necessary that the radiographer be able to compensate for changes in imaging system components, such as intensifying screens and grids.

Intensifying screen speed is directly related to density and inversely related to mAs. As screen speed increases, all other factors remaining constant, radiographic density increases. As screen speed increases, therefore, mAs must be decreased in order to maintain the original density.

For example, if 200 speed screens (having a factor of 1) were used with 20 mAs for a particular examination, what mAs would be required using 400 screens?

$$\frac{\text{screen speed factor 1}}{\text{screen speed factor 2}} = \frac{\text{mAs 1}}{\text{mAs 2}}$$

$$\frac{1}{0.5} = \frac{20}{x}$$

$$x = 10 \text{ mAs using 400 speed screens}$$

Grid selection is dependent on the part being radiographed and the desired film characteristics. As grid ratio increases, scattered radiation cleanup increases and, as a result, contrast increases.

Grid ratio is inversely related to radiographic density and directly related to mAs. As grid ratio increases, all other factors remaining constant, radiographic density decreases. As grid ratio increases, therefore, mAs must be increased to maintain the original radiographic density (Fig. 12–61). As discussed earlier in the chapter, conversion factors may be used when changing from nongrid to grid or from one grid ratio to another.

For example, 12 mAs was used with an 8:1 ratio grid for a particular exposure. It is desired to repeat the exposure using a 16:1

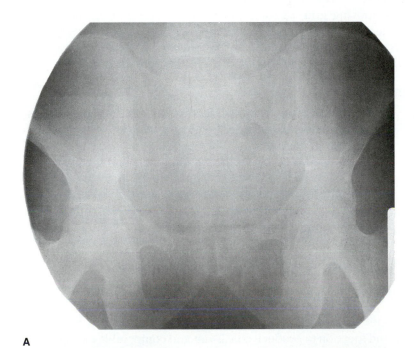

A

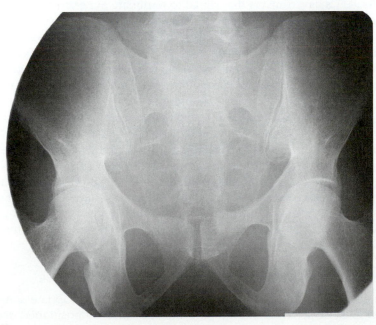

B

Figure 12–61. *Grids* are usually required for parts that generate large amounts of scattered radiation. **(A)** Made without a grid, using 40 mAs. **(B)** Made with a 12:1 grid and 200 mAs. Although a significant increase in exposure is required, the use of grids enables the production of diagnostic radiographs. (From the American College of Radiography Learning File. Courtesy of the American College of Radiology.)

ratio grid. What new mAs factor will be required to maintain the original radiographic density?

$$\frac{mAs_1}{mAs_2} = \frac{\text{conversion factor}_1}{\text{conversion factor}_1}$$

$$\frac{12}{x} = \frac{4}{6}$$

$$4x = 6(12)$$

$$4x = 72$$

$$x = 18 \text{ mAs using a } 16:1 \text{ grid}$$

These conversion factors allow for mAs compensation from nongrid to moving grid, or for changing from one grid to another, all other technical factors remaining constant. Because stationary grids are somewhat less efficient in the cleanup of scatter radiation, their use might require slight modification of the correction factor.

Summary

- **When selecting technical factors and radiographic accessories, consideration must be given to the patient's age, habitus, and pathology.**
- **Screen speed choice is dependent upon patient modifying factors (age, condition) and radiographic requirements (detail).**
- **The ratio of moving grids can differ from one radiographic room to another.**
- **Stationary grids are usually low ratio.**

V. AUTOMATIC EXPOSURE CONTROLS

A. TYPES

Automatic exposure controls (AECs) are used in today's x-ray equipment and function to produce consistent and comparable radiographic results. AECs have sensors that signal to terminate the exposure once a predetermined (known correct) exposure has been made.

In one type of AEC there is an *ionization chamber* just beneath the tabletop, *above* the cassette (Fig. 12–62). The part to be examined is centered to the sensor and radiographed. When a predetermined quantity of ionization has occurred (which equals the correct density), the exposure automatically terminates.

The other type of AEC is the *photomultiplier* type *(phototimer),* in which a small fluorescent screen is positioned *beneath* the cassette. When the exit radiation emerging from the patient exposes the image receptor and exits the cassette, the fluorescent screen emits light and charges a photomultiplier tube. Once a predetermined charge has been reached, the exposure is automatically terminated.

In either case, the manual timer should always be used as a *backup timer.* In case of AEC malfunction, the exposure would terminate, thus *avoiding patient overexposure and tube overload.*

B. POSITIONING ACCURACY

To achieve the expected radiographic density, the appropriate sensor(s) must be selected and the part must be correctly positioned directly above the sensor(s) and photocell(s).

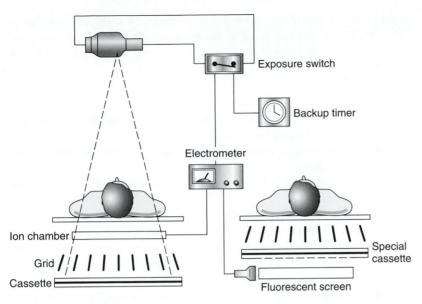

Figure 12–62. The two types of *automatic exposure devices* are the *ionization chamber* (left) and the *photomultiplier* (right). Note the *backup timer* that functions to terminate the exposure should the AEC fail to operate properly.

If a structure having less tissue density than the part of interest is positioned above the sensor, or if the sensor is not completely covered, the sensor will terminate the exposure sooner and the area of interest will be underexposed. Similarly, if the incorrect sensor for the anatomic part is selected, a density error will result.

On the other hand, if the sensor is positioned under a structure having greater tissue density than the part of interest (eg, if the center sensor is used for a PA chest image) the exposure will be greater than required and an overexposed radiograph will result.

Hence, although the exposure is "automatic," knowledge of anatomy and accurate positioning skills are essential to producing proper optical density.

C. PATHOLOGY

The presence of pathology often modifies tissue composition. Changes that occur are often spoken of as *additive* or *degenerative*. Additive pathology is that which makes tissues denser, requiring an increase in exposure factors (eg, ascites). Degenerative pathology involves deterioration of the part (eg, osteoporosis), and requires a decrease in exposure factors.

Because the function of an automatic exposure device is to "recognize" differences in tissue density and thickness, it will compensate for most pathologic changes by adjusting the mAs. In the event further compensation is necessary, most AECs have a *master density control* (on the control panel) that allows the radiographer to modify its output.

Normal exposure and density can usually be varied in increments of 25%, plus or minus. It must be noted that if a radiograph is overexposed because an exposure shorter than the *minimum reaction time* (shortest possible exposure) is required, a reduction in master density control will not resolve the situation. Rather, a lower mA station should be selected so that an exposure time within the machine's capability can be used.

Summary

- **The function of AECs is to produce consistent and comparable radiographic images.**
- **There are two types of AECs: ionization chamber and photomultiplier.**
- **Ionization chambers are located between the x-ray table and cassette.**
- **Photomultipliers are located beneath the cassette.**
- **Backup timers are used in conjunction with AECs and function to terminate the exposure in case of AEC malfunction.**
- **Minimum reaction time is the shortest exposure time possible with a particular AEC.**
- **The successful use of AECs requires accurate patient positioning and proper photocell/chamber selection.**
- **Pathologic conditions may be either additive or degenerative; correct use of the AEC will usually compensate for pathologic conditions.**
- **AECs have a density control, usually adjustable in increments of 25%.**

VI. TECHNIQUE CHARTS

A. *OPTIMAL AND FIXED KVP TECHNIQUE*

A *fixed kVp technique* chart specifies a particular kVp for each body part or type of examination. A kVp is selected that will provide adequate penetration and the appropriate scale of contrast. mAs is used to compensate for variation of patient size and condition.

B. *VARIABLE KVP TECHNIQUE*

In a *variable kVp technique* chart, the mAs is fixed and the kVp is increased as part thickness increases. For each cm increase in thickness, the kVp is increased by two. Accurate measurement with calipers is required.

The variable kVp technique chart is not frequently used today because it is associated with increased scattered radiation production and inconsistent contrast and density.

C. *VERSUS AECs*

Fixed kVp techniques are generally used with AECs. An optimum kVp for each body part (hip, IVU, sinuses, etc.) is selected and the exposure is automatically terminated once the predetermined correct exposure (mAs) has been reached.

D. *MEASUREMENT OF PART*

Accurate measurement of the part to be radiographed is essential with the *variable* kVp technique chart, because the kVp increases by two for every 1 cm increase in part thickness. *Fixed* kVp charts may

Fixed kVp Technique Chart

	Fixed kVp*	Grid
Extremities	55	No grid
Skull	75	Grid
Abdomen	75	Grid
Lateral Lumbar Region	90	Grid
Barium Studies	120	Grid
Chest Examinations	120	Grid

*For 3φ equipment factors; single φ will require approximately 12% higher kVp.

specify a specific kVp for the "small," "medium," or "large" patient, which corresponds to measurements within a particular range (eg, 10 to 12 cm = small; 13 to 15 cm = medium; 16 to 18 cm = large). Accurate measurement may be essential for the correct application of each method.

Structures radiographed using AECs do not require measurement, because the AEC automatically adjusts the exposure for tissue variations.

E. OTHER CONSIDERATIONS

Body position plays an important role in obtaining the expected radiographic results. For example, a well exposed radiograph of a normal adult abdomen measuring 24 cm in the recumbent AP position cannot be duplicated using the same factors if the patient is turned prone or positioned decubitus or erect.

A particular chest properly exposed on *inspiration* using a 14 × 17-inch cassette cannot be duplicated, without a change in factors, when the exposure is made on *expiration* or the field size is *collimated* to an 8 × 10-inch cassette.

A *plain* image of a particular abdomen requires different exposure factors from the same abdomen having a *barium* filled stomach.

Different exposures will be required for extremities with and without *casts*.

Body parts undergoing additive or destructive *pathologic changes* can require substantial exposure changes in order to maintain the desired density and contrast.

AECs will compensate for thickness and density differences (including those caused by position and respiration), pathologic changes, and beam restriction. However, it should be emphasized that the radiographer's skill and accuracy in *positioning* and *photocell selection* play an important role in the proper function of AECs.

Summary

- There are two types of technique charts: fixed kVp type and variable kVp type.
- The fixed kVp type chart uses an optimal kVp for each anatomic part.
- The advantage of the fixed kVp chart is consistency of radiographic contrast.
- The variable kVp type chart increases the kVp by two for each 1 cm increase in body thickness; thus accurate part measurement is necessary.
- AECs usually employ fixed kVp factors for consistent contrast, while varying the exposure and density.
- AECs will compensate for tissue thickness and density differences (including those caused by body position and respiration), pathologic changes, and beam restriction.
- The use of AECs requires accurate positioning and correct photocell selection.

Chapter Exercises

⭐ ***Congratulations!*** *You have completed the entire chapter. If you are able to answer the following group of very comprehensive questions, you should feel confident that you have really mastered this section. You can refer back to the indicated pages to check your answers and/or review the subject matter. For best results, be certain to complete this section before proceeding to the multiple choice questions!*

1. Define recorded detail; list other terms that can be used to refer to recorded detail ***(pp. 279, 280).***

2. To what does the term "resolution" refer; how is it measured and expressed ***(pp. 279–281)?***

3. Differentiate between *detail* and *distortion* ***(p. 280).***

4. What are the geometric factors affecting recorded detail ***(pp. 283, 286)?***

5. What is the relationship among OID, recorded detail, and magnification ***(p. 283)?***

6. What is the relationship among SID, recorded detail, and magnification ***(p. 283)?***

7. What are the two types of shape distortion? How can shape distortion be avoided ***(p. 280)?***

8. How is object unsharpness, with respect to its three-dimensional shape and OID, an inherent part of every radiographic image ***(pp. 284–285)?***

9. Distinguish between actual and effective/projected/apparent focal spot size; what is the line focus principle ***(pp. 286, 289)?***

10. How is actual focal spot size related to recorded detail? How does the size of the projected focus vary along the length of the image receptor ***(p. 286)?***

11. How are focal spot size and anode angle related to x-ray tube heat-loading capacity ***(p. 289)?***

12. Distinguish between voluntary and involuntary motion and discuss the most effective means of avoiding each ***(p. 291).***

13. Why is motion intentionally introduced in some radiographic examinations? Give some examples ***(p. 291).***

14. What is the relationship between the fluorescent light from intensifying screens and the total exposure received by the film emulsion ***(p. 295)?***

15. What is the purpose of a thicker *rear* intensifying screen *(p. 295, Figure 12–18)?*

16. Discuss how phosphor type and size, active or phosphor layer thickness, and reflective backing affect the speed on intensifying screens *(pp. 295, 296).*

17. What is lag or afterglow; how can it affect the radiographic image *(p. 296)?*

18. What are the three most commonly used rare earth phosphors *(p. 296)?*

19. What is the importance of spectral matching *(p. 296)?*

20. How is intensifying screen speed related to recorded detail? With what type of intensifying screens is quantum mottle usually associated *(pp. 296, 298)?*

21. What is the importance of screen and film contact? How is its accuracy tested *(pp. 298)?*

22. Define radiographic density; describe optical density (OD) *(p. 304).*

23. Describe how radiographic density and mAs are related to the intensity and exposure rate of the x-ray beam *(p. 304).*

24. What is the reciprocity law, and how is it related to radiographic density? Give examples *(p. 304).*

25. What change in mAs is required to make a perceptible change in radiographic density *(p. 306)?*

26. How is SID related to x-ray beam intensity and technical factors (specifically mAs)? What law expresses this relationship *(pp. 307, 308)?*

27. How is kVp related to x-ray beam intensity and radiographic density *(p. 310)?*

28. What is the 15% rule? Give examples *(p. 310).*

29. What is the relationship among radiographic density, mAs, and intensifying screen speed? Give examples *(p. 312).*

30. What three factors determine the quantity of scatter radiation produced? How can each be modified to limit the production of scattered radiation *(p. 313)?*

31. How do grids affect the amount of scattered radiation reaching the image recorder? How do they impact radiographic density *(p. 313)?*

32. What is a stationary grid? Give some examples of its use. What are its disadvantages *(p. 315)?*

33. What is a moving grid? How does its construction generally differ from the stationary grid? What is its advantage over a stationary grid *(p. 315)?*

34. Define convergence line; focusing distance; focal range; crossed grid *(p. 315)*.

35. Define grid cut-off; lateral decentering; focus–grid distance decentering *(p. 316)*.

36. Describe grid ratio, number of lead strips per inch, lead content; describe their relationship to *cleanup* and radiographic density *(pp. 317, 318)*.

37. Of what material(s) is grid interspace material usually made? How is each related to efficiency, patient dose, sturdiness *(p. 318)*?

38. Describe contrast improvement factor and selectivity *(p. 318)*.

39. Describe how the Bucky factor, or grid-conversion factor, can be used to determine the required mAs adjustment *(p. 319)*.

40. How can an air gap influence radiographic density *(p. 320)*?

41. What is inherent filtration? Of what does it consist *(p. 321)*?

42. What is added filtration? Of what does it consist *(p. 321)*?

43. What is the primary purpose of total filtration? What effect does it have on radiographic density *(p. 321)*?

44. Describe why and how compensating filters are used, how they affect radiographic density; give examples of common usage *(p. 321)*.

45. Describe how body position, condition, and pathology affect radiographic density *(pp. 323, 324)*.

46. Differentiate between and give examples of destructive and additive pathologic conditions *(p. 324)*.

47. How are different types of x-ray generators related to changes in radiographic density? How is mAs (or kVp) changed when changing from single-phase equipment to 3ɸ 6P or 3ɸ 12P equipment? Which technical factor is it preferable to change *(pp. 324, 325)*?

48. How can beam restriction affect radiographic density *(p. 327)*?

49. How can the anode heel effect impact radiographic density? Under what conditions is the heel effect most noticeable *(pp. 290, 327, 328)*?

50. How can automatic processing affect radiographic density *(p. 327)*?

51. What is the function of radiographic contrast? What are its two components *(p. 334)*?

52. Describe the difference between long-scale and short-scale contrast. What is the single most important technical factor regulating radiographic contrast *(pp. 335, 336–337)*?

53. What is subject contrast and how is it related to beam quality *(pp. 334, 337)?*

54. Describe the impact of scattered radiation on radiographic contrast; what is the most important way to limit the production of scattered radiation *(pp. 338, 339)?*

55. What kinds of pathologic conditions impact radiographic contrast *(p. 340)?*

56. How does the use of grids affect radiographic contrast *(pp. 341, 342)?*

57. Of what material(s) are film base and film emulsion made *(pp. 348, 349)?*

58. To what three sources is base-plus-fog attributable? What is the maximum permissible base-plus-fog density *(p. 349)?*

59. Explain what is meant by film latitude; give examples of uses for high-contrast film and low-contrast (latitude) film *(p. 349)*.

60. What do we call the study of film emulsion's response to exposure? How can this response be illustrated *(pp. 349, 350)?*

61. Draw a simple characteristic curve and label its toe, straight-line portion, shoulder, D_{max}, and solarization point *(p. 350)*.

62. Explain what is meant by exposure latitude; what technical factor regulates exposure latitude *(p. 351)*.

63. Describe the two types of AECs. Include in your description *(pp. 354–355):*

    (A) the location of each relative to the tabletop and cassette

    (B) operation of each and how exposure is terminated

64. Explain the importance of a backup timer used in conjunction with an AEC *(p. 354)*.

65. Explain the importance of proper AEC photocell selection; describe typical errors in photocell selection and the subsequent radiographic results *(p. 355)*.

66. Explain how to correct a radiographic image overexposed as a result of requiring an exposure shorter than the minimum reaction time *(pp. 355, 356)*.

67. Why are fixed kVp technique charts preferred over variable kVp technique charts *(p. 356)?*

68. Discuss why exposures made using an AEC do not require measurement of the part being examined *(p. 357)*.

69. Discuss why positioning accuracy is essential to proper function of the AEC *(p. 357)*.

A&U Chapter Review Questions

☆ *Congratulations!* *You have completed the last portion of this chapter. You may go on to the "Registry type" multiple choice questions that follow. For greatest success, be sure also to have first completed the short answer questions found before this section.*

1. The use of optimum kVp for small, medium, and large body parts is the premise of:
   (A) fixed kVp, variable mAs technique chart
   (B) variable kVp, fixed mAs technique chart
   (C) fixed mAs, variable body part technique
   (D) fixed mAs, variable SID technique

2. The function(s) of automatic beam limitation devices include:
   1. reducing the production of scattered radiation
   2. absorption of scattered radiation
   3. changing the quality of the x-ray beam
   (A) 1 only
   (B) 2 only
   (C) 1 and 2 only
   (D) 1, 2, and 3

3. Base plus fog is a result of
   1. blue-tinted base
   2. chemical development
   3. manufacturing
   (A) 1 only
   (B) 1 and 2 only
   (C) 1 and 3 only
   (D) 1, 2, and 3

4. The characteristic curve is used to illustrate the relationship between the:
   (A) source to image receptor distance and the resulting optical density
   (B) exposure reaching the phosphors and the resulting fluorescence
   (C) exposure given the film and the resulting optical density
   (D) kVp used and the resulting optical density

5. That portion of a characteristic curve generally representative of the useful radiographic density range is the:
   (A) toe portion
   (B) straight-line portion
   (C) shoulder portion
   (D) solarization point

6. Using the fixed mAs, variable kVp exposure factor technique, each centimeter increase in patient thickness requires what adjustment in technique?
   (A) increase 2 kVp
   (B) decrease 2 kVp
   (C) increase 4 kVp
   (D) decrease 4 kVp

7. Which of the following can be used to determine the sensitivity of a particular film emulsion?
   (A) characteristic curve
   (B) dose-response curve
   (C) reciprocity law
   (D) inverse square law

8. Film base is typically made of which of the following materials?
   (A) cellulose nitrate
   (B) cellulose acetate
   (C) polyester
   (D) glass

9. Which of the following chemicals is used in the production of radiographic film emulsion?
   (A) sodium sulfite
   (B) potassium bromide
   (C) silver halide
   (D) chrome alum

10. Which of the following pathologic conditions would require an increase in exposure factors?
    (A) pneumoperitoneum
    (B) obstructed bowel
    (C) renal colic
    (D) ascites

Answers and Explanations

1. (A) The optimum kVp (or fixed kVp) technique separates patients into small, medium, and large categories and assigns an optimum (or best) kVp for that particular body part. Patient thickness (cm measurement) determines mAs. This method of establishing exposure factors results in less variation in the scale of contrast than the variable kVp method of technique selection.

2. (A) Beam restrictors function to limit size of the irradiated field. In doing so, they limit the volume of tissue irradiated (thereby decreasing the percentage of scattered radiation generated in the part) and help reduce patient dose. Beam restrictors do not affect the quality (energy) of the x-ray beam—that is the function of kVp and filtration. Beam restrictors do not absorb scatter radiation—that is a function of grids.

3. (D) Every film emulsion has a particular base plus fog which should not exceed 0.2. Base density is a result of the manufacturing process (ie, environmental radiation) and the blue tint added to the base to reduce glare. The remaining fog density is a result of the chemical development process, when exposed silver bromide grains are converted to black metallic silver.

4. (C) The characteristic (or Hurter and Driffield [H&D]) curve is used to illustrate the relationship between the exposure given the film and the resulting density. The relationship between the source to image receptor distance and resulting density is expressed in the inverse square law of radiation. The effect of kVp on contrast can be illustrated using a penetrometer (aluminum step-wedge).

5. (B) A characteristic curve is the representation of a film emulsion's response to exposure by light or x-rays. Upon observation, it is seen that a characteristic curve does not begin at zero density. That is because an "unexposed" and processed film has a small base plus fog density (which should not exceed 0.2) because of base dye, environmental radiation fog during production, transportation and storage, and chemical fog from high processing temperatures. The initial ascent of the curve is called the "toe," and represents minimal density. The straight line portion of the curve represents the useful radiographic density range, lying approximately between densities 0.25 and 2.0. The characteristic curve levels off again at the "shoulder" portion of the curve, which represents maximum radiographic density (D_{max}). Past the shoulder is the solarization point, where further exposure would reverse image densities.

6. (A) Using the variable kVp method, a particular mAs is assigned to each body part. As part thickness increases, the kVp (penetration) is also increased. The body part being radiographed must be carefully measured and for each centimeter increase in thickness, 2 kVp is added to the exposure.

7. (A) The characteristic curve is used to show the relationship between the exposure given the film and the resulting film density. It can therefore be used to evaluate a particular film emulsion's response (speed, sensitivity) by determining how long it takes to record a particular density. A dose response curve is used in radiation protection and illustrates the quantity of dose required to produce a particular effect. The reciprocity law states that a particular mAs, regardless of the combination of mA and time, should produce the same degree of blackening. The inverse square law illustrates the relationship between distance and radiation intensity.

8. (C) Film base functions to support the silver halide emulsion. Today's film base is made of tough, nonflammable polyester. Cellulose nitrate was used in the past, but was highly flammable. Cellulose acetate was not flammable, but was not as durable as polyester. The earliest supports for emulsion were plates of glass (hence the term "flat *plate*").

9. (C) Film emulsion consists of silver halide crystals suspended in gelatin. Sodium sulfite is a film processing preservative and potassium bromide is a developer restrainer. Potassium and chrome alum are emulsion hardeners used in fixer solution.

10. (D) Because pneumoperitoneum is an abnormal accumulation of air or gas in the peritoneal cavity, it would require a decrease in exposure factors. Obstructed bowel usually involves distended, gas-filled bowel loops, again requiring a decrease in exposure factors. With ascites, there is an abnormal accumulation of fluid in the abdominal cavity, necessitating an increase in exposure factors. Renal colic is the pain associated with the passage of renal calculi; no change from the normal exposure factors is usually required.

Image Processing and Quality Assurance

I. FILM STORAGE CONSIDERATIONS

A. STORAGE CONDITIONS

The conditions under which x-ray film is stored can have considerable impact on the final radiographic image. The most common result of improper film storage is fog, which has a severely degrading effect on image quality.

1. Temperature and Humidity. Films should be stored at a temperature no greater than 70°F. Excessive heat can accelerate the deterioration process and cause film fog. Atmospheric *humidity* should be kept between 40% and 60%. Excessively low humidity is conducive to the production of *static electricity* discharge (Fig. 13–1). High humidity levels encourage the production of fog. An unopened (ie, *hermetically sealed*) bag of film protects the film from humidity but not excessive temperatures.

2. Chemicals and Radiation. Boxes of film must also be stored away from chemical fumes that can fog film emulsion. Film can be fogged if stored too close to radiographic rooms or radionuclides.

3. Expiration Dates. Each box of x-ray film is identified with an expiration date before which the film must be used in order to avoid age fog. When replenishing film supply, film boxes should be rotated so that the oldest film is used first. (Use the *fifo* system: first in, first out.)

4. Position of Film Boxes. Film boxes, should be stored in the upright position. If film boxes are stacked on one another, the sensitive emulsion (especially in the central portion) can be affected by pressure from the boxes above. *Pressure marks* (ie, areas of fog) are produced and result in *loss of contrast* in that area of the radiographic image. Larger size film boxes are particularly susceptible to this problem.

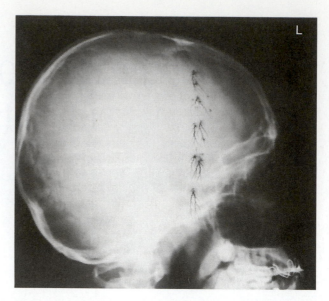

Figure 13–1. Plus-density artifact resulting from static electric discharge. (From Saia DA. *Appleton & Lange's Review for the Radiography Examination* (3rd ed). East Norwalk, CT: Appleton & Lange, 1997.)

5. Film Bin. The *film bin* is a light-tight storage area where opened boxes of film are available for reloading empty cassettes. If a single door separates the darkroom from exterior white light, it is wise to have an automatic interlock system in place that prevents opening of the darkroom door while the film bin is open.

B. SAFELIGHT ILLUMINATION

Adequate and safe darkroom lighting is an essential part of ensuring quality radiographic images. A source of white light is required for cleaning and routine maintenance. The white light often has a safety device to help prevent accidental film exposure. *Safelight* illumination must be appropriate for the type film used and bright enough to provide adequate illumination and still not expose the sensitive emulsions (exposed film emulsion is about eight times more sensitive than unexposed emulsion).

1. Types. A frequently used *safelight* is the Kodak Wratten Series 6B, a brownish *safelight filter,* with a 7.5- to 15-watt frosted light bulb placed 4 feet above the work surface. Another available safelight, which is somewhat brighter, is the Kodak GBX all-purpose filter, which provides a more reddish illumination. This type of filter is often placed in the darkroom so that its light is directed upward toward the ceiling and reflected back down, thus reducing the chance of safelight fog.

2. White Light Leaks. Routine darkroom maintenance includes regular cleaning of all surfaces and walls and checks for white light leaks. When checking for light leaks, all darkroom lights must be turned off, adequate time given for eyes to adjust to the darkness, then a careful visual inspection made for white light leaks.

Summary

- **Film should be stored in a cool and dry environment, under 70°F and between 40% and 60% humidity.**
- **Excessive temperatures cause film fog.**
- **Excessively low humidity encourages buildup of static electricity.**
- **Film should be stored away from radiation and chemicals.**
- **The film box expiration date should be noted, and oldest film used first.**
- **Film boxes should be stored upright to avoid production of pressure marks.**
- **Kodak Wratten Series 6B and GBX darkroom filters are the most frequently used.**
- **Safelights should be placed 4 feet from the work surface with 7.5- to 15-watt light bulbs.**

II. CASSETTES

A. ROUTINE CARE

Routine documented care of all imaging system components is part of an efficient *quality assurance* program.

Cassettes require care and maintenance inside and out. They should be stored upright, according to size (ie, 14" × 17", 10 " × 12", etc.) and speed (ie, 100, 400). Stacking cassettes on top of each other or jammed in a passbox renders the cassettes more susceptible to damage. Cassettes should be inspected visually for damage and cleanliness. The inside of cassettes should be cleaned regularly to keep them lint and dust-free; screens should be cleaned with special antistatic cleaner appropriate for the type screen used; incorrect cleaner can affect the speed of screens.

Screens must also be tested periodically for screen-film contact with a *wire-mesh test.* The cassette to be tested is placed on the x-ray table, the wire-mesh device on *top* of the cassette, and an exposure made of about 5 mAs (milliampere-seconds) and 40 kVp (kilovoltage peak). The processed film should be viewed at a distance of at least 6 feet. Any *blurry* areas are indicative of poor screen–film contact and representative of diminished image detail. The areas of poor contact will also exhibit an increase in density and loss of contrast.

B. ARTIFACTS

Radiographically speaking, an *artifact* is a fault, blemish, or aberration in an x-ray image. It can be the result of improper handling, automatic processing, or use of defective radiographic accessories.

Cassettes, screens, and film must be handled carefully to avoid leaving fingerprints or producing other film artifacts. Hands should be kept clean and dry, free from residue-leaving creams and powder from gloves. Film should be handled carefully by the corners when loading and unloading cassettes. The technologist should not *slide* film into or out of the cassette, as the friction can cause static electricity buildup. Cassettes should be numbered or otherwise identified so that artifact causing problems can be located and removed (Fig. 13–2).

Common Artifacts and Their Causes

Crescent (Kink) Marks Bending film sharply over finger

Minus Density, Pinhole Marks Dust on intensifying screens (see Fig. 13–2)

Static Electricity Low humidity, improper handling (see Fig. 13–1)

Fingerprints Body oils, other material on skin

Scratches Pressing film down on feed tray

Fog Damaged cassette; cracked safelight; bulb too bright; exposure to radiation; chemical fumes; illuminated clock or watch face; turning on white light before film is in processor; darkroom light leak

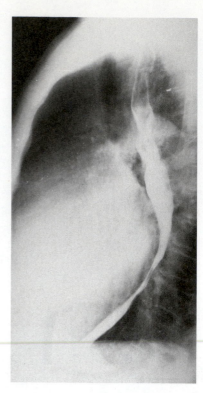

Figure 13–2. Dirty and dusty screens. Small particles of dust, or other foreign objects, on intensifying screens keep the fluorescent light from reaching the film emulsion, hence a clear (unexposed) area corresponds to each foreign particle. (From the American College of Radiology Learning File. Courtesy of the American College of Radiology.)

Summary

■ Cassettes should be stored upright according to size and speed.
■ Cassettes should be tested periodically for adequate screen-film contact.
■ Intensifying screens must be cleaned periodically with anti-static screen cleaner.
■ Inadequate cleaning can result in white pinhole type film artifacts.
■ Rough, improper handling or storage of cassettes can lead to damage resulting in poor screen-film contact.
■ Film must be handled carefully and properly to avoid artifacts such as static electricity, scratches, fog, or crescent marks.

III. IDENTIFICATION OF RADIOGRAPHS

A. *ESSENTIAL INFORMATION*

Every radiograph *must* (for *medicolegal* reasons) include certain specific patient information.

• Patient's name or identification number
• The side marker, right or left
• The examination date
• Name of the institution

Other pertinent information *may* be included.

• Patient's age or birthdate
• Attending physician
• Time of day

When multiple films are taken of a patient on the same day, it is important that the time the radiographs were taken be included on the film. This permits the physician to chronologically follow the patient's progress.

B. *TYPES OF SYSTEMS*

There are a number of *film identification* systems. Cassettes are purchased with a lead blocker in a specified corner to shield the underlying film from x-ray exposure. This unexposed corner of the film is then "flashed" with essential patient information. Some identification devices are used only in the darkroom because the film is removed from the cassette before the information is flashed onto it. Another type of film identification device allows recording of patient information in normal lighted conditions with the film inside the specially designed cassette.

Summary

■ Medicolegal implications require that every radiograph include the patient's name or identification number, left or right side marker, examination date, and name of institution.
■ When multiple films are taken of a patient the same day, the time of day should be indicated on the radiographs.

- **Some film identification systems can be used only in a darkroom.**
- **Other film identification systems use special cassettes and are used in daylight conditions.**

IV. AUTOMATIC FILM PROCESSING

Film emulsion consists of silver bromide (halide) crystals suspended in gelatin. Sensitization specks are added to increase the sensitivity of the silver salts. Positive silver ions form the inner portion of the emulsion, while the negative bromine ions form the outer layer. At the time of exposure, the outer, negative bromine ions are energized, and their valence electrons ejected and absorbed by the (now negatively charged) sensitivity speck. The inner, positive silver ions migrate to the negative charges and become metallic silver. Thus, the *latent* (exposed but invisible) *image* is formed. This is referred to as the Gurney–Mott theory of latent image formation. The development process transforms the latent image to a *manifest* (visible) black metallic silver *image*.

Automatic film processing is carried out by a machine that *transports* the x-ray film through the necessary chemical solutions, at the same time providing *agitation, temperature regulation,* and *chemical replenishment.* Within the processor are the *developer, fixer,* and wash tanks, followed by the dryer.

Rapid processing is accomplished by the use of increased solution temperatures, which requires that a *hardener* be added to the developer to control excessive emulsion swelling.

Each of the processor systems accomplishes specific functions; a basic understanding of these systems is required so that the processor can be used correctly and efficiently. A properly maintained and monitored processor will ensure consistent radiographs that will retain their quality images over a long period of time (archival quality).

A. CHEMISTRY OVERVIEW

1. Developer. The developer functions to convert the latent (invisible) image into the manifest (visible) silver image by *reducing the exposed silver bromide crystals to black metallic silver.* Important factors affecting the development process are *time* (length of development), *temperature* (of the developer solution), and solution *activity* (strength, concentration).

The developer solution has an *alkaline* nature for optimal function of the *reducing agents. Sodium* or *potassium carbonate* provides the necessary alkalinity and serves as an *activator* (or accelerator) by swelling the gelatin emulsion so that the reducing agents are better able to penetrate the emulsion and reach the exposed silver bromide crystals.

The *reducing agents* are *hydroquinone,* which works slowly to build up blacks in the film areas of greater exposure, and *phenidone,* which quickly produces the gray tones in areas of lesser exposure. With respect to sensitometry, hydroquinone controls the shoulder (D_{max}) of the characteristic curve, and phenindone controls the toe (D_{min}) area.

Advantages of Automatic Over Manual Processing

- Speed
- Convenience
- Consistency
- Reduced labor
- Improved archival quality

Developer Reduces Exposed Silver Crystals to Black Metallic Silver

Sodium and Potassium Carbonate Activator, accelerator: swells gelatin; provides alkaline medium.

Hydroquinone Reducing agent: works slowly; builds up black areas.

Phenidone Reducing agent: works quickly; produces gray tones.

Sodium Sulfite and Cycon Preservatives: prevent oxidation of developer.

Potassium Bromide Restrainer: anti-fog agent.

Glutaraldehyde Hardener: controls emulsion swelling.

Water Solvent.

The developer solution, particularly the hydroquinone, is especially sensitive to oxygen. If the developer oxidizes, it becomes weaker and less effective. The *preservative, sodium sulfite* or *cycon,* is added to the developer to prevent its rapid oxidation. The *solvent* for the concentrated chemicals is water, used to dilute the concentrate to the proper strength.

Rapid processing is achieved through the use of high temperatures that accelerate the development process; however, high temperatures can cause excessive emulsion swelling. Because excessive swelling can result in roller transportation problems a hardener, traditionally *glutaraldehyde,* is added to the developer to control the amount of emulsion swelling.

A *restrainer,* or antifog agent, is added to the developer to limit its activity to only the exposed silver crystals. The typical restrainer is *potassium bromide.* Without the restrainer the developing agents would attack the *unexposed* crystals, creating *chemical fog.* Potassium bromide is frequently referred to as "starter solution" because it is added only to fresh, new developer. As films are developed, bromine ions are released from the emulsion into solution; thus, potassium bromide is not found in replenisher solution.

Fixer Clears Film of Unexposed and Undeveloped Silver Bromide Crystals

Acetic Acid Activator: provides acid medium. Neutralizes any residual developer.

Ammonium Thiosulfate Fixing or clearing agent: removes unexposed and undeveloped silver.

Potassium Alum or *Aluminum Chloride* Hardening agent: shrinks, re-hardens emulsion for protection and archival purposes.

Sodium Sulfite Preservative: prolongs the effective life of the solution.

Water Solvent.

---

2. Fixer. The function of the fixer *(hypo)* is to clear the film of the unexposed, undeveloped silver bromide crystals. This process serves to protect the film from further exposure. The *fixing* or *clearing agent* is *ammonium thiosulfate.*

The fixer is an acidic solution that functions to neutralize any residual developer carried over and provide the required acid medium for the hardener. *Acetic acid* provides the required acidic medium.

The fixer contains a hardener whose function it is to shrink and reharden the gelatin emulsion, thus protecting it from abrasion and promoting *archival quality.* The most commonly used hardeners are *potassium alum* or *aluminum chloride.* Fixer preservative is the same as that found in the developer, that is, sodium sulfite.

3. Wash. The function of the wash is to rid the film of residual chemicals. Should chemicals remain in the emulsion (eg, as a result of defective wash cycle), the film will discolor with age. Since radiographic records are kept for a number of years, it is important that they have sufficient archival quality.

Cold-water processors are, in general, less efficient in removing chemicals than warm-water processors. Agitation during the wash process and large quantities of water help to rid the emulsion of chemical residue.

Summary

- Developer solution reduces the exposed silver bromide crystals to black metallic silver.
- The development process is greatly affected by development time and solution temperature and activity.
- Sodium or potassium carbonate provides the necessary alkalinity and functions as the solution activator by swelling the gelatin emulsion.
- Reducing agents are phenidone and hydroquinone.
- Sodium sulfite or cycon preserves the developer solution from excessive oxidation.

- **Glutaraldehyde is a hardener, added to developer solution to control excessive swelling.**
- **Potassium bromide serves as an antifog agent and restrains the developer from attacking the unexposed silver bromide crystals.**
- **Potassium bromide is starter solution, and is not required in replenisher solution.**
- **The fixing or clearing agent (ammonium thiosulfate) removes unexposed silver bromide crystals from the emulsion, preventing further exposure.**
- **Acetic acid provides the necessary acid medium for the fixer solution.**
- **Potassium alum or aluminum chloride serves to harden the film emulsion.**
- **The fixer preservative is sodium sulfite.**
- **Adequate washing of residual chemicals from the film emulsion is essential for good archival quality.**

B. TRANSPORT SYSTEM

The *transport system* functions to convey the film through the different processor sections by means of a series of rollers (Fig. 13–3) driven by gears, chains, and sprockets. This is accomplished without damage to the film and at a prescribed speed, which determines the length of time film spends in each solution. The roller system also provides constant, vigorous agitation of the solution at the film surface. The entire conveyance system consists of the *feed tray, crossover rollers, deep racks, turnaround assemblies,* and *receiving bin.*

Film is aligned against one side of the feed tray as it is introduced into the processor. A sensor initiates solution replenishment as the film enters, and replenishment continues as the length of the

> **Transport System Functions**
>
> - Conveys film through processor.
> - Establishes processing time (via roller speed).
> - Activates replenishment.
> - Agitates solution over film surface.
> - Provides squeegee action on film emulsion.

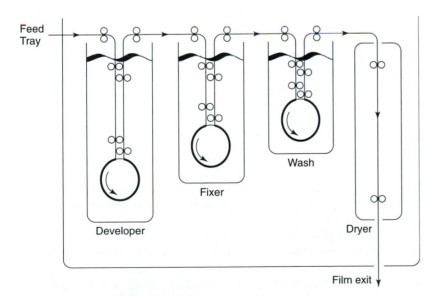

Figure 13–3. Major components of an automatic processor. A series of rollers conveys film through each processor section. (From Wolbarst AB. *Physics of Radiology.* East Norwalk, CT: Appleton & Lange, 1993.)

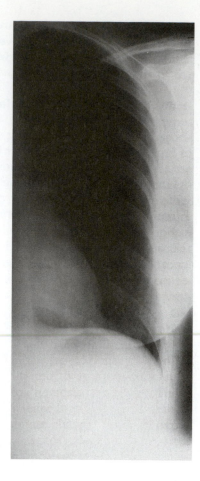

Figure 13–4. Because adjacent rollers are positioned closer together at their periphery, roller pressure on film emulsion is greater at film edges. This can cause a plus-density mottled appearance *(wet-pressure sensitization marks)* along film edges. If developer hardener or replenisher is insufficient, allowing excessive emulsion swelling, this artifact can occur across the length of the film. (From the American College of Radiology Learning File. Courtesy of the American College of Radiology.)

film passes the sensor. Films should be fed into the processor along their short edge; feeding the film in "the long way" leads to overreplenishment and increased radiographic density.

Crossover racks are out of solution and bridge the gaps between developer and fixer, fixer and wash, and wash and dry sections of the processor. Crossover rollers must be kept free of crystallized solutions that can cause film artifacts as the soft emulsion passes by (Fig. 13–4). The last set of rollers in each solution section has a *squeegee* action on film emulsion, thus removing excess solution before film enters the next tank.

When the processor is not in use for a period of time, it is advisable to leave the lid open so that moisture can escape. Because the crossover rollers are out of solution, chemicals carried onto them by film can crystallize and should be cleaned off before the processor is used again.

Turnaround assemblies are located at the bottom of the deep racks and serve to change the film direction as it changes from downward to upward motion. Guide shoes, or deflector plates, are also located where film must change direction. They will occasionally scratch film, leaving characteristic *guide-shoe marks,* when they require adjustment.

When returning rollers to the processor after cleaning, care must be taken to seat them securely in their proper position. Transport problems (processor jam-up) will result if racks are misaligned.

C. Replenishment System

As films travel from one processor solution section to another, chemical solution is carried away in the swollen film emulsion. It is the function of the processor *replenishment* system to keep solution tanks full. If solution level is allowed to lower, film immersion time decreases and radiographic density and contrast changes will occur. Transport problems can also arise from inadequate replenishment; that is, if insufficient developer replenisher, the inadequate addition of hardener will result in excessive emulsion swelling. The essentially "thicker" film has difficulty transporting between the closely distanced rollers.

As film travels through the fixer, it accumulates residual developer solution; fixer solution also accumulates unexposed silver cleared from the emulsion. Wash water accumulates fixer. In these ways, the activity of each solution is depleted through continual use. Diminished solution activity can have the same effects as low solution levels. The replenishment system assures that proper solution concentration is maintained.

D. Temperature Regulation

The temperature regulation system functions to control the temperature of each section of the automatic processor. Developer is the most important solution temperature to regulate; in a 90-second processor, developer temperature is usually maintained at 92° to 95°F. Once the correct developer temperature is established, it must be constantly maintained. Even a minor fluctuation (ie, 0.5°F) in developer temperature can cause a visible change in radiographic density and contrast.

Developer temperature is thermostatically controlled and developer solution is circulated through a heat exchanger under the fixer tank. Thus, the fixer temperature is regulated (in cold-water processors) by heat conducted from the developer solution. In older processors having stainless steel tanks, fixer temperature is regulated by heat convection from the neighboring developer solution.

E. Recirculation System

As replenishment chemicals are added to solution, the *recirculation system* provides agitation necessary for uniform solution concentration. As temperature adjustments are made, the recirculation system agitates solution to promote temperature uniformity. *Agitation* provided by the system also functions to keep fresh solution in contact with film emulsion. The recirculation system also functions to filter debris, such as gelatin particles, from the solutions.

F. Wash and Dryer Systems

Thorough removal of chemical solutions from the film emulsion is required for good *archival film quality* and is provided by the wash section of the automatic processor. Agitation of the water makes the process more efficient. Any residual chemicals will eventually result in film stain. *Residual fixer* will eventually stain the film a yellowish brown that ultimately obscures the image and diminishes the archival quality. Films can be tested (usually by the film manufacturer or distributor) to determine their degree of fixer retention.

The dryer section functions to remove water from the film by blowing warm, dry air over the film surface. Dryer temperature is usu-

---

Replenishment System Functions

- Maintain solution level.
- Maintain solution activity and concentration.

Temperature Regulation

- Especially important for developer solution.
- Developer heated by thermostat.
- Fixer/wash warmed by heat exchangers.

Recirculation System Functions

- Maintain uniform solution activity through agitation.
- Maintain uniform temperature through agitation.
- Keep fresh solution in contact with film emulsion.
- Provide filtration of processor debris.

Wash Functions

- Remove chemicals from emulsion.
- Contribute to archival quality.

Dryer Functions

- Air recirculation.
- Dry film.

Daily Monitoring and Maintenance Procedures

At Start-Up Time
Clean crossover and other out of solution rollers.
Check solution levels in processor tanks and replenisher tanks.
Process two to four *un*exposed 14″ × 17″ films to clean rollers.
Clean feed tray, receiver tray, and darkroom work surfaces.
Perform sensitometric tests.

At Shut-Down Time
Another sensitometric test may be done.
Clean crossover and other out of solution rollers.
Leave lid open 1″ to allow escape of moisture.

---

ally 120° to 130°F, sufficient to shrink and dry the emulsion without being excessive. Excessive heat and overdrying can cause film damage. If films emerging from a properly heated dryer are damp, the problem may be excessive emulsion swelling and water retention as a result of inadequate developer or fixer replenisher (hardener).

G. SILVER RECOVERY

X-ray film is expensive and represents a large part of a radiology department annual budget. About half of the film's silver remains in the emulsion after exposure and processing. The other half (unexposed silver) is removed from the film during the fixing process and most of it is recoverable through *silver recovery* methods. A drain is connected to the fixer tank and fixer is allowed to flow directly into a *silver recovery unit* or to a large centrally located receptacle.

Silver recovery is desirable for financial and ecological reasons. Fixer silver is toxic to the public water supply and environmental legislation makes persons responsible for its direct passage into sewer lines, or other means of improper disposal, subject to severe fines and penalties.

There are three types of silver recovery methods. Used fixer enters a *metallic displacement* (or metallic replacement) cartridge and metallic silver is precipitated onto the steel wool within. This method of silver recovery is most useful for low-volume locations.

Electrolytic silver recovery units (cells) pass an electric current through the fixer solution, causing silver to be plated onto the cathode cylinder of the unit. The silver is periodically removed by scraping it from the stainless steel cathode. Electrolytic cells are best used in locations having medium to high volume.

There are a number of chemicals that will *precipitate* metallic silver. In the presence of one of these chemicals (eg, sodium borohydride), metallic silver falls to the bottom of the tank and forms a sludge. This method of silver recovery is generally used only by large institutions having large, centralized receptacles or by professional silver dealers, who employ special techniques for separating the sludge or removing the entire tank.

H. PROCESSOR MAINTENANCE

The biggest advantage of automatic processors is their contribution to radiographic consistency. Testing and monitoring procedures serve to indicate potential problems before they arise. Developer, fixer, and wash temperature should be checked twice a day. *Preventive maintenance* is frequently provided for by a commercial cleaning and parts replacement service.

Sensitometry is the measure of film response to exposure and processing. A particular box of film is designated for testing purposes only, and a special device *(sensitometer)* is used to precisely and consistently expose the film. Once the film is processed and its densities read (with a *densitometer*) and compared to known correct readings, any variation in film density must be due to processor variation.

If solution levels in processor and replenisher tanks are frequently low, a bigger problem may exist and should be brought to the attention of the processor service company. *Preprocessed* films should *not* be used to clean rollers, because they may contain residual fixer which will contaminate the developer solution.

The more effective the processor quality control program, the less troubleshooting will be required. Nevertheless, it is important that the radiographer be able to recognize and resolve some common processor problems.

I. TROUBLESHOOTING: COMMON PROCESSOR PROBLEMS AND THEIR CAUSES

Transport Problems (Jam-Ups)
- Inadequately maintained (dirty) rollers
- Too rapid film feeding, overlapping
- Misaligned crossover or other racks
- Inadequate developer replenisher (hardener)

Excessive Density (Processor Related)
- Developer temperature elevated
- Insufficient dilution of developer

Inadequate Density (Processor Related)
- Developer temperature too low
- Excessive dilution of developer

Damp Films
- Dryer temperature too low
- Faulty dryer blower
- Inadequate fixing
- Inadequate developer replenisher (hardener)

Fog (Darkroom Related)
- Unsafe safelight
- Contaminated developer
- Outdated film
- Improper film storage conditions
- Darkroom light leak

J. PROCESSING DIGITAL IMAGES

The processing of digital images is very different from processing conventional screen-film images. Digital imaging will be reviewed in detail in *Part V: Equipment Operation and Maintenance*. Any conventional screen–film image can be scanned and digitized by a special film digitizer unit.

Computed radiography uses special detector plates inside cassettes to record the radiologic image. No film is used, hence the term *filmless radiography*. A cassette is exposed just like a conventional screen–film cassette. Upon exposure, a latent image is produced on the image detector plate. The image plate (IP) is placed in a special processor and scanned with a laser to obtain the pixel data, which can then be displayed on a monitor as the visible image.

Using a *picture archiving and communications system* (PACS), and *teleradiology*, digital images can be sent anywhere there is the equipment to receive and display them.

Interpretation of digital images can be made from the display monitor ("soft copy display") or "hard copies" can be made on film using a multiformat camera or laser printer. A *multiformat camera* can place several images on a film by taking pictures of the display screen. A *laser camera* records the displayed image by exposing a film with laser light; it can also record several images on one film. The multiformat camera or laser printer is connected to an automatic processor for immediate processing and interpretation.

Chapter Exercises

⭐ ***Congratulations!*** *You have completed the entire chapter. If you are able to answer the following group of very comprehensive questions, you should feel confident that you have really mastered this section. You can refer back to the indicated pages to check your answers and/or review the subject matter.*

1. What are the ideal conditions for x-ray film storage *(p. 365)?*

2. Describe the possible effect of excessive temperature; of very low humidity *(p. 365).*

3. Describe how each of the following can affect radiographic film *(pp. 365–367):*

    A. chemical fumes

    B. radiation

    C. storage past the expiration date

    D. stacking boxes of film upon each other

    E. film bin or darkroom with light leaks

    F. safelight too close to work bench

    G. too high wattage safelight

4. Explain correct care of cassettes; intensifying screens *(p. 367).*

5. How can suspected flaws in film–screen contact be detected *(p. 367)?*

6. List at least five radiographic artifacts and identify their cause *(p. 367).*

7. What information *must* every radiographic image include? Describe two types of film identification systems *(p. 368).*

8. Define latent image; manifest image *(p. 369).*

9. List five advantages of automatic processing over manual processing. What modification of manual processing helps achieve rapid processing *(p. 369)?*

10. What is the main function of the developer solution? What are the three important factors in the development process *(pp. 369, 370)?*

11. Identify the chemical associated with each of the following developer constituents and describe its function(s) *(pp. 369, 370):*

    A. reducing agents (two)

    B. preservative

    C. activator and accelerator

    D. restrainer

    E. hardener

    F. solvent

12. What are the main functions of the fixer solution *(p. 370)?*

13. Identify the chemical associated with each of the following fixer constituents and describe its function(s) *(p. 370):*

    A. fixing and clearing agent

    B. activator

    C. hardener

    D. preservative

    E. solvent

14. List the order in which film travels through each of the four sections of the automatic processor *(p. 371).*

15. List five functions of the transport system. What can result from transport problems *(p. 371)?*

16. Describe the appropriate care of crossover racks *(p. 372).*

17. Describe the location of the rollers having squeegee action and explain their purpose *(p. 372).*

18. What is the usual cause of wet-pressure sensitization marks occasionally found along film edges *(p. 372, Figure 13–4)?*

19. Name and describe the location of the structures that function to guide film in the proper direction through the processor roller systems *(p. 372).*

20. What are the two functions of the processor replenishment system? What can be the result of inadequate replenishment *(p. 373)?*

21. Describe the importance of temperature-regulation systems in automatic processing *(p. 373).*

22. List four functions of the processor recirculation system *(p. 373).*

23. What are the functions of the processor wash and dry sections? What can result from an inadequate wash process? Inadequate drying *(pp. 373, 374)*

24. Explain the economic and ecologic importance of silver recovery *(p. 374).*

25. Describe the three types of silver recovery methods *(p. 374).*

26. Describe the start-up and shutdown procedures recommended for daily processor maintenance *(p. 374).*

27. List at least 10 common radiographic problems associated with processing and identify their cause *(p. 375).*

28. Describe what is meant by the term "filmless radiography" *(p. 375).*

29. Name and describe the two devices that can be used to record hard copies of digital images *(p. 375).*

A&U Chapter Review Questions

1. The developer temperature in a 90-second automatic processor is usually about:
   - (A) 75° to 80°F
   - (B) 80° to 85°F
   - (C) 85° to 90°F
   - (D) 90° to 95°F

2. Conditions contributing to poor radiographic archival quality include:
   1. fixer retention
   2. insufficient developer replenishment
   3. poor storage conditions
   - (A) 1 only
   - (B) 3 only
   - (C) 2 and 3 only
   - (D) 1, 2, and 3

3. The amount of replenishment solution added to the automatic processor is determined by:
    1. size of the film
    2. position of film on tray feeding into processor
    3. length of time required for film to enter processor
    (A) 1 only
    (B) 1 and 2 only
    (C) 1 and 3 only
    (D) 1, 2, and 3

4. The device used to give a predetermined exposure to a film to test its response to processing is called the:
    (A) sensitometer
    (B) densitometer
    (C) step wedge
    (D) spinning top

5. The cause of films coming from the automatic processor still damp can be:
    (A) air velocity too high
    (B) unbalanced processing temperatures
    (C) insufficient hardening action
    (D) excessive hardening action

6. Which of the following chemicals functions to reduce exposed silver halide grains to black metallic silver?
    (A) phenindone
    (B) sodium thiosulfate
    (C) sodium sulfide
    (D) sodium carbonate

7. The conversion of the invisible latent image into a visible manifest image takes place in the:
    (A) developer
    (B) stop bath
    (C) first half of the fixer process
    (D) second half of the fixer process

8. Which of the following can result from poor storage or handling practices?
    1. film fog from outdated film
    2. film fog from exposure to excessive temperatures
    3. film fog from exposure to chemical fumes
    (A) 1 only
    (B) 1 and 2 only
    (C) 2 and 3 only
    (D) 1, 2, and 3

9. Which of the following devices functions to produce hard copies of digital images?
   1. digitizer
   2. laser printer
   3. multiformat camera
   (A) 1 only
   (B) 1 and 2 only
   (C) 2 and 3 only
   (D) 1, 2, and 3

10. Crescent-shaped crinkle mark artifacts on a film are caused by:
    (A) improper film storage
    (B) improper film handling
    (C) exposure to white light
    (D) exposure to excessive humidity

Answers and Explanations

1. (D) The advantages of automatic processors are quicker, more efficient operation and consistent results. Quicker operation is attained with increased solution temperatures. The usual temperature of a 90-second developer is 90 to 95°F. Excessively high developer temperature can cause chemical fog.

2. (D) The archival quality of a film refers to its ability to retain its image for a long period of time. Many states have laws governing how long a patient's medical records, including films, must be retained. Very importantly, they must be retained in their original condition. Archival quality is poor if radiographic films begin to show evidence of stain after being stored for only a short time. Probably the most common cause of stain, and hence poor archival quality, is *retained fixer within the emulsion*. Fixer may be retained because of poor washing, or because there was insufficient hardener (underreplenishment) in the developer, thus permitting fixer to be retained by the swollen emulsion. A test for quantity of retained fixer in film emulsion is often included as part of a quality control program. Stain may also be caused by poor storage conditions. Storage in a hot, humid place will cause even the smallest amount of retained fixer to react with silver, causing stain.

3. (D) When a film first enters the processor from the feed tray, a microswitch signals the replenishment pump to begin sending replenisher solution into the processor. Replenishment continues until the microswitch senses the end (edge) of the film and terminates pump action. So, as long as film is being fed into the processor, replenishment solution will be added. There is, therefore, more replenisher added with larger size films. There is also more replenisher added when rectangular films are fed into the processor "the long way" because the processor is sensing, for example, 17 inches of film rather than 14 inches of film. Film should be put through the processor consistently according to the particular department's preference or routine. A change in film direction can lead to over- or underreplenishment and, hence, a change in film density.

4. (A) To test a film's response to processing, the film must first be given a predetermined exposure with a *sensitometer*. The film is then processed and the densities are read using a *densitometer.* Any significant variation from the expected densities is further investigated. A step wedge is used to evaluate the effect of kVp on contrast, and a spinning top test is used to check timer accuracy.

5. (C) If the fixer fails to sufficiently reharden the gelatin emulsion, water will remain within the still swollen emulsion. The dryer mechanism will be unable to completely rid the emulsion of wash water, and the film will emerge from the processor damp and tacky. On the other hand, excessive hardening action may produce brittle radiographs. High air velocity usually encourages more complete drying. Unbalanced processing temperatures can result in blistering of the emulsion.

6. (A) Developer reduces exposed silver crystals to black metallic silver. *Hydroquinone* is a reducing agent that works slowly and builds up black areas. *Phenindone* is also a reducing agent that works quickly and produces gray tones. *Sodium and potassium carbonate* are activators that serve to swell gelatin and provide the necessary alkaline medium. *Sodium sulfite and cycon* are preservatives that prevent oxidation of developer.

Fixer functions to clear film of unexposed and undeveloped silver halide grains. *Ammonium or sodium thiosulfate* are fixing or clearing agents that remove unexposed and undeveloped silver. *Sodium sulfite* is the preservative that prolongs the effective life of the solution.

7. (A) The invisible silver halide image is composed of exposed silver grains. These are "reduced" to a visible black metallic silver image in the developer solution. The fixer solution functions to remove unexposed silver halide crystals from the film.

8. (D) All of those effects listed can result from poor storage practices. Film should be rotated with the oldest being used first to avoid fog from outdated film. By protecting film from chemical fumes and from excessive temperatures, fogging of the sensitive emulsion is prevented.

9. (C) A conventional screen–film image can be scanned and digitized by a special machine called a *film digitizer.* Interpretation of a digital image can be made from the display monitor ("soft copy display") or "hard copies" can be made on film using one of two devices: a multiformat camera or a laser printer. A *multiformat camera* can place several images on a film by taking pictures of the display screen. A *laser camera* records the displayed image by exposing a film with laser light; it can also record several images on one film. The multiformat camera or laser printer is connected to an automatic processor for immediate processing and interpretation.

10. (B) An *artifact* is an unnatural feature on a radiograph. Several kinds of artifacts can be produced from careless handling during production of a radiographic image. A crinkle mark appears as a crescent shaped artifact and is a result of bending the film sharply, as over one's finger when removing from the cassette. Improper storage conditions, exposure to light, and excessive humidity are also harmful to film emulsion and can cause fogging of the film.

Evaluation of Images

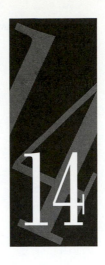

I. EVALUATION STANDARDS AND IMAGE CHARACTERISTICS

A. OVERVIEW

It is important to look at radiographic images with a critical eye, evaluating each of the components that contribute to their overall quality. The goal is to have as much information as possible, transferred as accurately as possible, from the part being radiographed to the image recorder.

B. RECORDED DETAIL AND DISTORTION

The radiograph should illustrate maximum transference of information without visible loss of image detail as a result of patient motion, excessive OID (object-to-image-receptor distance), insufficient SID (source-to-image-receptor distance), inappropriate screen and film combination, or focal spot size. There should not be evidence of shape distortion as a result of improper alignment of x-ray tube, part, and film.

C. RADIOGRAPHIC DENSITY AND CONTRAST

There should be adequate *background optical density* and a *scale of grays* sufficient to make various *tissue densities* visible.

D. GRID SELECTION AND USE

A *grid ratio* should be used that is appropriate for the kVp (kilovoltage peak) level employed. X-ray tube centering, angulation, and SID should be suitable for the particular type grid used.

E. FILM IDENTIFICATION

All essential medicolegal information should be visible on each radiograph: patient name or identification number, side marker, date, and institution.

F. COLLIMATION AND SHIELDING

To ensure patient protection, there must be visible evidence of *collimation*. *Shielding* should be evident when the reproductive organs are in the collimated primary beam, or within 5 cm of it, when the patient has reproductive potential, and when diagnostic objectives permit.

G. DEMONSTRATION OF STRUCTURES

The radiograph must include the anatomic *areas of interest* in the desired position and projection.

II. IDENTIFYING AND CORRECTING ERRORS

It is essential that the radiographer be aware of the impact each of the imaging components has on the finished radiographic image. The radiographer must be able to recognize and correct imaging errors.

Each radiograph should be evaluated according to the standards addressed above. If the image is suboptimal in any category, steps must be taken to determine the cause, correct the error, and ensure that the error will not be repeated.

It is impossible to address and illustrate here all possible errors in technical factor selection, equipment use and positioning, patient variables, artifacts, and processing. Some have been illustrated in earlier portions of this volume and others are illustrated here. Patient positioning errors are addressed in Part II. Try to identify the illustrated error, then check your answer with that given in the caption.

A. TECHNICAL FACTOR SELECTION (SEE FIGS. 14–1 THROUGH 14–3)

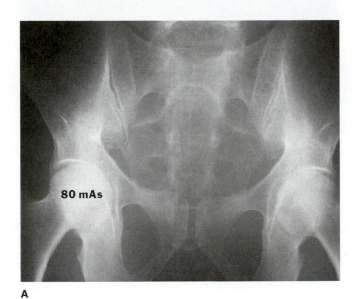

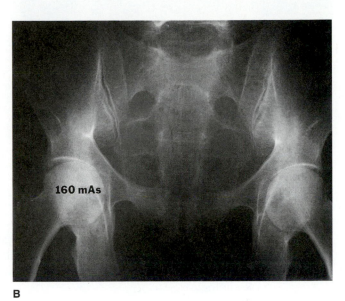

A   **B**

Figure 14–1. *Excessive optical density*; improper selection of *mAs* (milliampere-seconds). Both images were made at 100 cm SID using 75 kVp. **(A)** Image correctly exposed at 80 mAs. **(B)** Image exposed at 160 mAs demonstrates excessive density. (From the American College of Radiology Learning File. Courtesy of the American College of Radiology.)

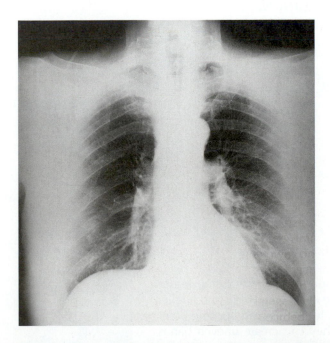

Figure 14–2. *High contrast* as a result of insufficient *kVp*. (From the American College of Radiology Learning File. Courtesy of the American College of Radiology.)

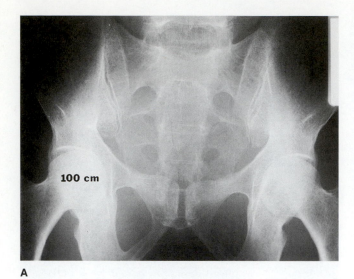

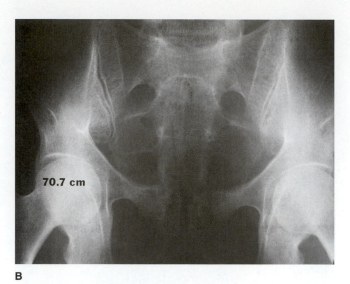

A   B

Figure 14–3. **(A)** X-ray beam intensity at a given point is dependent upon the distance from its source. Optical *density increases* in image **(B)** as a result of *decreased SID*. (From the American College of Radiology Learning File. Courtesy of the American College of Radiology.)

B. EQUIPMENT USE AND POSITIONING (SEE FIGS. 14–4 THROUGH 14–9)

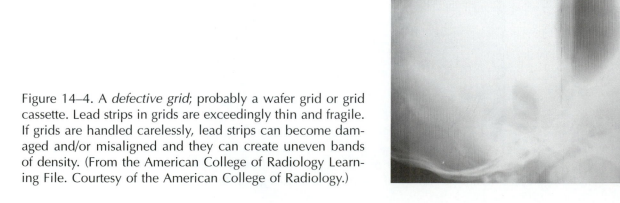

Figure 14–4. A *defective grid*; probably a wafer grid or grid cassette. Lead strips in grids are exceedingly thin and fragile. If grids are handled carelessly, lead strips can become damaged and/or misaligned and they can create uneven bands of density. (From the American College of Radiology Learning File. Courtesy of the American College of Radiology.)

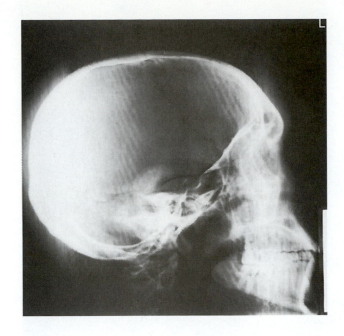

Figure 14–5. *Inverted focused grid.* If a focused grid is placed upside down, the divergent x-ray beam will be absorbed by the grid's lead strips (everywhere but the grid's central portion, where grid lines are vertical). See density versus grids section of Chapter 12. (From Saia DA. *Appleton & Lange's Review for the Radiography Examination,* 2nd ed. East Norwalk, CT: Appleton & Lange, 1997.)

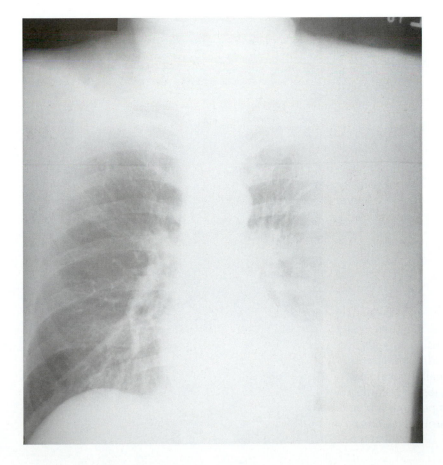

Figure 14–6. *Off focus and lateral decentering* errors. Notice the asymmetric cut-off from right to left (see density versus grids section of Chapter 12). (From the American College of Radiology Learning File. Courtesy of the American College of Radiology.)

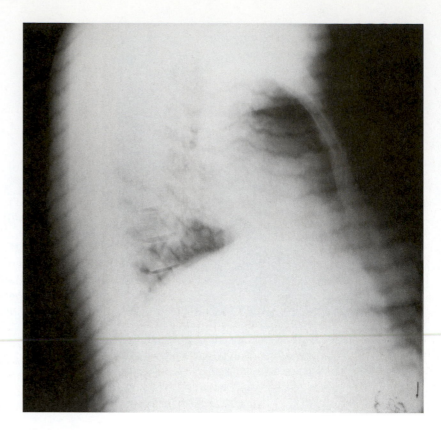

Figure 14–7. *Moiré effect.* This is a classic example of the effect of *superimposing two linear grids*, that is, a grid cassette placed in a Bucky tray. When the lead strips are aligned in the same direction, yet not exactly superimposed, this unmistakable moiré pattern occurs. (From the American College of Radiology Learning File. Courtesy of the American College of Radiology.)

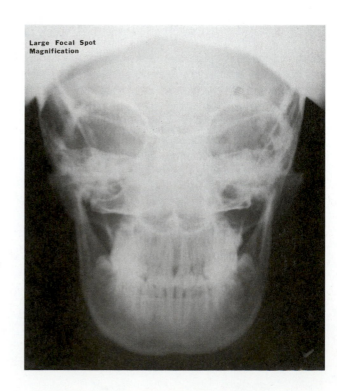

Figure 14–8. *Magnification* image performed using *large focal spot.* Magnification studies can yield useful information about tiny details *only* if a *fractional* (0.3 mm or smaller) focal spot is used. Use of a larger focal-spot size causes loss of recorded detail as a result of increased visualization of penumbra blur. (From the American College of Radiology Learning File. Courtesy of the American College of Radiology.)

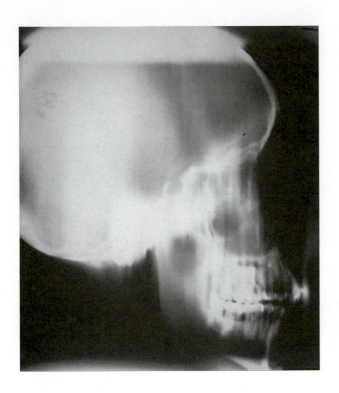

Figure 14–9. *Tomographic streaking.* Longitudinal streaking can be very pronounced in *linear tomography* when the dominant anatomic lines parallel tube motion. Placing the x-ray tube motion and dominant lines at right angles to each other, or using an appropriate tube motion (with pluridirectional tomographic equipment), can remedy the situation. (From the American College of Radiology Learning File. Courtesy of the American College of Radiology.)

C. PATIENT VARIABLES (SEE FIGS. 14–10 THROUGH 14–15)

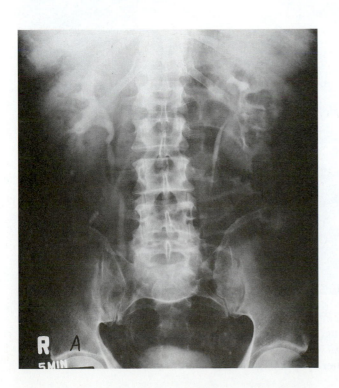

Figure 14–10. *Involuntary motion* on right (ureter) caused by *peristalsis.* Use of the shortest possible exposure time is the best way to avoid loss of detail caused by involuntary motion. (From the American College of Radiology Learning File. Courtesy of the American College of Radiology.)

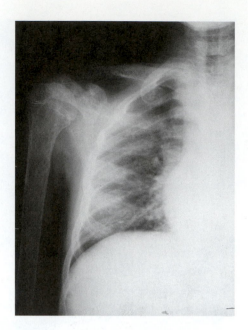

Figure 14–11. *Osteoporotic* bone as a result of thalassemia (Cooley's or Mediterranean anemia) requires *reduction of technical factors.* (From the American College of Radiology Learning File. Courtesy of the American College of Radiology.)

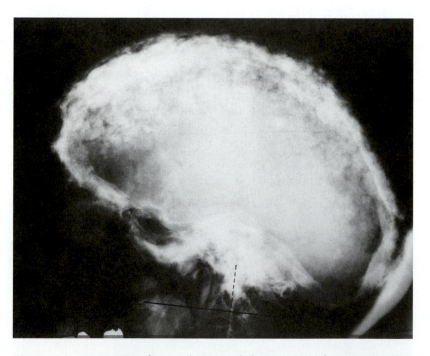

Figure 14–12. *Paget's disease* (osteitis deformans) is characterized by bone thickening, and therefore requires an increase in technical factors. (From the American College of Radiology Learning File. Courtesy of the American College of Radiology.)

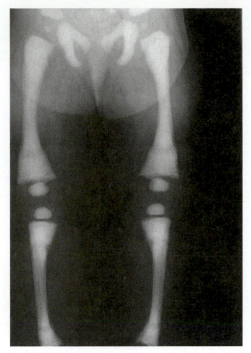

A

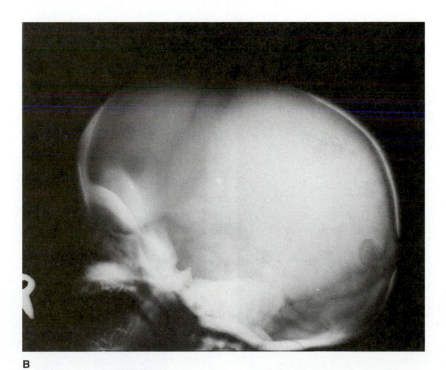

B

Figure 14–13. *Osteopetrosis* (Albers-Schönberg, or marble-bone, disease) is characterized by *increased bone density*, requiring an appropriate *increase in technical factors*. (From the American College of Radiology Learning File. Courtesy of the American College of Radiology.)

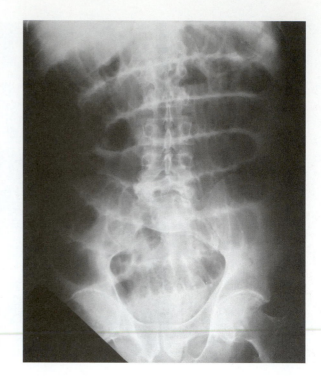

Figure 14–14. Pathology such as *increased amounts of air* can require decrease in technical factors. (From the American College of Radiology Learning File. Courtesy of the American College of Radiology.)

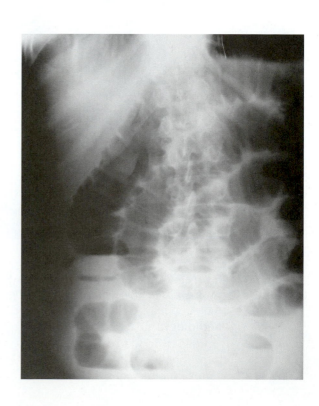

Figure 14–15. A change in *body position* from recumbent to erect will require an increase in technical factors. (From the American College of Radiology Learning File. Courtesy of the American College of Radiology.)

D. IDENTIFICATION OF ARTIFACTS

Many *artifacts* are produced by misuse of imaging equipment, as discussed in section B. Several others, having various origins, are illustrated in Figures 14–16 through 14–26. Artifacts can be classified as *exposure* artifacts (ring on finger, hair braids, etc.), *handling* artifacts (crinkle or crescent marks, fingerprints, etc.), or *processor* artifacts (guide-shoe marks, pi lines, etc.).

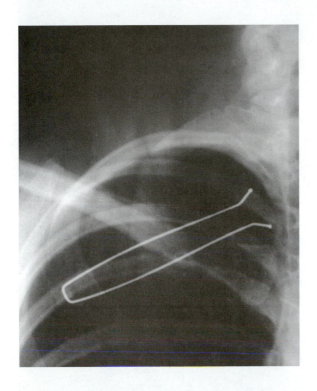

Figure 14–16. Hairpin and braid artifacts. (From the American College of Radiology Learning File. Courtesy of the American College of Radiology.)

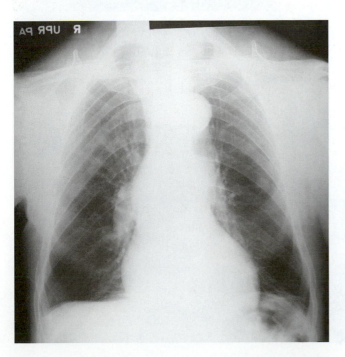

Figure 14–17. The suspicious *coin lesion* seen in the mid–left-lung field was discovered to be a *wad of chewing gum* placed there for safekeeping during this radiographic examination!! (From the American College of Radiology Learning File. Courtesy of the American College of Radiology.)

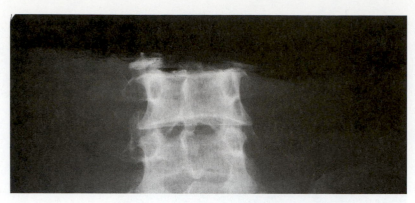

Figure 14–18. *Light leak.* Fogging from *exposure to white light,* such as film bin exposure resulted in exposed upper edge of film. (From the American College of Radiology Learning File. Courtesy of the American College of Radiology.)

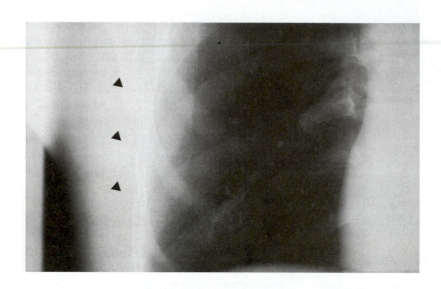

Figure 14–19. *Safelight fog.* Notice the fingers imaged in the soft tissues of the right thorax. This was probably caused by an unsafe safelight over the processor feed tray. The safelight wattage may be too great, or the safelight may be positioned too close to the feed tray. (From the American College of Radiology Learning File. Courtesy of the American College of Radiology.)

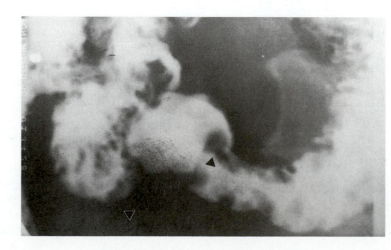

Figure 14–20. *Fingerprints.* Notice that the fingerprints are black (mid-right edge of film). If developer solution is on fingers while handling film, silver grains will be *overdeveloped* (black). If oils from the skin are deposited on the film during handling, developer will be prevented from reaching the silver grains and the fingerprints will be white (*undeveloped*). (From the American College of Radiology Learning File. Courtesy of the American College of Radiology.)

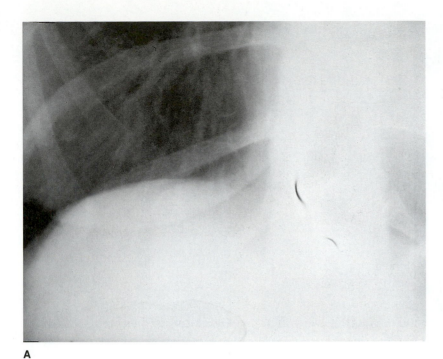

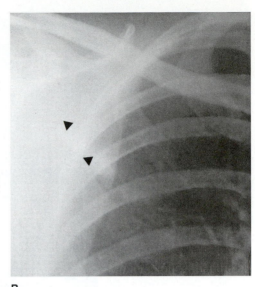

B

A

Figure 14–21. *Sensitized and desensitized marks.* **(A)** Typical, obvious *sensitized* (plus density) crescent (kink) mark caused by bending the film sharply *after* exposure. **(B)** Less-obvious *desensitized diffuse* (minus density) area (near the axillary border of fourth and fifth ribs) is caused by bending the film *before* exposure. Both of these artifacts are caused by *pressure on the film emulsion.* (From the American College of Radiology Learning File. Courtesy of the American College of Radiology.)

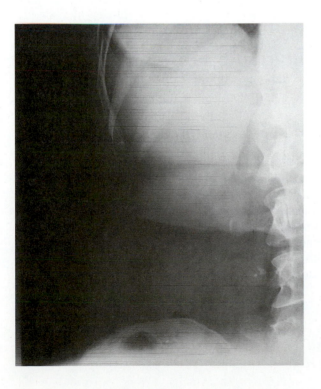

Figure 14–22. *Scratches.* Notice that the scratches are varied and irregular, unlike processor scratches, which are usually uniform and regularly spaced. These scratches were probably made by *sliding one film from a box of tightly packed films.* (From the American College of Radiology Learning File. Courtesy of the American College of Radiology.)

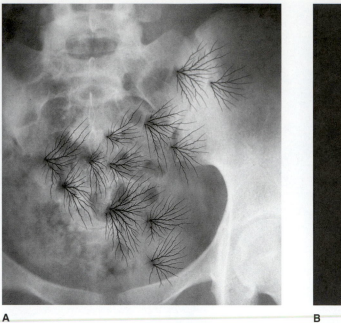

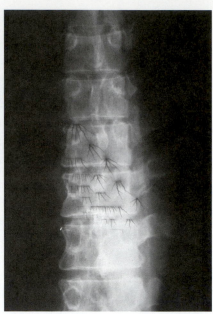

A

B

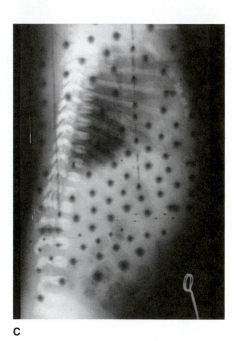

C

Figure 14–23. *Static electrical discharge.* **(A)** *Tree* static. **(B)** *Crown* static. **(C)** *Smudge* static. Static electricity artifacts are caused by *low humidity and improper handling* of films, and can obscure diagnostic information. Darkroom personnel should avoid clothing made of *synthetic materials* and screens should be cleaned with special antistatic screen cleaner. Most importantly, because *friction between film and screen* causes static buildup, it is essential not to slide film in and out of cassettes. (From the American College of Radiology Learning File. Courtesy of the American College of Radiology.)

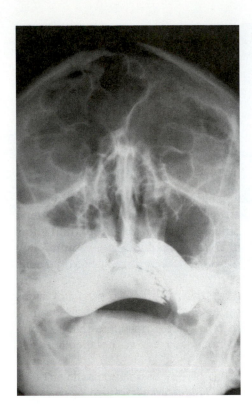

Figure 14–24. *Dentures artifact.* (From the American College of Radiology Learning File. Courtesy of the American College of Radiology.)

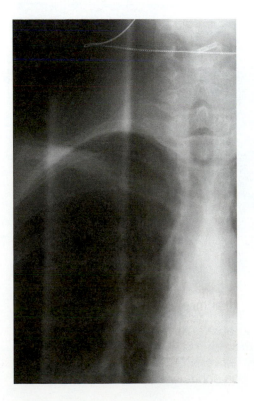

Figure 14–25. Neck chain held in patient's mouth, but (magnified) *IV pole* left between patient and x-ray tube!! (From the American College of Radiology Learning File. Courtesy of the American College of Radiology.)

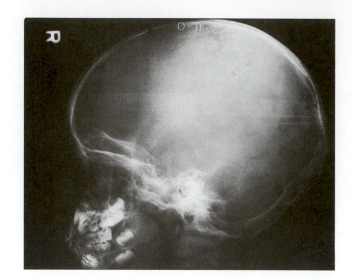

Figure 14–26. *Tape* used for immobilization is often imaged and can obscure bony detail. (From the American College of Radiology Learning File. Courtesy of the American College of Radiology.)

E. PROCESSING ERRORS AND MALFUNCTION
(SEE FIGS. 14–27 THROUGH 14–34)

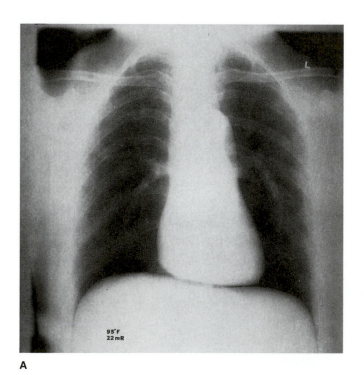

A

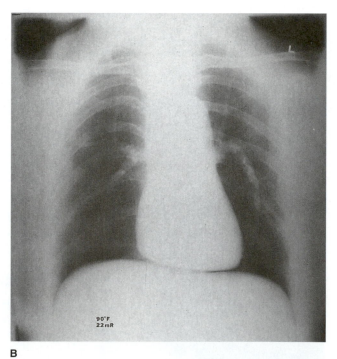

B

Figure 14–27. **(A)** Film received adequate development at 95°F and exhibits satisfactory density. **(B)** Film received insufficient development at 90°F and exhibits inadequate density caused by *underdevelopment.* Developer *activity is retarded by too low a temperature.* (From the American College of Radiology Learning File. Courtesy of the American College of Radiology.)

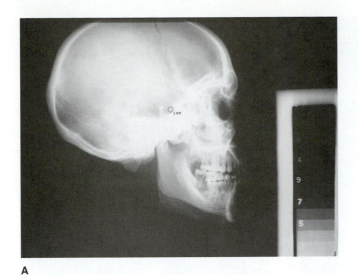
A

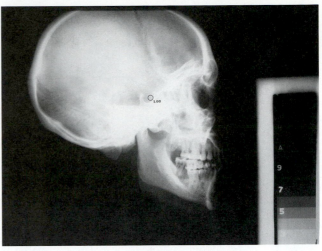
B

Figure 14–28. *Underreplenishment.* The only differences between films **(A)** and **(B)** are replenishment rate and mAs. *Notice the difference in exposure factors required to reproduce identical density: film* **(A)** *at 37 mAs; film* **(B)** *at 50 mAs.* While film **(A)** replenishment rate was 150 cc per 14 × 17-inch film, film **(B)** replenishment rate was 30 cc per 14 × 17-inch film. Underreplenishment leading to underdevelopment (and a "light" film) was *compensated for by an increase in mAs.* This problem was common before automatic processing. Today's quality control measures make this an unlikely occurrence. (From the American College of Radiology Learning File. Courtesy of the American College of Radiology.)

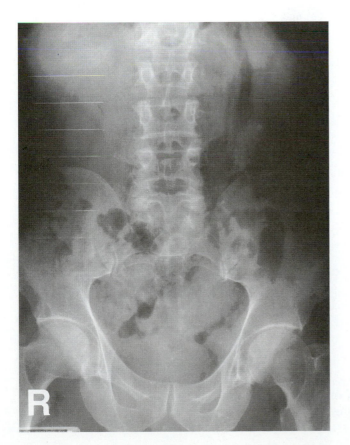

Figure 14–29. *Minus-density artifacts* (scratches), running in the direction of film travel, caused by *misaligned guide shoes.* (From Saia DA. *Appleton and Lange's Review for the Radiography Examination,* 2nd ed. East Norwalk, CT: Appleton & Lange, 1997.)

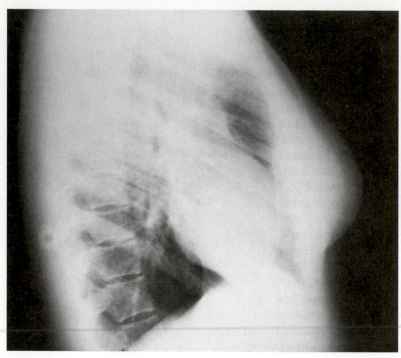

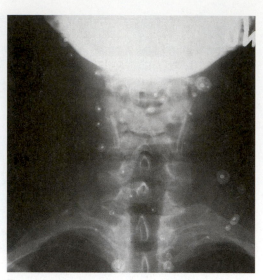

A

Figure 14–30. *Chemicals splashed on film before development.* **(A)** Film (across midthorax: anterior chest wall, in heart, soft tissue posterior chest) illustrates *fixer* splash. **(B)** *Developer* splash. (From the American College of Radiology Learning File. Courtesy of the American College of Radiology.)

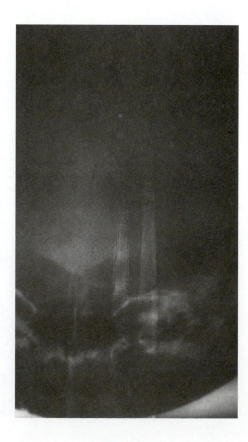

Figure 14–31. *Underdeveloped areas caused by fixer spill* on processor feed tray. (From the American College of Radiology Learning File. Courtesy of the American College of Radiology.)

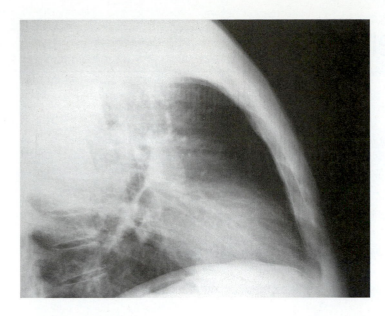

Figure 14–32. *Dirty-roller artifact.* Notice that the artifact is most apparent on the leading edge of the film (anterior chest) and diminishes with the film travel (as the film "cleans" the roller). (From the American College of Radiology Learning File. Courtesy of the American College of Radiology.)

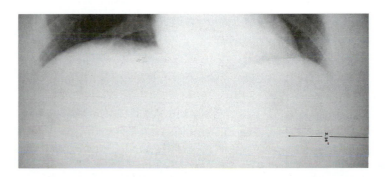

Figure 14–33. A *pi line* is a plus-density artifact occurring 3.14 inches from the film edge. (From the American College of Radiology Learning File. Courtesy of the American College of Radiology.)

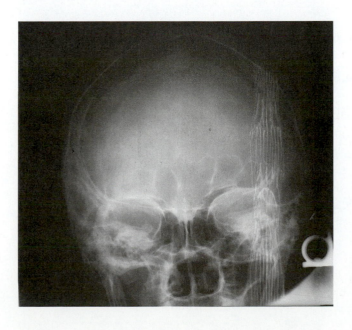

Figure 14–34. Artifact was caused by partially *crystallized fixer* on the edge of the developer-fixer crossover roller. (From the American College of Radiology Learning File. Courtesy of the American College of Radiology.)

Chapter Exercises

⭐ ***Congratulations!*** *You have completed this chapter. If you are able to answer the following group of very comprehensive questions, you should feel confident that you have mastered this section.*

1. Evaluate radiographs, assessing them for:

    A. recorded detail and distortion *(pp. 383, 388, Figure 14–8; 389, Figure 14–10)*

    B. radiographic density and contrast, including structural considerations *(pp. 383, 385–386, Figures 14–1 to 14–3)*

    C. film and screen combinations *(p. 383)*

    D. grid selection and use *(pp. 383, 386–387, Figure 14–4 to Figure 14–6)*

    E. film identification *(p. 383)*

    F. beam restriction *(p. 384)*

    G. patient shielding *(p. 384)*

    H. proper use of AEC *(pp. 254–255)*

    I. positioning accuracy, including structural considerations *(pp. 384, 390–392, Figure 14–11 to Figure 14–15)*

    J. evidence of artifacts *(p. 393, Figure 14–16 and 14–17)*

    K. processing malfunctions or errors *(pp. 394–395, Figure 14–18 to Figure 14–22)*

2. Determine the cause(s) of any problem(s) your evaluation has uncovered and discuss recommendations for corrective action.

part

V

Equipment Operation and Maintenance

Radiographic and Fluoroscopic Equipment

15

I. TYPES OF EQUIPMENT

The various kinds of x-ray machines are generally named according to the x-ray energy they produce or the specific purpose(s) for which they are designed, for example, mammographic unit, head stand, tomographic equipment, mobile unit, 150-kVp (kilovoltage peak) chest unit, 1200 mA (milliampere) general diagnostic unit, digital fluoroscopy (DF), or computed radiography (CR).

A. FIXED

Most x-ray equipment is *fixed*, or stationary, that is, it is installed in a particular place and cannot be moved. Most general radiographic and fluoroscopic equipment in the radiology department is fixed.

B. MOBILE

Mobile x-ray equipment is designed for patients who are unable to travel to the radiology department, for example, the very ill, incapacitated patients, and patients in surgery. Mobile equipment is available for radiographic and/or fluoroscopic x-ray procedures.

C. DEDICATED

X-ray equipment that is designed for a specific purpose or type of examination is referred to as *dedicated equipment*. Examples of dedicated equipment are head units, mammography equipment, chest units, and tomographic equipment.

D. DIGITAL/ELECTRONIC

Computed radiography and digital fluoroscopy units are examples of equipment whose images can be manipulated and stored for transfer via electronic means and/or printed as hard copies.

II. X-RAY TRANSFORMERS AND RECTIFIERS

Fundamental to the study of x-ray equipment is a basic understanding of magnetism and electricity. The relationship between magnetism and electricity is central to the operation of many x-ray circuit components; therefore, it is important to review these concepts prior to reviewing x-ray circuit components.

Generators function to change mechanical energy to electrical energy (whereas *motors* convert electrical energy to mechanical energy). Electrical current flowing through a conductor in only one direction and with constant magnitude, is called *direct current* (DC). A familiar source of direct current is the *battery*.

Electricity is more efficiently transported over long distances at low current and high voltage values to avoid excessive power loss (according to the power, or heat, loss formula: $P = I^2R$). Most applications of electricity require the use of *alternating current* (AC), in which the amplitude and polarity of the current vary periodically with time (Fig. 15–1). AC consists of sinusoidal waves. One *wave-*

Alternating Current Amplitude and Polarity Vary Periodically

- Amplitude and polarity vary periodically.
- **Wavelength:** Distance between 2 consecutive crests; one positive and one negative half cycle.
- **Crest:** Positive half cycle peak.
- **Trough:** Negative half cycle peak.
- **Amplitude:** Maximum height of the wave.
- **Frequency:** Number of cycles per second.
- **Hertz:** Unit of frequency.

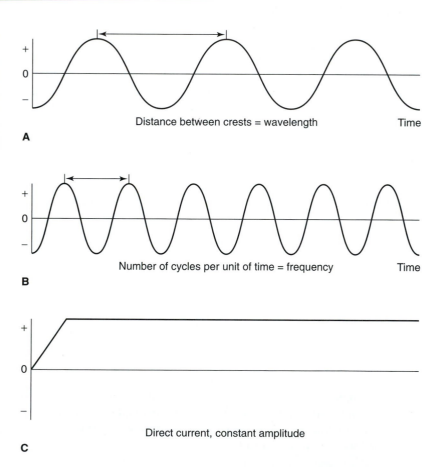

Figure 15–1. Alternating and direct current waveforms. **(A)** Alternating current (AC), low frequency. **(B)** High frequency AC. Compare the distance between crests and troughs in **(B)** with those in **(A)**. **(C)** Direct current, like that supplied by a battery, is characterized by constant amplitude (peak potential).

length consists of two half-cycles: a *positive half-cycle* and a *negative half-cycle*. A wavelength is defined as the distance between two consecutive *crests*. A crest is the positive half-cycle peak and a *trough* is the negative half-cycle peak. The maximum height of the wave/impulse is referred to as its *amplitude*, and represents electrical potential, or voltage. *AC is therefore characterized by varying amplitude and periodic reversal of polarity.* The number of cycles per unit of time (eg, second) is called *frequency* (Fig. 15–1) and its unit of measure is the *hertz* (Hz). In the United States, AC is generated at 60 Hz or cps (cycles per second), that is, 60 cycles (60 positive half-cycles and 60 negative half-cycles) occur each second. One half second, therefore, would include 30 cycles (1/2 × 60 = 30); consequently, 4 cycles represent a 4/60 or 1/15 second time interval.

X-rays are produced when high-speed electrons are suddenly decelerated upon encountering the tungsten atoms of the anode. To produce x-rays of diagnostic value, high voltage must be available. To produce high-quality radiographs, a selection of x-ray energy levels (kVp) must be available. The use of alternating current and electromagnetic principles are fundamental to the operation of the high voltage transformer and the autotransformer. These are the x-ray circuit devices responsible, respectively, for producing the required high voltage and permitting a selection of kilovoltages.

It has long been known that there is an important relationship between magnetism and electricity. Famous scientists, including Volta, Oersted, Lenz, and Faraday, worked various experiments demonstrating the relationship, making important observations, and formulating principles that explain the operation of electromagnetic devices.

Faraday's observation that a *magnetic field* will induce an electric current in a conductor if there is motion of either the magnetic field or the conductor (Fig. 15–2), is the fundamental principle of operation of the high voltage *transformer*. If a coiled conductor is supplied with an alternating current, a magnetic field expands and collapses around the coil, accompanying the peaks and valleys of the AC waveform. If a second coiled conductor is placed near, but not touching, the first (primary) coil, the moving magnetic field will interact similarly with the second coil and an electric current will be induced in it. Thus, the moving magnetic field from the primary coil can be used to induce a current in another circuit with whom it has no physical connection; this is called *mutual induction*. An alternating current, producing a continuously moving magnetic field, is necessary for mutual induction to occur.

A conductive wire shaped into a coil is called a *helix*, a helix supplied with a current is a *solenoid*. If an iron core is inserted within the coil, a simple *electromagnet* is formed and the magnetic lines of force are intensified. Thus, a transformer's conductor is frequently coiled around an iron core to increase its efficiency.

Summary

- ■ **X-ray equipment may be described as either fixed or mobile.**
- ■ **X-ray equipment designed for a particular purpose (eg, mammographic, head, chest units) is called dedicated.**

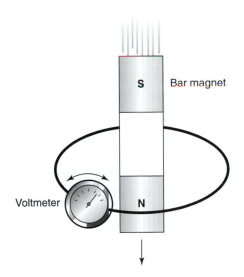

Figure 15–2. Electromagnetic induction. An electric current will be induced in a conductor whenever there is relative motion between a conductor and magnetic field; that is, if a conductor moves through a magnetic field, if a magnetic field moves across a conductor, or if the magnetic field is constantly changing (as in AC). (From Wolbarst AB. *Physics of Radiology.* East Norwalk, CT: Appleton & Lange, 1993.)

- A generator converts mechanical to electrical energy; a motor converts electrical to mechanical energy.
- Electricity is transported over long distances at high voltage and low current values to minimize energy loss, according to the heat loss formula: $P = I^2R$.
- Alternating current is characterized by constantly changing polarity and amplitude.
- A coil of wire is a helix; supplied with current it is a solenoid; with an iron core it is the simplest type of *electromagnet*.
- X-ray transformers operate on the principle of *mutual induction*.

Types of Energy Loss Inherent in All Transformers

- *Copper losses* are caused by the resistance to current flow that is characteristic of all conductors and are reduced by using larger *diameter* conductive wire.
- *Hysteresis losses* are a result of the continually changing magnetic domains of the core material (as a result of changing polarity of AC) and can be reduced by using core material of greater *permeability* (eg, silicon).
- *Eddy current* losses are a result of small currents (eddy currents) built up in the core material as a result of the continually changing magnetic fields. Eddy current losses are reduced by *laminating* the core material; any currents generated can travel only the small distance between laminations and, therefore, represent a smaller energy loss.

A. HIGH-VOLTAGE TRANSFORMERS

X-ray transformers are used to increase the incoming voltage to the more useful *kilovoltage* required for x-ray production. Transformers that increase voltage are called *step-up transformers* or high voltage transformers. The degree to which transformers increase voltage is determined by their *turns ratio*, that is, the number of turns in the secondary (high voltage) coil compared to the number of turns in the primary (low voltage) coil; the higher the ratio, the greater the voltage increase. As voltage increases, however, current decreases proportionally according to the (*transformer law*) equations that follow.

$$\frac{V_S}{V_P} = \frac{N_S}{N_P} \qquad \frac{N_S}{N_P} = \frac{I_P}{I_S}$$

Notice that the relationship between the turns ratio and the *voltage* is a *direct one*, while there is an *inverse* relationship between the turns ratio and *current*. So, as voltage increases, current decreases proportionally.

For example, if a particular x-ray transformer has a turns ratio of 500 to 1 and is supplied with 50 amps and 220 volts, what is its kVp and mA output?

$$\frac{x}{200} = \frac{500}{1} \qquad\qquad \frac{500}{1} = \frac{50}{x}$$

$$x = (500)(220) \qquad\qquad 500x = 50$$

$$x = 110,000 \text{ volts} = \textit{110 kVp} \qquad x = 0.1 \text{ amp} = \textit{100 mA}$$

Transformers can also be the *step-down* type, like that found in the x-ray filament circuit.

Although transformers operate at approximately 95% efficiency, energy loss varies according to transformer design. An *open-core* transformer consists of two parallel iron cores with conductive windings; however, a loss or leaking away of magnetic flux occurs at the ends of the iron cores. A *closed-core* transformer (Fig. 15–3) consists of a ring-shaped core of iron that serves to reduce leakage flux energy loss. A *shell* type transformer has a central partition, effectively dividing it into two halves. The transformer primary and secondary coil are wound around the center bar (but not touching each other) and this arrangement serves to reduce energy loss still further.

B. AUTOTRANSFORMERS

The x-ray circuit transformer is a *fixed*-ratio transformer, that is, the turns relationship is constant. How, then, are we able to have a selection of kilovoltages from which to choose? It is through the use of an *autotransformer*, which sends the correct amount of *voltage* to the primary of the high-voltage transformer to be stepped up to the required *kilovoltage* level.

The autotransformer consists of an iron core with a single coil wrapped around it (that serves as its primary and secondary winding) and operates on the principle of *self-induction.* Each coil turn has a contact or tap. A movable contact (corresponding to the kV selector dial on the control panel) makes connection with the appropriate tap on the autotransformer. The voltage sent to the primary coil of the high voltage transformer depends upon the number of coils "tapped." For example, a particular autotransformer has 2000 windings and is supplied with 220 volts. If 500 windings are tapped, what voltage is sent to the primary of the step-up transformer? The solution can be determined by using the *autotransformer law* (which is the same as the transformer law).

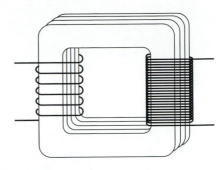

Figure 15–3. The *closed-core* transformer reduces loss of magnetic flux. Note the *laminated* silicon steel that serves to reduce *eddy-current* losses. (Modified from Wolbarst AB. *Physics of Radiology.* East Norwalk, CT: Appleton & Lange, 1993.)

$$\frac{V_S}{V_P} = \frac{N_S}{N_P}$$

$$\frac{x}{220} = \frac{500}{2000}$$

$$2000x = (500)(220)$$

$$2000x = 110{,}000$$

$$x = 55 \text{ volts sent to primary coil of step-up transformer}$$

Summary

- High-voltage (step-up) transformers function to provide the necessary kilovoltage for x-ray production.
- As the high-voltage transformer steps up voltage to kilovoltage, it proportionally steps down current according to the primary to secondary turns ratio and the transformer law.
- The transformer and autotransformer laws are expressed by the following equations.

$$\frac{V_S}{V_P} = \frac{N_S}{N_P} \qquad \frac{N_S}{N_P} = \frac{I_P}{I_S}$$

- Step-down transformers are also called filament transformers; they function on the same principles as step-up transformers, and are placed in the filament circuit.
- Transformers can be designed as open core, closed core, or shell type.
- Transformers are approximately 95% efficient.
- Types of transformer losses include copper losses, eddy current losses, and hysteresis losses.
- The autotransformer, operating on the principle of self induction, functions to provide a selection of kilovoltages.
- Both the transformer and autotransformer require AC for operation.

C. RECTIFICATION

Some x-ray circuit devices, such as the transformer and autotransformer, will operate only on AC. The efficient operation of the x-ray tube, however, requires the use of unidirectional current, so current must be *rectified* before it gets to the x-ray tube. The process of full wave *rectification* changes the negative half-cycle to a useful positive half-cycle.

An x-ray circuit rectification system is located between the secondary coil of the high-voltage transformer and the x-ray tube. Rectifiers are solid state diodes made of *semiconductive materials* such as silicon, selenium, or germanium that conduct electricity *in only one direction.* Thus, a series of rectifiers placed between the transformer and x-ray tube function to change alternating current to a more useful unidirectional current.

Although rectification remedies the changing polarity problem of single-phase AC, the problem of constantly varying amplitude remains. The continually changing voltage from zero to maximum potential and back to zero produces a pulsating beam of x-rays having a wide range of energies. *Three-phase rectification* superimposes three AC waveforms, each separated from the other two by 120 degrees and resulting in a nearly constant potential waveform. Whereas *single-phase rectification* produces a waveform having 100% "ripple" (ie, 100% drop in potential between pulses), the three-phase waveform exhibits only a slight drop between pulses (Fig. 15–4).

Three-phase/6-pulse rectification presents a 13% ripple; 3-phase/12-pulse presents only a 4% ripple. The average beam energy therefore increases. For example:

1φ 2p − 100 kVp − approximately 70 keV (kiloelectron volt) beam

3φ 6p − 100 kVp − approximately 95 keV beam

3φ 12p − 100 kVp − approximately 98 keV beam

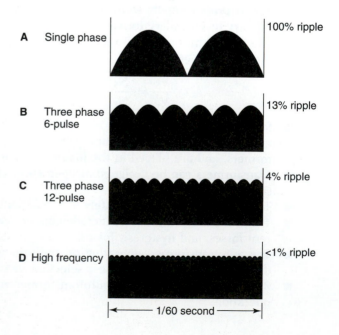

Figure 15–4. **(A)** Single-phase, full-wave rectified wave form. Note the 100% voltage ripple as each pulse starts at 0 potential, makes its way to 100%, and returns to 0 potential. **(B)** The three-phase/six-pulse waveform exhibits a 13% voltage drop between peak potentials. **(C)** Three-phase/12-pulse has only a 4% voltage drop between peak potentials. **(D)** High-frequency generators are most efficient and produce a less than 1% voltage ripple. (From Wolbarst AB. *Physics of Radiology.* East Norwalk, CT: Appleton & Lange, 1993.)

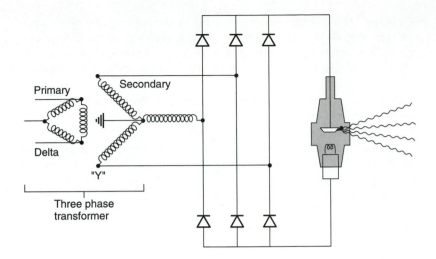

Figure 15–5. A simplified diagram of the secondary (high voltage) side of a 3φ 6p rectified x-ray circuit. 3φ equipment requires the use of three autotransformers (not shown) and one transformer having three windings arranged in *delta* and *star* (or wye) configuration. (From Wolbarst AB. *Physics of Radiology.* East Norwalk, CT: Appleton & Lange, 1993.)

Three-phase rectification requires the use of *three autotransformers* (one for each incoming current) and *one transformer* having three windings. A transformer winding can be arranged in either *star* (wye) or *delta* configuration (Fig. 15–5).

Remember that a change in technical factors is required when changing among Sφ to 3φ 6p to 3φ 12p rectified equipment.

Comparison of Technical Factors Required		
Single φ	3φ 6p	3φ 12p
x mAs	2/3*x* mAs	1/2*x* mAs

Summary

- **The x-ray tube operates most efficiently on unidirectional current.**
- **The rectification system changes AC to unidirectional current and is located between the secondary coil of the high-voltage transformer and the x-ray tube.**
- **Rectifiers are solid state diodes made of semiconductive materials such as silicon, selenium, or germanium that permit the flow of electricity in only one direction.**
- **3φ rectification uses three alternating currents out of phase with each other by 120 degrees.**
- **In 3φ rectification, only the peak values of the waveform are used, thus creating a nearly constant potential current.**
- **3φ rectification may be 6 pulse (13% ripple) or 12 pulse (4% ripple), depending on the number of rectifiers employed.**
- **3φ rectified equipment requires three autotransformers and one high-voltage transformer.**
- **3φ high-voltage transformer windings are arranged in either star (wye) or delta formation.**

III. THE X-RAY TUBE

X-rays are produced when high-speed electrons emitted from the cathode filament are suddenly decelerated as they encounter tungsten atoms of the x-ray tube anode or target.

1. *Bremsstrahlung* ("Brems") or "braking" *radiation*:

A high-speed electron, passing through a tungsten atom is attracted and "braked" (ie, slowed down) by the positively charged nucleus, and therefore is deflected from its course with a resulting loss of energy. *This energy loss is given up in the form of an x-ray photon* (see Fig. 8–4). The electron may not give up all its kinetic energy in one such interaction; it may go on to have several more interactions deeper in the target, each time giving up an x-ray photon having less and less energy. This is one reason the x-ray beam is heterogeneous (ie, has a spectrum of energies). Brems radiation comprises 70 to 90% of the x-ray beam.

2. *Characteristic radiation:*

In this case, a high-speed electron encounters the tungsten atom and ejects a K shell electron (Fig. 8–5A), leaving a vacancy in the K shell (Fig. 8–5B). An electron from the adjacent shell (that is, the L shell) fills the vacancy and in doing so *emits a K characteristic ray* (Fig. 8–5C). The energy of the characteristic ray is equal to the difference in energy between the K and L shell.

A. COMPONENT PARTS

X-ray tubes are used for both radiographic and fluoroscopic purposes. Their basic components are the *anode* (positive electrode) and *cathode* assembly (negative electrode), enclosed within an evacuated glass envelope (Fig. 15–6).

The *glass envelope* enclosure creates a *diode* (two electrodes) tube somewhat reminiscent of early radio and television tubes. The x-ray tube glass enclosure, however, is made of glass that is extremely heat resistant to maintain the necessary *vacuum* for the production of x-rays. Should the vacuum begin to deteriorate, air molecules within the tube would collide with, and decelerate, the high-speed electrons traveling to the anode, thus diminishing the

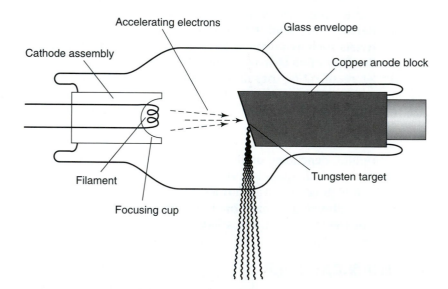

Figure 15–6. A simplified illustration of a *stationary* anode x-ray tube. The tungsten target is embedded in a solid block of copper that serves to conduct heat away from the tungsten and into the oil coolant that surrounds the glass envelope. Most x-ray tubes today use *rotating* anodes as a means of more even heat distribution. (From Wolbarst AB. *Physics of Radiology.* East Norwalk, CT: Appleton & Lange, 1993.)

production of x-rays. Air within the glass envelope is referred to as a "gassy tube," and will eventually cause oxidation and burnout of the cathode filament.

The cathode assembly consists of one or more *filaments*, their supporting wires, and a *focusing cup*. The filament is a fine (approximately 0.2-mm diameter), 1- to 2-cm coil of tungsten wire that, when heated to incandescence by about 4 amps of current, boils off (ie, liberates) outer shell tungsten electrons. This event is called *thermionic emission*. Most x-ray tubes actually have two or more filaments and are called *double-focus tubes*. The typical x-ray tube has two filaments, one small and one large, to direct electrons to either the small or large anode focal spot. Each filament is closely embraced by a negatively charged molybdenum focusing cup that serves to direct the electrons toward the anode.

As the filament boils off electrons, small quantities of tungsten can be vaporized and deposited on the inner surface of the glass envelope. If tungsten is deposited on the port window, it acts as a filter and reduces the intensity of the x-ray beam; it can also affect the tube vacuum and ultimately lead to tube failure.

The filament is heated with the required 3 to 5 amps and 10 to 12 volts by the *filament circuit*. The filament current is kept at a standby quantity until the rotor is activated; at that time the *filament booster circuit* brings it up to the level required for exposure. The rotor switch should not be activated for extended periods because the filament current is at maximum potential and tungsten vaporization can increase. Extended activation can also result in bearing damage and decreased tube life.

The anode is a 2- to 5-inch diameter molybdenum or graphite disc with a beveled edge. The beveled surface has a *focal track* of tungsten and rhenium alloy. The anode rotates at about 3600 rpm (high-speed anode rotation is about 10,000 rpm), so that heat generated during x-ray production is evenly distributed over the entire track. *Rotating anodes* can withstand delivery of a greater amount of heat for a longer period of time than *stationary anodes*.

The anode is made to rotate through the use of an *induction motor*. An induction motor has two main parts, a *stator* and a *rotor*. The stator is the part located outside the glass envelope and consists of a series of electromagnets occupying positions around the stem of the anode. The stator's electromagnets are supplied with current and the associated magnetic fields function to exert a drag or pull on the rotor within (Fig. 15–7).

Tungsten (W) is usually chosen as target material because of its *high atomic number* (Z 74), *high melting point* (3410°C), and *thermal conductivity* (equal to that of copper). The high atomic number serves to increase the efficiency of x-ray production; its high melting point makes it resistant to pitting and cracking; its thermal conductivity helps it dissipate the heat produced during x-ray production. Rhenium is added to further resist anode pitting at high temperatures (Fig. 15–8).

Summary

- **X-rays (Brems and characteristic) are produced by the abrupt deceleration of high-speed electrons by tungsten atoms within the target (anode).**

Characteristics of Tungsten (W) as Target Material

- High atomic number (74) increases x-ray production.
- High melting point (3410°C) to resist pitting and cracking.
- Thermal conductivity for heat dissipation.

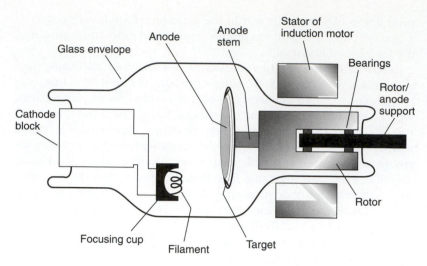

Figure 15–7. The component parts of a rotating anode x-ray tube. Note the position of the stator and rotor. Note the beveled edge of the anode, forming the focal track, and the position of the filament directly across from the rotating focal track. (Modified from Wolbarst AB. *Physics of Radiology*. East Norwalk, CT: Appleton & Lange, 1993.)

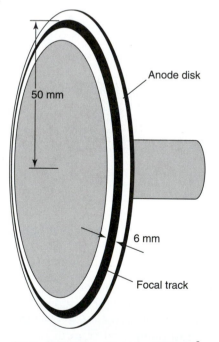

Area = (6 mm)(2π · 50 mm) = 1900 mm²

Figure 15–8. A typical rotating anode. The anode disc is usually made of molybdenum and has a beveled edge containing a "band" of tungsten/rhenium alloy that forms the focal track. (Modified from Wolbarst AB. *Physics of Radiology*. East Norwalk, CT: Appleton & Lange, 1993.)

- **The x-ray tube is a diode; that is, it has a negative electrode (cathode) and a positive electrode (anode).**
- **The x-ray tube's electrodes are enclosed within a vacuum glass envelope; a "gassy" tube produces x-rays less efficiently and results in filament oxidation, or burnout.**
- **The cathode assembly consists of tungsten filament(s) with supporting wires and a (negatively charged) molybdenum focusing cup.**
- **Most x-ray tubes have at least two filaments, one for each focal spot.**
- **Heating of the filament to incandescence (with 3 to 5 amps, 10 to 12 volts) and subsequent "boiling off" of electrons is called thermionic emission.**
- **The anode is a 2- to 5-inch molybdenum or graphite disc with a peripheral focal track of tungsten and rhenium alloy.**
- **Tungsten is the target material of choice because of its high atomic number, high melting point, and thermal conductivity; rhenium helps prevent pitting.**
- **An induction motor, consisting of stator and rotor, rotates the typical anode approximately 3600 rpm.**

The production of x-rays involves the generation of significant amounts of heat; *only 0.2% of the kinetic energy of the electron stream is converted to x-rays*, the rest of the energy is converted to *heat*. Because heat can be very damaging to the x-ray tube and its efficient operation, several features are incorporated to expedite its dissipation. The *thermal conductivity* of tungsten is one feature; however, most cooling is a result of heat diffusion to the oil that surrounds the x-ray tube. If large quantities of heat were continually directed to a single stationary small spot, that spot would be subjected to all the heat generated and would suffer more abuse and subsequent damage. The focal track of the rotating anode serves to spread generated heat over a large area. The width of the focal track on the anode's beveled edge is approximately 6 mm. Rotating anodes having a diameter of 2 to 5 inches will, therefore, provide significant surface area for the production and dissipation of heat.

The width of the beveled focal track is referred to as the *actual* focal spot size. A distinction is made between the actual focal spot and the *effective*, projected, or apparent focal spot. The actual focal spot size is the width of the finite area on the tungsten target that is actually bombarded by electrons from the filament. The effective, projected, or apparent focal spot is the *foreshortened* size of the focus as it is projected down toward the image receptor, that is, as it would be seen looking up into the x-ray tube (Fig. 15–9). This is called line focusing or the *line-focus principle*. The effective focal spot size is also affected by the degree of focal track bevel, or anode angle. Anode angles are usually 5 to 20 degrees. Anode angle also has a significant effect on the severity of the heel effect. The line focus principle and the *anode heel effect*, and their effects on radiographic quality, are discussed more fully in Part IV. When specifying focal spot size, it is the effective focal spot size that is quoted. We often

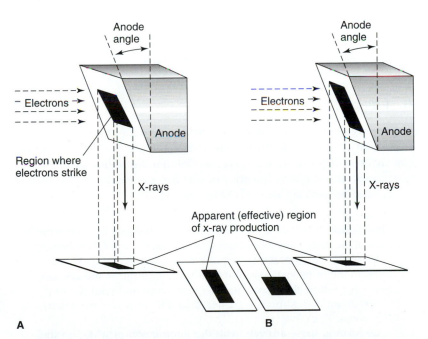

A   **B**

Figure 15–9. Line focus principle. Note how foreshortening of the actual focal spot impacts the effective (projected or apparent) focal spot. **(A)** A square actual focal spot produces a rectangular effective focal spot. **(B)** An elongated actual focal spot produces a square effective focal spot. As the anode *angle* is made smaller, the actual focal spot may be made larger while a small effective focal spot is still maintained. (From Wolbarst AB. *Physics of Radiology.* East Norwalk, CT: Appleton & Lange, 1993.)

speak of "double focus" x-ray tubes, meaning that a small (eg, 0.6 mm) and a large (1.2 mm) focal spot is available to choose from. These x-ray tubes actually have only one focal track, a portion of it is used for the small focus setting. It is more accurate to say that these are *double filament* tubes, for there are two filaments?the smaller one is activated when the small focal spot is selected, and the large one is activated for the large focal spot.

The amount of heat produced at the target is expressed in terms of *heat units* (HU). Exposure factor selection has a significant effect on the production of heat as expressed in the following equation.

$$HU = mA \times s \times kVp \text{ (single phase)}$$

For example:

300 mA, 0.4 second, 80 kVp = 9600 HU

300 mA, 0.2 second, 92 kVp = 5520 HU

Thus, a greater number of heat units are produced with higher mAs and lower kVp exposure factors. A *correction factor* is added to the equation when using three-phase equipment.

$$HU = mA \times s \times kVp \times 1.35 \text{ (3}\phi\text{ 6p)}$$

$$HU = mA \times s \times kVp \times 1.41 \text{ (3}\phi\text{ 12p)}$$

For example:

300 mA, 0.4 second, 80 kVp (3ϕ 6p) = 12,960 HU

300 mA, 0.4 second, 80 kVp (3ϕ 12p) = 13,536 HU

B. OPERATION

Each x-ray tube has its own *tube rating chart* and *anode cooling curve* that illustrate safe tube *heat limits* and the particular *cooling characteristics* of the anode. It is essential that the radiographer know how to use these charts in order to use the x-ray tube properly and safely, and to prolong its useful life (Fig. 15–10).

> *For example:* What is the maximum safe kVp that may be used with each of the three x-ray tubes using 200 mA and 0.2 second exposure?
> Do this for each of the x-ray tubes illustrated: Find the exposure time on the horizontal axis, follow it up until it meets the 200 mA line, then follow that across to the vertical axis and read the kVp.
> A = about 147 kVp; B = greater than 150 kVp (off the chart); C = about 57 kVp.
> Comparing these answers with the information provided in the legend for Figure 15–10, it can be seen that the *size of the focal spot* and the *type of rectification* significantly impact heat loading characteristics of an x-ray tube.

Next, refer to the anode cooling curve. For example, if the x-ray tube were saturated with 1,300,000 HU, it would take 30 minutes to cool down to 300,000 HU. How long would it take to cool from 700,000 HU to 450,000 HU? (Answer: Approximately 10 minutes.)

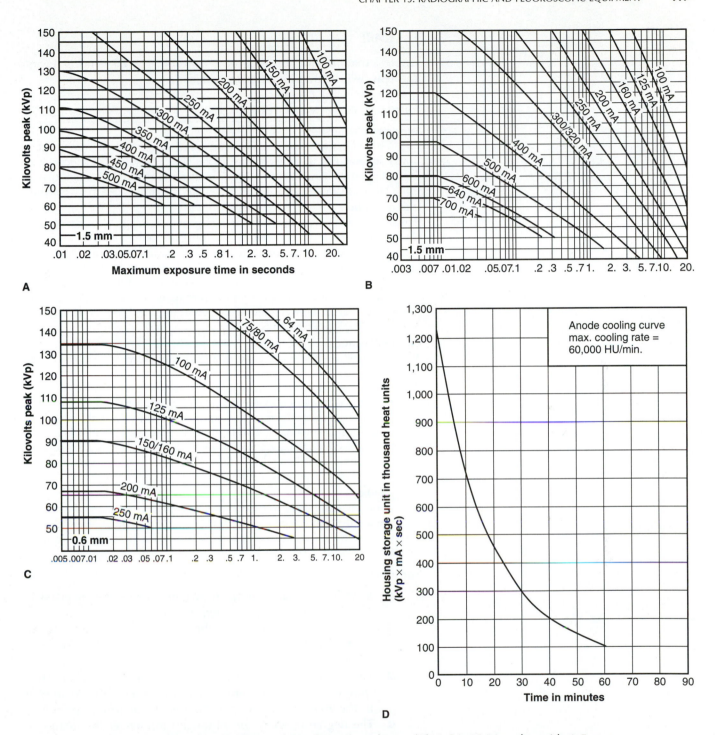

Figure 15–10. Three radiographic tube rating charts. **(A)** A Sφ 60-Hz tube with 1.5-mm focal spot. **(B)** A 3φ 60-Hz tube with 1.5-mm focal spot. **(C)** A 3φ 60-Hz tube with 0.6-mm focal spot. **(D)** An anode cooling curve illustrates the cooling characteristics of the x-ray tube. (Reproduced with permission of General Electric Company.)

C. CARE

Careless treatment or abuse of the x-ray tube, as well as normal wear and tear, will lead to its ultimate demise.

SOME CAUSES OF X-RAY TUBE FAILURE

Vaporized Tungsten

As a result of thermionic emission, quantities of tungsten can be vaporized and deposited on the inner surface of the glass envelope. When deposited on the port window, tungsten acts as a filter and reduces the intensity of the beam; it can also alter the tube vacuum and finally lead to tube failure.

Pitted Anode

Exposures made exceeding the tube rating create enough excessive heat to produce many small melts, or pits, over the surface of the focal track. X-ray photons are absorbed by these surface irregularities and, consequently, x-ray intensity is reduced. Extensive *pitting* also results in *vaporized* tungsten deposited on the inner surface of the tube window that acts as an additional filter and further reduces beam intensity. Arcing can occur between the filament and tungsten deposit, resulting in a cracked glass envelope.

Cracked Anode

A single, large, excessive exposure to a cold anode can be severe enough to crack the anode: the large dose of heat creates sudden expansion of the cold anode. It is therefore advisable to practice tube *warm-up procedures*, as suggested by the manufacturer, prior to starting the day's examinations or after the tube has not been used for several hours. Typical warm-up procedure consists of two exposures made using 100 mA, 2-second exposure, and 70 kVp. The long 2-second exposures distribute heat over the entire surface of the anode and promote uniform thermal expansion of the anode.

Gassy Tube

If the tube vacuum begins to deteriorate, air molecules collide with and decelerate the high speed electrons, thus decreasing the efficiency of x-ray production. The condition is referred to as a "gassy tube," and eventually causes oxidation and burnout of the cathode filament.

Summary

- **Most of the energy used to produce x-rays is converted to heat; only 0.2% is converted to x-rays.**
- **Heat is damaging to x-ray tubes; x-ray tubes are surrounded with oil to carry heat away from the anode (also for insulating purposes).**
- **The width of the focal track is identified as the *actual focal spot;* its bevel (angle) projects a smaller, *effective focal spot* to the image receptor according to the line-focus principle.**
- **The degree of anode bevel (angle) influences the degree of *heel effect;* the smaller the angle, the more pronounced the heel effect.**
- **Heat units (HU) are used to express the degree of accumulation of anode heat and are determined by mA × time × kVp; the correction factor for 3ϕ 6p is 1.35 and for 3ϕ 12p, it is 1.41.**
- **Excessive heat loading will cause accelerated tube aging and failure as a result of conditions such as pitted or cracked anode, gassy tube, or vaporized tungsten.**
- **Tube rating charts and anode cooling curves must be used to determine safe exposures and heat loading.**

IV. THE RADIOGRAPHIC CIRCUIT

The x-ray circuit can be divided into three portions.

1. The *low-voltage*, or *primary, circuit* contains most of the devices found on the control console.
2. The *filament circuit* varies the current sent to the filament in order to provide the required mA value.
3. The *high-voltage*, or *secondary, circuit* includes the high-voltage transformer, rectification system, and x-ray tube.

A. PRIMARY CIRCUIT COMPONENTS

PRIMARY OR LOW VOLTAGE CIRCUIT DEVICES

Main Switch and Circuit Breakers
These are usually located on a wall in or near the x-ray room (Fig. 15–11). Circuit breaker switches must be closed to energize the equipment.

Autotransformer
The autotransformer is a variable transformer that operates on AC and enables the radiographer to select kilovoltage. The function and operation of the autotransformer was discussed earlier in this section.

kV Selector
This is used by the radiographer to choose the kilovoltage, often as kV major (in increments of 10) and kV minor (in increments of 2). In doing so, the appropriate number of coils (representing volts) on the autotransformer are selected by the movable contact.

Line-Voltage Compensator
This functions to automatically adjust for any fluctuations in incoming voltage supply. A uniformly consistent and accurate voltage supply is

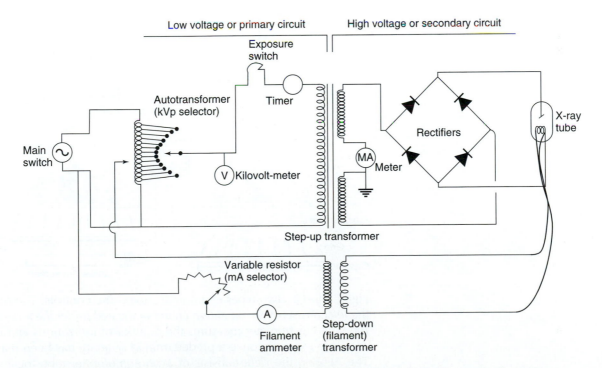

Figure 15–11. Simplified x-ray circuit. High-voltage current from the secondary transformer coil is rectified before it reaches the x-ray tube.

required for predictable radiographic results. A small variation in voltage entering the primary transformer coil voltage represents a much larger variation as it leaves the secondary coil. The control consoles of some older x-ray units were equipped with line-voltage compensators that were adjustable by the radiographer, but in equipment manufactured today, the process takes place automatically within the machine.

Timer

Timers function to regulate the length of x-ray exposure. Very simple timers such as the mechanical, synchronous, and impulse timers are rarely used in x-ray equipment manufactured today because they do not permit very fast, accurate exposures. *Mechanical timers* are capable of exposures only as short as 1/4 second; *synchronous timers* as short as 1/60 second. *Impulse timers* are more accurate and capable of exposures as short as 1/120 second.

The *electronic timer* used in x-ray equipment manufactured today, is somewhat complex and based on a capacitor-resistor circuit. Electronic timers are very accurate and capable of rapid exposures as short as 1 millisecond (ie, 1/1000 or 0.001 second).

The *milliampere-second timer* (mAs timer) monitors the product of mA and time and terminates the exposure when the desired mAs has been reached. Milliampere-second timers are found on some mobile x-ray units. They are also found on some older fixed x-ray units and display the mAs exposure value when exposure time is too short to permit the actual mA to register on the mA meter.

Another type of timer is the automatic exposure device (AED), or *automatic exposure control* (AEC), which functions to produce consistent radiographic results (Fig. 15–12). AECs have sensors that

---

Types of X-Ray Timers

- Mechanical
- Synchronous
- Impulse
- Electronic
- mAs
- AEC (photomultiplier or ionization chamber)

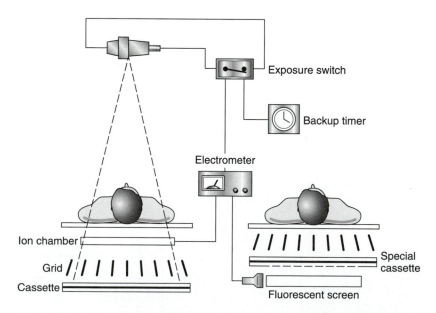

Figure 15–12. Two types of automatic exposure controls. The AEC on the *left* consists of an *ionization chamber* located *under the x-ray table-top*. The electrometer measures the number of ionizations and terminates the exposure once a predetermined quantity has been reached. The AEC on the *right* consists of a *photomultiplier* tube located *behind the cassette.* Note that a backup timer is in place to terminate the exposure, should the AEC fail to do so.

signal to terminate the exposure once a predetermined, known correct, exposure has been reached.

One type of AEC, the *ionization chamber*, is located just beneath the tabletop, above the x-ray cassette. The part being radiographed is centered to the sensor and exposed. When the predetermined quantity of air ionization has occurred within the chamber, as measured and determined by an electrometer, the exposure is automatically terminated.

Another type of AEC is the *photomultiplier* (*phototimer*), located behind the cassette. The phototimer consists of a special fluorescent screen that, when activated by x-ray, produces light and charges a photomultiplier tube. When the correct charge has been reached, as determined by the electrometer, the exposure is automatically terminated. Special cassettes, having very little foil backing, are often used with phototimers.

A *backup timer* (the manual timer) is used to protect the patient from excessive exposure and x-ray tube from damage should the AEC fail to operate properly. Additional discussion of AECs can be found in Part IV.

X-ray timer malfunction can cause undesirable fluctuation in radiographic density. If the timer terminates the exposure too soon, the radiograph will be underexposed; if the exposure is delayed in terminating, the radiograph will be overexposed. The radiographer should be able to perform a *spinning-top test* to evaluate timer accuracy (Figs. 15–13 and 15–14).

A simple spinning top consists of a circular steel or lead disc with a small hole in its periphery. The disc is mounted on a base that allows the disk to revolve freely. The device is placed on a cassette, the spinning top is set in motion, and an exposure made using the exposure time station to be evaluated.

Recall that with single-phase equipment there are 120 useful x-ray impulses per second using *single-phase full-wave rectified* current. If the x-ray timer is set to use some portion of the impulses,

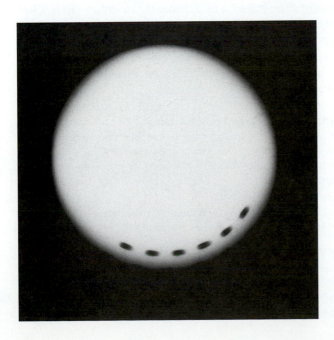

Figure 15–13. The spinning top test was made using 1/20 (0.05) second exposure and correctly produced 6 dots.

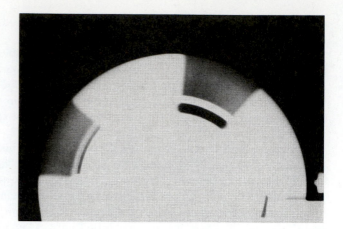

Figure 15–14. Synchronous spinning top test. An exposure was made using 1/12 (0.083) second. The resulting image correctly demonstrates a 30-degree arc. (From Saia DA. *A&L Review for the Radiography Examination*, 4th ed. East Norwalk, CT: Appleton & Lange, 2000.)

eg, 1/4 second, then one fourth of the 120 impulses should be recorded on film if that time station is accurate. Thus, the film should show 30 dots. A minor discrepancy usually indicates a *timer malfunction*; exactly one-half the correct number of dots indicates a *rectifier problem*. If an exposure of 1/10 second is made, 12 dots should be recorded, and so on. Simply multiply the number of impulses per second (120 in the case of Sϕ full-wave rectified equipment) by the exposure time. In the unlikely event that *half-wave rectified* equipment is being tested, the exposure time is multiplied by 60 (useful impulses/second).

Because most x-ray equipment manufactured today is three-phase, a slightly different approach must be taken when evaluating these timers. Because *three-phase full-wave rectified* equipment produces a *ripple wave*, that is, almost constant potential, the standard spinning top test does not demonstrate impulses; rather, a *solid arc* is recorded. The use of a *synchronous* (motorized) *spinning top* (or oscilloscope) is required. The exposure is made at the time station to be evaluated and the resulting radiograph demonstrates a solid arc. If the exposure time made was 1 second, an entire circle (360 degrees) should be demonstrated. For exposure times less than 1 second, the corresponding portion of a circle should be recorded. For example, an exposure made at 1/4 second should record a 90-degree arc (ie, 1/4 of a 360-degree circle); at an exposure of 1/10 second, a 36-degree arc should be recorded.

Primary Coil of the High-Voltage Transformer
The primary coil of high voltage transformer is the final component of the primary, or low-voltage, circuit. The low voltage entering the primary coil is stepped up to high kilovoltage in the secondary coil by means of mutual induction.

Exposure Switch
The exposure switch is a remote control switch that functions to start the x-ray exposure (the timer terminates the exposure).

B. FILAMENT CIRCUIT COMPONENTS

The filament circuit is responsible for supplying low voltage current (3 to 5 amps, 10 to 12 volts) to the filament of the x-ray tube. Because the incoming voltage (110 to 220 volts) is greater than that required, a *step-down transformer* is placed in the filament circuit to make the required voltage adjustment. A *rheostat*, or other type of *variable resistor*, is placed in the filament circuit to adjust amperage and corresponds to the *mA selector* on the control console.

C. SECONDARY CIRCUIT COMPONENTS

SECONDARY OR HIGH-VOLTAGE CIRCUIT DEVICES

Secondary Coil of High Voltage Transformer
This carries the required high voltage for x-ray production (and proportionally smaller current value).

mA Meter
This is located at the midpoint of the secondary transformer coil. Because it is grounded, it can be safely placed in the operator's console. The mA meter displays the tube current value.

Rectifiers
The *rectification* system of diodes is located between the secondary coil of the high-voltage transformer and the x-ray tube. Recall from earlier discussion that it functions to change alternating current to unidirectional pulsating current. Current pulsations decrease with solid-state three-phase rectification (3ϕ 6p rectification has a 13% ripple; 3ϕ 12p has a 4% ripple).

X-ray Tube
The x-ray tube is the final device in the secondary circuit. The filament of its negative electrode, the cathode, is heated by its own circuit to produce *thermionic emission*. As high voltage is applied, the thermionic electron cloud is driven to the anode target. The rapid deceleration of electrons, and their interaction with tungsten atoms of the target, results in an energy conversion to heat and x-rays (99.8% heat, 0.2% x-rays).

D. CIRCUITRY OVERVIEW OF A SINGLE EXPOSURE

1. X-ray machine is turned on. This activates the filament circuit and heats the x-ray tube filament (10 to 12 volts; 3 to 5 amps).
2. If the machine has been off overnight, warm-up exposures are made to warm the anode throughout (anode cracking can occur when surface heat is applied to a cold anode).
3. Appropriate exposure factors are chosen on the control panel (machines having a line-voltage compensator on the control panel should be adjusted to compensate for any incoming voltage fluctuation).
4. The rotor/exposure switch is a two-step button and should be depressed completely in one motion; the first click heard after partial depression is the induction motor bringing anode rotation up to speed. At this time, the filament is heated to maximum (thermionic emission) and produces an electron cloud.
5. Upon complete depression of the rotor/exposure switch, the exposure is made. The moment the exposure button is depressed the voltage selected by the autotransformer is sent to the step-up transformer where it is converted to the high voltage (kV) and low amperage (mA) required. This high voltage current then passes through the rectification system which changes AC to pulsating DC.

6. The applied high voltage (potential difference) propels the electron cloud to the anode where interactions between the high speed electrons and tungsten target atoms converts electron kinetic energy to (99.8%) heat energy and (0.2%) x-ray photon energy (see *x-ray production* details in Chapter 8).

E. COMPUTED RADIOGRAPHY

Computed radiography is also referred to as *filmless radiography* because a photostimulable phosphor plate (image plate [IP] or storage plate) is used as the image receptor. The IP looks very similar to a traditional radiographic cassette, is used in the same way, and is available in similar sizes. Instead of the traditional intensifying screens and film, the computed radiography cassette contains an image plate coated with europium-doped barium fluorohalide crystals. When the IP receives image-forming remnant x-ray photons, the x-ray energy is absorbed, changed to visible light, and stored (hence the term *storage plate*). This stored energy represents the latent image. The IP is placed in the computed radiography scanner. Here a helium-neon laser beam scans the IP and the stored energy is released as blue-violet light (phosphostimulated luminescence [PSL]). This light signal (representing the latent image) is transferred to an *analog-to-digital converter* (*ADC*) which converts the signal to a digital (electrical) one. The resulting digital information can now be displayed on a monitor, electronically transmitted, manipulated, and stored efficiently (archived). After the reading process has been completed, the image data stored on the IP is *erased* by exposing the IP to high intensity light and the IP is ready for reuse.

The following is an overview of how we use computers to represent data, and the factors that influence image characteristics.

Computer System. The computer system consists of the *hardware*, which is any physical component of the computer, and the *software*, which is a set of instructions or program to operate the computer.

The hardware consists of input and output devices. These devices allow information to be put into a computer and allow information to be directed outside the computer. The *central processing unit* (CPU) is the primary control center for the computer consisting of a control unit, arithmetic unit, and memory. The speed is measured in "millions of instructions per second" (MIPS). Most desktop computer speeds are given in MHz. The *memory* is solid state. It is used by the computer during execution of a program. There are two types of memory. The first is *RAM*, or random access memory. This memory is volatile and will lose all information when the computer is turned off unless previously saved. Read only memory, or *ROM*, is memory that is hard wired into the computer, which means it stays in the computer even when the computer is turned off. ROM usually contains the booting instructions.

The software is a set of instructions the computer uses to function effectively, known as a program. Computer programmer languages include, but are not limited to:

- Fortran: Formula translation. Used mainly in science and engineering applications.
- Basic: A beginners all-purpose language with symbolic instructions and code.

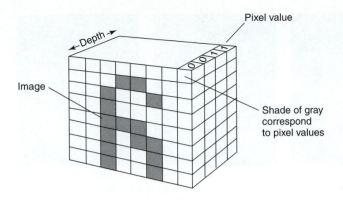

Figure 15–15. A digital image may be likened to a three-dimensional object made up of many small cubes, each containing a binary digit or bit. The image is seen on one surface of the block, whose depth is the number of bits required to describe each pixel's gray level.

- Cobol: Common business-oriented language.
- Pascal: High-level mathematics.

Binary Numbers. The computer hardware interprets all information as a simple "yes" or "no" decision. Current "on" implies "yes" and current "off" implies "no." This is symbolically represented with digits 1 and 0. A *bit* in computer terminology refers to an individual one or zero and is a single bit of information. A *byte* is equal to 8 bits, and a word is equal to 16 bits or 2 bytes.

Image Storage. Image storage is located in a *pixel* (Fig. 15–15), which is a two-dimensional "picture element." Pixels are measured in the "XY" direction.

The third dimension in the matrix of pixels is the depth which together with the pixel is referred to as the *voxel* (Fig. 15–16). The voxels are measured in the "Z" direction. The depth of the block is the number of bits required to describe the gray level that each pixel can take on. This is known as the *bit depth*.

The *matrix* is the number of pixels in the XY direction. *The larger the matrix size, the better the image resolution* (Fig. 15–17).

Typical image matrix sizes used in radiography are:

- Nuclear medicine   128 × 128
- Digital subtraction angiography
  (DSA) (Fig. 15–18)   1024 × 1024
- CT   512 × 512
- Chest radiography   2048 × 2048

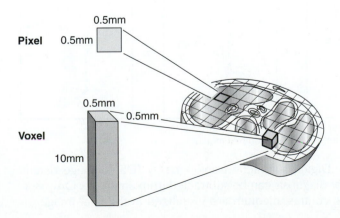

Figure 15–16. The third dimension in the matrix of pixels is the depth, which together with the pixel is referred to as the voxel (volume element).

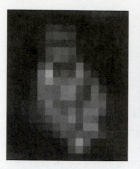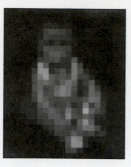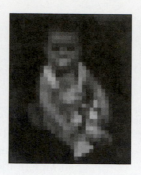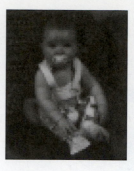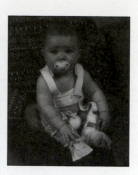

Figure 15–17. The matrix is the number of pixels in the XY direction. The larger the matrix size the better the image resolution.

A digital image is formed by a *matrix* of *pixels* in rows and columns. A matrix having 512 pixels in each row and column is a 512 × 512 matrix. The term *field of view* is used to describe how much of the patient (eg, 150-mm diameter) is included in the matrix. The matrix or field of view can be changed without affecting the other, but changes in either will change pixel size. As in traditional radiography, *spatial resolution* is measured in line pairs per mm (*lp/mm*). As matrix size is increased, there are more and smaller pixels in the matrix therefore improved resolution. Fewer and larger pixels results in a poor-resolution "pixelly" image, that is, one that you can actually see the individual pixel boxes (Fig. 15–17).

One of the most important factors to consider in computed radiography is the ability to transmit images over distances, known as *teleradiography*. The amount of information transferred per unit time is known as the baud rate and is in units of bits per second.

> Example: A network is capable of transmitting data at a rate of 9600 baud. If each pixel has a bit depth of 8 bits how long will it take to transmit a 512 × 512 image?
> Solution:
>
> (512 × 512 pixels)(8 bits/pixel)/9600 bits/second = 128 seconds.

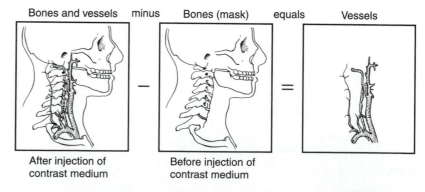

Figure 15–18. Digital subtraction angiography (DSA). Image details not required for diagnosis can be subtracted from an image. Only vessels containing contrast medium are visualized in the final image.

There are three possible means of image transmission. *Telephone wires* offer low transmission speed while using a modem. *Coaxial cable* will transmit at approximately 100 MBaud. Finally, there are *fiber-optic cables* that are unaffected by electrical fields and therefore have less error than cables or wires with electrical signals.

Another advantage of computed radiography is the ability to *manipulate the image after exposure*. Image manipulation postprocessing can be used for *noise reduction*, *contrast modification*, *image subtraction* (Fig. 15–18), and *windowing*. Image subtraction is used primarily in angiography to remove superimposed bone structures on contrast-filled vessels.

The digital images' *scale of contrast*, or *contrast resolution*, can be changed electronically through leveling and windowing of the image. The *level control* determines the *central or mid density* of the scale of contrast, while the *window control* determines the *total number* of densities or grays (to the right and left of the central or mid-density).

Windowing is a process of changing the contrast and density setting on the finished image. The window *width* controls the *number* of shades of gray in the image, while the window *level* corresponds to the *density* in the *center* of the window (the midpoint of the contrast scale). Narrower windows result in higher (shorter scale) contrast. Pixel values *below* the window range will be displayed as *black*, while pixel values *above* the window range will be displayed as *white*. Pixel values between the two limits are spread over the full scale of gray.

Applications for computed imaging include the following.

- CT scanning
- Nuclear medicine
- Magnetic resonance imaging
- Ultrasonography
- DSA (see Fig. 15–18)

Summary

- The x-ray circuit has three major portions: the primary, or low-voltage, side; the filament circuit; and the secondary, or high-voltage, side.
- Most of the control console devices are in the primary circuit.
- Primary circuit devices include the main switch and circuit breaker; the autotransformer and kV selector; line-voltage compensator; timer; primary coil of the high-voltage transformer; and exposure switch.
- The line-voltage compensator automatically adjusts for any fluctuations in the incoming electrical supply.
- The timer regulates the length of the x-ray exposure; types of timers include mechanical, impulse, synchronous, mAs timer, electronic timer, and AEC.
- There are two types of AECs: the photomultiplier (phototimer), located behind the cassette, and the ionization chamber, located above the cassette.
- A back-up timer terminates the exposure should the AEC fail, thereby functioning to protect the patient and x-ray tube from excessive exposure.

- Timer accuracy can be tested with a spinning-top test: a simple spinning top for single-phase equipment and a synchronous spinning top for three-phase equipment.
- Single-phase spinning-top tests show a series of dots, each representing an x-ray impulse.
- Three-phase spinning top tests show a solid arc exposure?a portion of a circle (measured in degrees) representative of a portion of a second.
- A step-down transformer and rheostat are placed in the filament circuit to supply the x-ray tube with low-voltage current.
- Secondary circuit devices include the secondary coil of the high-voltage transformer, mA meter, rectifiers, and x-ray tube.
- The grounded mA meter displays the tube current value on the control console.
- Rectifiers are located between the transformer's secondary coil and the x-ray tube; they function to change AC to unidirectional current.
- There are two types of computer memory: RAM and ROM.
- A two-dimensional picture element is a *pixel*; a three-dimensional picture element is a *voxel*.
- Computed radiography enables image manipulation *after* exposure.
- *Windowing* is the process of changing contrast and density on the finished image; window *width*, which controls the *number* of grays, and window *level*, which corresponds to the *density* in the *center* of the window.

V. THE FLUOROSCOPIC SYSTEM

Fluoroscopic x-ray examinations are used to study the dynamics of various parts in *motion*. Fluoroscopy was performed almost exclusively in the very early days of radiology, because of the lack of dependable x-ray tubes and image recording systems (Fig. 15–19). In

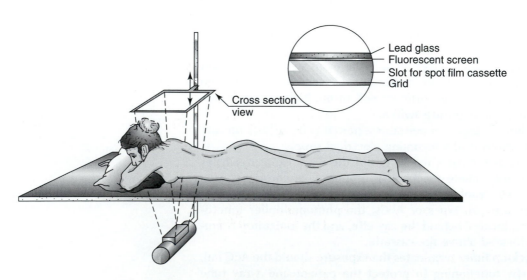

Figure 15–19. Basic early fluoroscope.

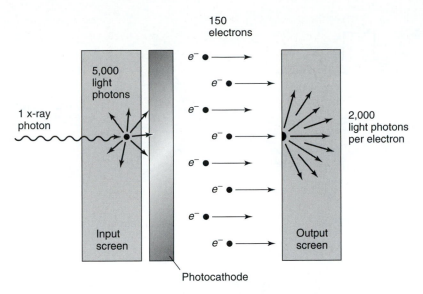

Figure 15–20. Conceptualization of relationship and function of an image intensifier input screen, photocathode, and output screen. For every one x-ray photon interacting with the input screen, 5000 fluorescent light photons are emitted. Note the close (but not touching) relationship between the input screen and photocathode for maintenance of resolution. The light photons interact with the photocathode and about 150 electrons are emitted by the photoemissive metal. The photoelectrons then interact with the output screen and 2000 fluorescent light photons are emitted for every electron.

the late 1940s and early 1950s, image intensification was developed and served to provide much brighter images at lower exposures. Present day *image intensifiers* (II) brighten (intensify) the conventional, or "dark," fluoroscopic image 5000 to 20,000 times. Today's fluoroscopic procedures are much safer (lower exposure) and brighter; the fluoroscopic image can be photographed still or moving (cine or videotape), or viewed with a television camera and projected onto a nearby or remote television monitor.

A fluoroscope has two principle components, an x-ray tube and a fluorescent screen, attached at opposite ends of a *C-shaped arm* (Figs. 15–20; 15–21A).

Fluoroscopic x-ray tubes are standard rotating anode tubes, usually installed under the x-ray table, but operated at much lower tube currents than radiographic tubes. Over-the-table fluoroscopic x-ray tubes result in higher radiation exposure to personnel than under-the-table x-ray tubes. Instead of the 50 mA to 1200 mA used in radiography, fluoroscopic tubes are operated at currents that range from *0.5 mA to 5.0 mA* (averaging 1 to 3 mA).

Patient dose is much higher in fluoroscopic than radiographic procedures because of the considerably shorter source-to-object distance (SOD) used in fluoroscopy. Fluoroscopic *entrance exposure* is significantly greater than exit exposure as a result of attenuation processes within the patient.

For radiation protection purposes, the fluoroscopic tabletop exposure rate must not exceed *10R/minute* and all fluoroscopic equipment must provide *at least 12 inches* (30 cm), and preferably 15 inches

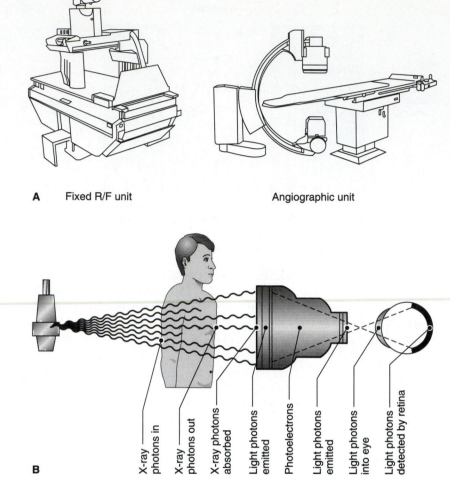

A Fixed R/F unit

Angiographic unit

B

X-ray photons in

X-ray photons out

X-ray photons absorbed

Light photons emitted

Photoelectrons

Light photons emitted

Light photons into eye

Light photons detected by retina

Figure 15–21. **(A)** *C-arm*: A fluoroscope has two principle components, an x-ray tube and a fluorescent screen, attached at opposite ends of a C-shaped arm. **(B)** Transition of x-ray photons emerging from x-ray tube, through part under study, into image intensifier, to human eye. (B is modified from Wolbarst AB. *Physics of Radiology*. East Norwalk, CT: Appleton & Lange, 1993.)

(38 cm), between the x-ray source (focal spot) and the x-ray tabletop. Positioning the image intensifier *closer* to the patient *decreases the SID* and *decreases patient dose*. Patient dose decreases because as the SID is *decreased* the number of x-ray photons at the input phosphor *increases*; this results in the automatic brightness control *decreasing the mA* to compensate for the increase in x-ray photons.

A *5-minute timer* is used to measure accumulated fluoroscopic examination time and make an audible sound or interrupt exposure after 5 minutes of fluoroscopy. X-ray production is usually activated by a foot switch (*dead-man switch*), thus leaving the fluoroscopist's hands free to handle the carriage and position and palpate the patient. The fluoroscopic tube is usually equipped with electrically driven collimating *shutters*. Leaded glass provides shielding from radiation passing through the intensifying screen and the image intensifier is lead lined. A *Bucky slot cover* and *protective curtain* also help reduce exposure to the fluoroscopist.

Many fluoroscopes are equipped with a *spot film* device to record fluoroscopic images. To expose a spot film, a motor is activated that brings a cassette from a lead lined compartment within the carriage over into the fluoroscopic field between the intensifying screen and grid (Fig. 15–21A). The fluoroscopic x-ray tube current then automatically increases to a conventional radiographic level of about 300 mA or more for the cassette exposure. The lead shutters usually adjust automatically but may be operated manually.

Summary

- **Fluoroscopes are used to examine moving parts and are often equipped with a device to take cassette-loaded spot films.**
- **A fluoroscope has two major parts: an x-ray tube and a fluorescent screen, attached at opposite ends of a C-shaped arm.**
- **The fluoroscopic tube is usually located (at least 12 inches) under the x-ray table and operated at 1 to 3 mA; mA automatically increases for cassette-loaded spot films.**
- **Fluoroscopic patient dose depends on exposure rate, tissue thickness or density, and length of exposure.**
- **Fluoroscopic patient dose decreases as the image intensifier is moved closer to the patient.**
- **Many guidelines regulate the operation of fluoroscopic equipment because of the unavoidably high patient dose inherent in fluoroscopic procedures (because of the short focus-to-patient distance).**
- **Image intensifiers brighten the conventional, dark fluoroscopic image 5000 to 20,000 times.**

A. THE IMAGE INTENSIFIER

The fluorescent layer of early conventional (or "dark") fluoroscopic screens was made of *zinc cadmium sulfide* (Patterson B-2 screen). The *input screen* of today's image intensifier tube is made of a thin layer of *cesium iodide*, is 5 to 12 inches in diameter, and slightly convex in shape.

Cesium iodide is much more efficient than zinc cadmium sulfide because it absorbs, and converts to fluorescent light, a greater number of the x-ray photons striking it. For each absorbed x-ray photon, approximately 5000 light photons are emitted. This fluorescent light strikes a *photocathode* made of a photoemissive metal. A number of electrons are subsequently released from the photocathode and focused toward the output side of the image tube. Although this step actually represents a *deamplification*, it has very little effect on the end result. A thin (0.2-mm) layer of glass or other transparent material is placed between the input screen and photocathode to prevent chemical reaction between the two; otherwise, the two must be as close as possible for maximum transfer of accurate information.

The electrons emitted from the photocathode are focused toward the output end of the tube by negatively charged *electrostatic focusing lenses*. They then pass through the neck of the tube where they are accelerated through a potential difference of 25,000 to 35,000 volts and strike the small (0.5- to 1-inch) fluorescent *output screen* that is mounted on a flat glass support (see Fig. 15–20; 15–22).

The entire assembly is enclosed within a 2- to 4-mm thick vacuum glass envelope. The glass is then coated to prevent the entry of

Some Radiation Safety Features of Fluoroscopic Equipment

- Maximum of 5 mA
- 12 inches minimum between focal spot and table top
- 10 R/min maximum tabletop exposure
- 5-minute cumulative timer
- Dead-man switch
- Automatic collimation
- Bucky-slot cover
- Protective curtain

light. The glass tube is enclosed within a metal housing that functions to attenuate magnetic fields from outside the tube that would distort the electron paths within.

For there to be undistorted focusing of electrons onto the output screen, each electron must travel the same distance; thus the slight curvature of the input screen.

There are several occasions of information transfer within the image intensifier: from x-ray beam to input screen, from input screen to photocathode, from photocathode to electron beam, from electron beam to output screen, and from output screen to the human eye (see Fig. 15–20). Thus, an electrical image is transformed to a light image, then back to an electron image, and finally back to a light image.

Electrons from the photocathode are accelerated as they travel toward the output screen. The gain in brightness achieved by the image intensifier is the result of this *electron acceleration (flux gain)* and *image minification. Flux gain* is defined as the ratio of light photons at the output phosphor to the number at the input phosphor. A typical image intensifier has a flux gain of approximately 50.

The image produced on the input screen of the image intensifier is reproduced as a minified image on the output screen. Because the output screen is much smaller than the input screen, the amount of fluorescent light emitted from it per unit area is significantly greater than the quantity of light emitted from the input screen. This process is referred to as *minification gain,* and is equal to the ratio of the diameters of the input and output screens squared.

$$\text{minification gain} = \left(\frac{\text{input screen diameter}}{\text{output screen diameter}} \right)^2$$

For example, the minification gain for an image intensifier with an input screen of 11 in and output screen of 1 in is 121.

$$\text{minification gain} = \left(\frac{11''}{1''} \right)^2$$

$$\text{minification gain} = 121$$

The total *brightness gain* of an image intensifier is the product of flux gain and minification gain.

$$\text{total brightness gain} = \text{flux gain} \times \text{minification gain}$$

For example, the total brightness gain for an image intensifier with a flux gain of 50 and minification gain of 121 is 6050.

$$\text{total brightness gain} = 50(121)$$

$$\text{total brightness gain} = 6050$$

The brightness, resolution, and contrast of an intensified image are greatest in the center of the image. Because the exposure rate is reduced at the periphery of the input screen, and because there is less-than-exact peripheral electron focusing from the photocathode, brightness, resolution, and contrast are reduced (up to 25%) toward the periphery; this characteristic of image intensifiers is called *vignetting.*

Input screen diameters of 5 to 12 inches are available. Although smaller-diameter input screens improve resolution, they do not permit viewing of large patient areas.

A type of image distortion, called *pincushion distortion,* is common to intensified images and is caused by the curvature of the in-

---

Comparisons Between Large and Small Fields of View and Modes

Larger Field of View
- More minification
- Focal point closer to output screen
- Less magnification of perceived image
- Brighter image and less exposure required

Smaller Field of View
- Less minification
- Focal point farther from output screen
- More magnification of perceived image
- Less brightness and more exposure required.

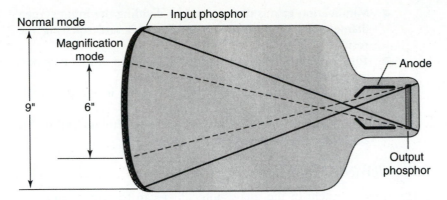

Figure 15–22. As field of view (patient area/normal vs magnification mode) decreases, magnification of the output screen image increases and contrast and resolution improve. Note that the focal point on the 6-inch field, or mode, is further away from the output phosphor; therefore the output image appears magnified. Because less minification takes place in this instance, the image is not as bright. Exposure factors are automatically increased to compensate for the loss in brightness. (Reproduced with permission from RA Fosbinder, CA Kelsey. *Essentials of Radiologic Science.* New York: McGraw-Hill, 2002.

put screen and diminished electron focusing precision at the image periphery.

There will always be some degree of magnification in image intensification (just as in radiography); the degree depends on the distance of the image intensifier from the patient.

Dual- and triple-field image intensifiers are available that permit magnified viewing of fluoroscopic images. Magnified images are reduced in brightness unless the mA is automatically increased when the image intensifier is switched to the magnification mode (Fig. 15–22).

Summary

- The basic parts of the image intensifier are the input screen, photocathode, electrostatic focusing lenses, accelerating anode, and output screen, within a vacuum glass envelope.
- The process of energy conversion within the image intensifier is from electrical to light, to electrical, and back to light.
- Cesium iodide is the preferred phosphor for the image intensifier's input screen; for each x-ray photon it absorbs, it emits approximately 5000 light photons.
- Light photons strike the photocathode, which releases a number of electrons that are directed toward the neck of the image intensifier by the negatively charged focusing lenses.
- The input screen and photocathode are slightly curved so that each electron travels the same distance to the output phosphor, to prevent distortion.
- Electrons are accelerated by the anode's 25 to 30 kV potential, thus making the output image brighter (flux gain).
- The electrons strike the output screen and are converted to a much brighter, smaller (minification gain), and inverted fluorescent image.

- **Minification gain is determined by dividing the input screen diameter by the output screen diameter and squaring the result.**
- **Total brightness gain is equal to the product of flux gain and minification gain.**
- **Diminished resolution and contrast at the image periphery is called vignetting.**
- **Magnification results in some loss of brightness and mA is automatically increased to compensate.**

B. VIEWING SYSTEMS

The optical system of the image intensifier can transfer the output screen image to a mirror viewing apparatus. Mirror viewing offers good resolution, but its disadvantages include limited viewing by one person at a time and limited fluoroscopist movement. In comparison, closed *circuit television fluoroscopy* is far more convenient, allows the fluoroscopist freedom of movement, and permits simultaneous viewing by a number of people.

As body areas of different thicknesses and density are scanned with the image intensifier, image brightness and contrast require adjustment. The *automatic brightness control* functions to maintain constant brightness and contrast of the output screen image, correcting for fluctuations in x-ray beam attenuation with adjustments in kVp and/or mA. There are also brightness and contrast controls on the monitor that the radiographer can regulate. Positioning the image intensifier *closer* to the patient *decreases the SID* and *decreases patient dose.* Patient dose decreases because as the SID is *decreased* the number of x-ray photons at the input phosphor *increases*; as a result, the automatic brightness control *decreases the mA* to compensate for the increase in x-ray photons.

The image on the output screen can be transferred via a television camera to a display *monitor.* The image intensifier output screen image is *coupled* via a *television camera* or a *charge-coupled device* (CCD) for viewing on a display monitor. This is an example of closed circuit TV. The *vidicon* and *Plumbicon* are currently the most frequently used (analog) television cameras. They are about 6 inches long and 1 inch in diameter.

When output screen light strikes the CCD cathode, a proportional number of electrons are released by the cathode and *stored as digital values* (hence, *digital* fluoroscopy) by the CCD or converted directly to conventional television signals. The CCD's rapid discharge time virtually eliminates image lag and is particularly useful in high speed imaging procedures such as cardiac catheterizations. CCD cameras are replacing analog cameras in newer fluoroscopic equipment.

C. RECORDING SYSTEMS

In addition to being transmitted to nearby or remote monitors, the image can be recorded on *videotape* or *cine* film. Television monitors do not offer the very good image resolution obtained from the image intensifier, so film recording systems such as spot film cameras and cine cameras are used to record high resolution images directly from the image intensifier (see Fig. 15–22).

1. Cinefluorography. The fluorescent image on the image intensifier's output screen can be photographed with a 16 mm or 35 mm movie camera. Approximately 85 to 95% of the light from the image intensifier's output screen is transmitted to the cine camera when it is in use. The rest of the light is used for television monitor viewing. During *cinefluorography*, x-ray exposure is on only when the film is in proper position for exposure (ie, no exposure during film movement between frames). *Grid-controlled x-ray tubes* are used to synchronize x-ray exposure with proper film position. Cine "flickering" is noticeable only with frame rates below 30 frames per second.

Film used in cine cameras must be sensitive to the fluorescent light emitted by the output screen. *Panchromatic* film is sensitive to all wavelengths (ie, colors) of visible light; *orthochromatic* film is sensitive to all but red light. These are the two film types most often used in cine cameras. Higher quality images are obtained with 35 mm film (rather than 16 mm) because the film size is four times greater than 16 mm frames; however, for that same reason, 35 mm film requires greater patient exposure and is more expensive. Another reason patient dose is significantly greater in cinefluorography than in routine image-intensified fluoroscopy is because the output screen image must be bright enough to expose the cine film (hence, increased mA). Typical doses measured at the image intensifier input phosphor are approximately 10 microR/frame.

2. Spot Films. Spot films in 70 mm, 90 mm, and 105 mm sizes can be made from the image on the output screen of the image intensifier. This method of recording static (still) images has gained wide acceptance over the cassette-loaded spot filming procedures (taken from the input screen of the image intensifier). The film used for spot-film cameras is less expensive, easier to store, can be exposed in rapid succession, and requires less patient exposure. Typical doses measured at the image intensifier input phosphor are approximately 50 to 100 microR/spot film. Image quality is slightly less than that of

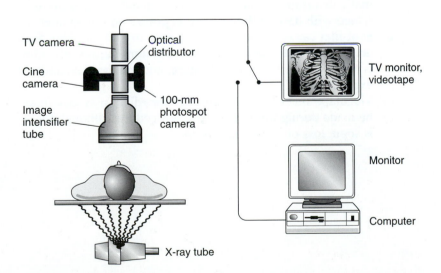

Figure 15–23. Image intensified fluoroscopic unit with several ancillary imaging devices.

cassette-loaded spot films (9 × 9-inch cassette), whose typical doses measured at the image intensifier input phosphor are approximately 300 to 400 microR/film.

3. Video Recording.

Fluoroscopic procedures can also be recorded on videotape. The most significant advantage of videotape recordings is that it allows *immediate* playback of dynamic (motion) images (eliminating film processing). Other advantages include the availability of sound and capabilities of playing at slower speeds and viewing single frames. Its biggest disadvantage is loss of some resolution with regular VHS equipment. High-resolution systems (VHS-S) require the use of high-resolution accessories such as high-resolution cameras and monitors, and thus provide a superior image quality. New video disc recorders are similar to videotape machines, sharing all their advantages and having the added advantage of improved image quality (resolution).

Summary

- **The optical system transfers the output screen image to either mirror viewing or television monitor (via Plumbicon or vidicon camera).**
- **Television monitor viewing is more practical and convenient, though it involves some loss of image quality.**
- **Automatic brightness control automatically adjusts kVp or mA; brightness and contrast controls are also available for adjustment on the TV monitor.**
- **The output screen image is usually coupled to the television camera via a series of complex and precisely adjusted lenses and mirror.**
- **When used in conjunction with cine and spot-film cameras, the largest portion of the output screen light is diverted to the spot film or cine camera; the remainder goes to the television monitor.**
- **Cineradiographic film is either 16 mm or 35 mm panchromatic or orthochromatic film; better quality images are obtained with 35 mm, but patient exposure dose is greater.**
- **Spot-film cameras use 70 mm, 90 mm, or 105 mm film, and are preferable to cassette-loaded spot films because the film is more economical, easier to store, and requires less patient exposure.**
- **Videotape recordings, permitting immediate playback, may be made during the fluoroscopic procedure, although there is some loss of image resolution.**

Chapter Exercises

 Congratulations! *You have completed your review of the entire chapter. If you are able to answer the following group of very comprehensive questions, you should feel confident that you have really mastered this section. You can refer back to the indicated pages to check your answers and/or review the subject matter.*

1. Define and give examples of dedicated x-ray equipment *(p. 405)*.

2. Distinguish between an AC and DC waveform *(p. 406)*.

3. Discuss the following characteristics of AC: amplitude, polarity, wavelength, and frequency *(p. 406)*.

4. Define helix, solenoid, electromagnet *(p. 407)*.

5. Describe the function of the transformer and identify the principle on which it operates *(p. 408)*.

6. Using the transformer law, determine the voltage and current delivered to the x-ray tube *(p. 408)*.

7. Identify four types of x-ray transformer construction *(p. 408)*.

8. Describe three types of transformer energy losses and methods by which they can be reduced *(p. 408)*.

9. Describe the function of the autotransformer and identify the principle on which it operates *(p. 409)*.

10. Using the autotransformer law, determine the voltage sent to the transformer primary *(p. 409)*.

11. Identify the type current required for operation of the transformer and autotransformer *(p. 409)*.

12. Define the function of the generator; motor *(p. 406)*.

13. Describe the rectification process *(p. 410)*.

14. Identify and give examples of the type of material of which solid state diodes are made *(p. 410)*.

15. Differentiate among single-phase, 3-phase/6-pulse, and 3-phase/12-pulse waveforms *(p. 410).*

16. Identify the pulse ripple for single phase, 3-phase/6-pulse, and 3-phase/12-pulse rectification *(p. 410).*

17. Identify the number of autotransformers and transformers required for three-phase rectification *(p. 411).*

18. Identify the two types of transformer winding configurations *(p. 411).*

19. List the three basic component parts of the x-ray tube *(p. 412).*

20. Discuss the importance of the evacuated glass envelope *(p. 412).*

21. Identify the component parts of the cathode assembly *(p. 413).*

22. Describe thermionic emission *(p. 413).*

23. Describe how a double or dual focus tube differs from a single focus tube *(pp. 413, 416).*

24. Explain why x-ray tube inherent filtration increases as the x-ray tube ages *(p. 413).*

25. Identify the current and voltage required by the filament circuit *(p. 413).*

26. Discuss why prolonged periods of rotor activation should be avoided *(p. 413).*

27. Describe the construction of the anode *(p. 413).*

28. Discuss the composition and function of the anode focal track *(p. 413).*

29. Discuss the value of anode rotation (versus stationary anode) *(p. 413).*

30. Identify the device responsible for anode rotation and its two major parts *(p. 413).*

31. Identify two characteristics of tungsten that make it a desirable target material *(p. 413).*

32. Describe the line focus principle; distinguish between actual and effective focal spot *(p. 415).*

33. Describe the anode heel effect; relate it to focal track bevel (anode angle) *(p. 415).*

34. Discuss why heat removal mechanisms are important in x-ray tube construction; give examples of heat reduction features *(p. 416).*

35. Determine heat units for $S\phi$, 3ϕ 6p, and 3ϕ 12p x-ray equipment *(p. 416).*

36. Determine safe exposure limits using tube rating charts and anode cooling curves *(pp. 416–417)*.

37. Discuss at least three causes of x-ray tube failure *(p. 418)*.

38. Identify the three portions of the x-ray circuit *(p. 419)*.

39. Identify the components of the primary, or low voltage, circuit *(pp. 419–422)*.

40. Describe the various types of x-ray timers and identify their accuracy *(pp. 420–421)*.

41. Describe the two types of AECs and identify the location of each *(pp. 420–421)*.

42. Discuss the importance of a back up timer *(p. 421)*.

43. Describe the tests used to evaluate Sϕ and 3ϕ timers *(pp. 421, 422)*.

44. Evaluate Sϕ and 3ϕ timer tests for accuracy *(pp. 421, 422)*.

45. Identify the function of the rheostat and transformer in the filament circuit *(p. 423)*.

46. Identify and describe the components of the secondary, or high-voltage, circuit *(p. 423)*.

47. Explain the function of fluoroscopy *(pp. 428, 429)*.

48. Identify the usual location of the fluoroscopy tube *(p. 429)*.

49. Identify the fluoroscopic mA range of operation *(p. 429)*.

50. List at least six fluoroscopic equipment features designed to reduce patient and personnel exposure *(pp. 429, 430)*.

51. Explain why fluoroscopic exposure dose is greater than radiographic dose *(p. 429)*.

52. Identify, with respect to the image intensifier (II), the:

    A. composition of the input screen, and its characteristics and advantages *(p. 431)*

    B. action of the photocathode *(p. 431)*

    C. function of the electrostatic focusing lenses *(p. 431)*

    D. function and potential difference of the accelerating anode *(p. 431)*

    E. function and size of the output screen *(p. 431)*

    F. two components of total brightness gain *(p. 432)*

53. Determine minification gain *(p. 432)*.

54. Define vignetting *(p. 432)*.

55. Discuss advantages and disadvantages of magnified images *(p. 433)*.

56. Identify ways in which the fluoroscopic image can be recorded *(pp. 434–436)*.

57. Identify by what means the image intensifier compensates for varying body thicknesses *(p. 434)*.

58. Define what is meant by coupling *(p. 434)*.

59. Identify the monitor controls regulatable by the radiographer *(p. 434)*.

60. Compare television monitor resolution with that of spot films *(pp. 435, 436)*.

61. Identify the sizes of cine film available and compare each with regard to patient dose and image quality *(p. 435)*.

62. Differentiate between panchromatic and orthochromatic film *(p. 435)*.

63. Identify the spot film sizes available and relate each to patient dose and image quality *(p. 435)*.

64. Describe the advantages and disadvantages of videotape image recording *(p. 436)*.

65. Describe *matrix, pixel,* and *voxel* and how they are related to *resolution. (pp. 425, 426)*

66. Describe how *windowing* (width and level) affects the contrast and density of the diagnostic image. *(p. 427)*

A&U Chapter Review Questions

1. Advantages of digital radiography (computed radiography) include all of the following, *except* the ability to:
   (A) compensate for exposure factors
   (B) make changes in contrast characteristics
   (C) improve geometric detail
   (D) store images in binary form

2. A three-phase timer can be tested for accuracy using a synchronous spinning top. The resulting image looks like a:
   (A) series of dots or dashes, each representative of a radiation pulse
   (B) solid arc, the angle (in degrees) representative of the exposure time
   (C) series of gray tones, from white to black
   (D) multitude of small mesh-like squares of uniform sharpness

3. In the production of Bremsstrahlung radiation, the incident electron:
   (A) ejects an inner shell tungsten electron
   (B) ejects an outer shell tungsten electron
   (C) is deflected with resulting energy loss
   (D) is deflected with resulting energy increase

4. Which of the following will occur as a result of decreasing the anode target angle?
   1. anode heel effect will be less pronounced
   2. effective focal spot size will decrease
   3. greater photon intensity toward the cathode side of the x-ray tube
   (A) 1 only
   (B) 1 and 2 only
   (C) 2 and 3 only
   (D) 1, 2, and 3

5. Which of the following image matrix sizes will result in the best resolution?
   (A) 128 × 128
   (B) 512 × 512
   (C) 1089 × 1089
   (D) 2048 × 2048

6. The device used to ensure reproducible radiographs, regardless of tissue density variations, is the:
   (A) phototimer
   (B) penetrometer
   (C) grid
   (D) rare earth screen

7. Narrower, or smaller, window control settings in digital imaging result in:
   (A) lower contrast
   (B) higher contrast
   (C) higher resolution
   (D) lower resolution

8. If the primary coil of the high voltage transformer is supplied by 220 volts and has 150 turns, and the secondary coil has 75,000 turns; what is the voltage induced in the secondary coil?
   (A) 75 kilovolts
   (B) 110 kilovolts
   (C) 75 volts
   (D) 110 volts

9. Which of the following circuit devices operate(s) on the principle of self induction?
   1. autotransformer
   2. choke coil
   3. high-voltage transformer
   (A) 1 only
   (B) 1 and 2 only
   (C) 2 and 3 only
   (D) 1, 2, and 3

10. Which of the following statements regarding transformer laws is (are) correct?
    1. the voltage and current values are increased with a step-up transformer
    2. the voltage is directly related to the number of turns in the two coils
    3. the product of voltage and current in the two circuits must be equal
    (A) 1 only
    (B) 1 and 2 only
    (C) 2 and 3 only
    (D) 1, 2, and 3

Answers and Explanations

1. (C) All other factors can be changed in the computer to manipulate the image. Geometric detail is only controlled by source-to-image-receptor distance (SID), object-to-image-receptor distance (OID), and focal spot size. These factors are fixed during the x-ray exposure.

2. (B) When a spinning top is used to test the efficiency of a single-phase timer, the result is a *series of dots* or dashes, with each dot or dash representing a pulse of radiation. With full-wave rectified current, and a possible 1/20 dots (pulses) available per second, one should visualize 12 dots at 1/10 second, 24 dots at 1/5 second, 6 dots at 1/20 second, and so on. But because three-phase equipment is almost constant potential, a synchronous spinning top must be used, and the result is a *solid arc* (rather than dots). The number of degrees formed by the arc is measured and equated to a particular exposure time. A multitude of small mesh-like squares describes a screen contact test. An aluminum step-wedge (penetrometer) may be used to demonstrate the effect of kVp on contrast (demonstrating a series of gray tones from white to black), with a greater number of grays demonstrated at higher kVp levels.

3. (C) Bremsstrahlung (or Brems) radiation is one of the two kinds of x-rays produced at the tungsten target of the x-ray tube. The incident high speed electron, passing through a tungsten atom, is attracted by the positively charged nucleus; therefore it is *deflected from its course with a resulting loss of energy*. This energy loss is given up in the form of an x-ray photon.

4. (C) Target angle has a pronounced geometric effect on the effective, or projected, focal spot size. As target angle *decreases* (ie, gets steeper or smaller), the effective (projected) focal spot becomes smaller. This is advantageous because it will improve radiographic detail without creating a heat-loading crisis at the anode (as would be the case if the actual focal spot size were reduced to produce a similar detail improvement). There are disadvantages, however. With a smaller target angle the anode heel effect increases; photons are more noticeably absorbed by the "heel" of the anode, resulting in a smaller percentage of x-ray photons at the anode end of the x-ray beam and a concentration of x-ray photons at the cathode end of the radiograph.

5. (D) A digital image is formed by a *matrix* of *pixels* in rows and columns. A matrix having 512 pixels in each row and column is a 512 × 512 matrix. As in traditional radiography, *spatial resolution* is measured in line pairs per mm (*lp/mm*). As matrix size is increased, there are more and smaller pixels in the matrix, which means improved resolution. Fewer and larger pixels results in a poor resolution "pixelly" image, that is, one that you can actually see the individual pixel boxes (see Fig. 15–16).

6. (A) Radiographic reproducibility is an important concept in producing high-quality diagnostic films. Radiographic results should be consistent and predictable, not only in positioning accuracy but with respect to exposure factors as well. Automatic exposure devices (phototimers and ionization chambers) automatically terminate the x-ray exposure once a predetermined quantity of x-ray has penetrated the patient, thus ensuring consistent results.

7. (B) One advantage of computed radiography is the ability to *manipulate* the image after exposure. Image manipulation post-processing can be used for *noise reduction, contrast modification, image subtraction,* and *windowing.* The digital images' *scale of contrast* can be changed electronically through leveling and windowing of the image. The *level control* determines the *central or mid-density* of the scale of contrast, while the *window control* determines the *total number* of densities/grays (to the right and left of the central or mid-density.

Windowing is a process of changing the contrast and density setting on the finished image. The window *width* controls the *number* of shades of gray in the image, while the window *level* corresponds to the *density* in the *center* of the window (the midpoint of the contrast scale). Narrower windows result in higher (shorter scale) contrast. Pixel values *below* the window range will be displayed as *black,* while pixel values *above* the window range will be displayed as *white.* Pixel values between the two limits are spread over the full scale of gray.

8. (B) The high-voltage, or step-up, transformer functions to *increase voltage* to the necessary kilovoltage. It *decreases the amperage* to milliamperage. The amount of increase or decrease *depends on the transformer ratio,* that is, the number of turns in the primary coil to the number of turns in the secondary coil. The transformer law is as follows:

To Determine Secondary V	**To Determine Secondary I**
$\dfrac{V_S}{V_P} = \dfrac{N_S}{N_P}$	$\dfrac{I_S}{I_P} = \dfrac{V_P}{V_S}$

Substituting known values:

$$\frac{x}{220} = \frac{75{,}000}{150}$$

$$150\,x = 16{,}500{,}000$$

$$x = 110{,}000 \text{ volts } (= 110 \text{ kV})$$

9. (B) The principle of self induction is an example of the second law of electromagnetics (Lenz's Law) which states that an induced current within a conductive coil will oppose the direction of the current that induced it. It is important to note that self induction is a characteristic of alternating current *only.* The fact that alternating current is constantly changing direction accounts for opposing currents set up in the coil. Two x-ray circuit devices operate on the principle of self induction: The *autotransformer* operates on the principle of self-induction and enables the radiographer to vary the kilovoltage. The *choke coil* also operates on the principle of self-induction; it is a type of variable resistor that may be used to regulate filament current. The high-voltage transformer operates on the principle of mutual induction.

10. (C) Transformers are used in the x-ray circuit to change the value of the supplied voltage to a value appropriate for the production of x-rays. Although the incoming voltage supply may be 220 volts, thousands of volts are required for the production of x-rays. A step-up transformer consists of two coils, a primary and a secondary, in close proximity to each other (eg, side by side). As the primary coil is supplied with AC, a magnetic field rises up around the coil and proceeds to "cut" the secondary coil. Because the current supply is AC, the magnetic field is constantly expanding and contracting (rising and falling) and continuously "cutting" the secondary coil. This interaction between magnetic field and conductive coils induces a current in the secondary coil *proportional to* the number of turns in the secondary coil. As the number of turns in the secondary coil increases, so does the induced voltage. However, because we cannot just create energy, only change its form, *the amperage in the second coil is proportionally less.* For example, if the voltage in the secondary coil increased 10 times, the current would decrease by a factor of 10. Therefore, in keeping with the law of conservation of energy, the product of the voltage and current in one coil must equal the product of voltage and current in the second coil.

Standards of Performance and Equipment Evaluation

16

National Council on Radiation Protection and Measurements (NCRP) Report no. 102 serves as a guide to good medical radiation practices by describing the federal regulations on equipment design, performance, and use. Manufacturers of x-ray equipment must follow guidelines that state maximum x-ray output at specific distances, total quantities of filtration, positive beam limitation, and other guidelines. Radiographers must practice safe principles of operation; *preventive maintenance* and *quality control* checks must be performed at specific intervals to ensure continued safe equipment performance.

Radiologic quality control involves monitoring and regulating the variables associated with image production and patient care. Every radiologic facility today must establish quality control (QC) guidelines and conduct quality control programs to provide a consistent standard of care. A properly documented, ongoing, and effective QC program is required by hospital accrediting agencies and state departments of health.

The rationale behind QC is that a radiographic imaging system performing in an erratic and undependable manner results in repeat exposures, thus contributing to unnecessary patient dose and uneconomical use of time, equipment, and supplies. *Radiographic quality control* is an organized and methodical evaluation of imaging components from the x-ray tube to the automatic film processor, with the purpose of decreasing repeat exposures, thereby decreasing patient radiation exposure and increasing cost-effectiveness. The *frequency of testing* ranges from daily processor checks to quarterly, semiannual, and annual equipment performance testing. Processor QC was discussed in Chapter 13.

The position of QC technologist is an increasingly important one requiring advanced knowledge and skills. In recognition of this, the ARRT has implemented an advanced certification examination in QC.

The QC program requires the combined efforts of the radiographer, QC technologist, service engineers, and medical physicist. The radiographer must be alert to any equipment malfunctions or unusual occurrences and report them to the QC technologist without delay. The QC technologist, service engineer, and medical physicist are re-

445

Elements of a Typical Quality Control Program

- Timer accuracy testing
- mA (milliampere) linearity testing
- kVp (kilovoltage peak) accuracy testing
- HVL (half-value layer) testing
- Exposure reproducibility testing
- Focal spot size test
- X-ray beam/light field/Bucky tray alignment evaluation
- Intensified screen cleaning and testing
- Illuminator cleaning and evaluation
- Automatic processor maintenance and control
- X-ray evaluation of lead aprons and gloves

sponsible for equipment testing, correlation of test results, any necessary corrections or modifications, and accurate documentation of their activities.

I. EQUIPMENT CALIBRATION

A. KVp

Kilovoltage accuracy is essential to achieve the desired radiographic contrast. *Calibration* of kVp (kilovoltage peak) was formerly evaluated using a Wisconsin test tool and cassette. The digital kVp test meters used today are more convenient and simple to use. When various kilovoltages are tested in the normal diagnostic range (40 to 150 kVp), the selected kV and actual kV value should not differ by more than 5 kVp or 10% for general diagnostic equipment and by 1 kVp or 5% for mammography equipment (Fig. 16–1).

B. MA

The accuracy of individual mA (milliampere) stations is related to *patient dose* and is essential for production of expected radiographic *density* levels.

An *aluminum step-wedge* (penetrometer) can be used to evaluate each mA station. A series of exposures is made at a particular kVp *using the same mAs (milliampere-seconds) value at each mA station,* with exposure time adjusted to maintain a constant mAs. The resulting step-wedge images should be identical. Performance of this

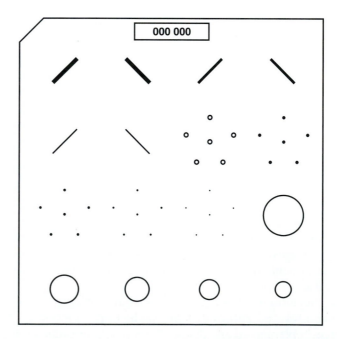

Figure 16–1. A mammographic phantom contains mylar fibers, simulated masses, and specks of simulated calcifications. American College of Radiology accreditation criteria states that a minimum of 10 objects (4 fibers, 3 specks, 3 masses) must be visualized on test films. (Courtesy of Gamex/RMI.)

test on properly calibrated equipment is a good illustration of the *reciprocity law. Linearity* of mA is frequently evaluated using a digital dosimeter (ionization chamber). Exposures are made at a particular mAs with various combinations of mA and time; x-ray output is measured in mR/mAs, and should be accurate to within 10%.

C. TIMER

Timer accuracy is related to patient dose and the production of expected radiographic densities, and should be tested at least on an annual basis. *Spinning top tests,* for determination of timer accuracy, were described in Chapter 15. The use of the digital dosimeter, however, is favored by many as a more simple and accurate measure of timer accuracy. The selected exposure time should be within 5% of the actual exposure time. Similar tests are used to evaluate the accuracy of automatic exposure devices (AECs).

D. REPRODUCIBILITY

This test should be performed annually and evaluates *consistency* of x-ray tube output. A particular group of technical factors is selected and a series of consecutive exposures (at least five) are made. The factors are changed between exposures and then changed back to the original technique. The digital radiation meter should register radiation output that does not vary more than 5%. If a radiographer notices an exposure fluctuation while using a particular group of technical factors, the *reproducibility* test is performed using those factors, but alternately changing to other technical factors between exposures.

E. HALF-VALUE LAYER

Half-value layer (HVL) testing provides *beam-quality* information that is different from that obtained from kVp testing. HVL is defined as the *thickness of any absorber that will reduce x-ray beam intensity to one-half its original value.* HVL is determined by measuring the beam intensity without an absorber, then recording the intensity as successive millimeters of aluminum are added to the radiation field. HVL is influenced by the type of rectification, total filtration, and kVp. An x-ray tube HVL should remain almost constant. If HVL decreases, it is an indication of a decrease in the actual kVp. If the HVL increases, it indicates the deposition of vaporized tungsten deposits on the inner surface of the glass envelope (as a result of tube aging) or an increase in the actual kVp.

F. FOCAL SPOT SIZE

Focal spot size accuracy is related to the degree of *geometric blur,* that is, edge gradient or penumbra. Manufacturer tolerance for new focal spots is a surprisingly large 50%; that is, a 0.3-mm focal spot may actually be 0.45 mm (that can significantly impact magnification radiography). Additionally, the focal spot can increase in size as the x-ray tube ages; hence the importance of *testing* newly arrived focal spots and periodic testing to monitor focal spot changes.

Focal spot size can be measured with a *pinhole camera, slit camera,* or *star-pattern*–type *resolution device.* The pinhole camera is rather difficult to use accurately and requires the use of excessive tube (heat) loading. With a slit camera, two exposures are made; one measures the length of the focal spot, the other measures the width. The star pattern, or similar resolution device, can measure focal spot size as a function of geometric blur and is readily adaptable in a QC program to monitor focal spot changes over a period of time. It is recommended that focal spot size be checked on installation of a new x-ray tube and annually thereafter.

II. RADIOGRAPHIC AND FLUOROSCOPIC ACCESSORIES

A. CASSETTES

The exterior of all cassettes should be checked periodically for damage and signs of wear. Loose latches or hinges, damaged frames, or deteriorated felt or sponge should be repaired or replaced.

B. INTENSIFYING SCREENS

Intensifying screens should first be visually inspected for abrasions, stains, and other signs of wear. Screens need regular periodic cleaning according to the manufacturer recommendations. In general, a nonabrasive, lint-free cloth is used with a special antistatic screen cleaner. Care must be taken not to use excessive solution and to allow the screens to dry thoroughly before use.

Adequate screen care includes periodic *screen–film contact tests* using the special wire-mesh test device. The cassette to be tested is placed on the x-ray table, the wire-mesh device on top of the cassette, and an exposure made of approximately 5 mAs and 40 kVp. The processed film should be viewed at a distance of at least 6 feet. Any blurry areas are indicative of poor screen to film contact and representative of diminished image detail. Cassettes having areas of poor screen and film contact must be repaired or replaced, as poor contact will seriously impair *recorded detail*.

Grid cassettes should be evaluated periodically to identify any damage to the fragile lead strips within. The film loaded grid cassette is slightly exposed, just enough to make the lead strips visible. The processed radiograph is examined for any areas of uneven density or evidence of damaged, misaligned lead strips.

C. ILLUMINATION

One of the most frequently overlooked components of an adequate QC program is radiographic illumination. Radiographic density and contrast can be significantly misrepresented on illuminators providing different degrees of brightness. A radiographic image viewed by the QC technologist in the processor room can look very different on the radiologist's illuminator. A simple light meter, held the same distance from each illuminator (approximately 3 feet), will reveal any differences in illumination.

Illuminator surfaces need to be cleaned periodically to remove buildup of dust and grime. When one bulb in a bank of illuminators requires changing, *all* the bulbs should be changed to guarantee uniform brightness.

D. LEAD APRONS AND GLOVES

Personal fluoroscopic shielding apparel such as lead aprons, gloves, and thyroid shields should be *fluoroscoped annually* to detect any cracks that may have developed in the leaded vinyl.

Proper care is required to help prolong the useful life of lead apparel. If soiled, it can be cleaned with a damp cloth. Lead aprons should not be folded or carelessly dropped to the floor, for that facilitates the development of cracks in the leaded vinyl. Lead aprons and gloves should be hung on appropriate racks when not in use.

Summary

- **The function of QC is to provide consistent high quality radiographs, thus reducing patient dose and increasing cost effectiveness.**
- **QC programs involve evaluation and documentation of all imaging components from the x-ray tube to automatic processor.**
- **Kilovoltage accuracy can be determined using a Wisconsin test cassette or digital meter, and must be accurate to within 5 kVp (plus or minus 10%).**
- **Milliamperage accuracy is determined using an aluminum step wedge or digital dosimeter, and must be accurate to within 10%.**
- **Timer accuracy is evaluated using a manual spinning top (for Sϕ) or synchronous spinning top (for 3ϕ), and must be accurate to within 5%.**
- **Reproducibility refers to tube output consistency, and must not vary more than 5%.**
- **HVL is tested periodically to evaluate x-ray beam quality; HVL should remain almost constant.**
- **Focal spot size is tested by using a pinhole camera, slit camera, or star test pattern on installation and every year thereafter.**
- **Cassette exteriors and interiors should be inspected periodically.**
- **Intensifying screens must be cleaned regularly and screen and film contact tests performed periodically.**
- **Grid cassettes should be tested for damaged lead strips.**
- **Illuminators must be cleaned and checked for uniformity.**
- **Lead gloves and aprons must be fluoroscoped annually to detect any cracks; they should be properly hung when not in use.**

Chapter Exercises

 Congratulations! *You have completed your review of the entire chapter. If you are able to answer the following group of very comprehensive questions, you should feel confident that you have really mastered this section. You are then ready to go on to "Registry-type" questions that follow. For greatest success, do not go to these multiple choice questions without first completing the short answer questions below.*

1. Describe the value of a QC program *(p. 445)*.

2. Identify the method used for kV calibration and the required degree of accuracy *(p. 446)*.

3. Describe the method of evaluating mA calibration using an aluminum step-wedge *(p. 446)*.

4. Describe how mA *linearity* is usually evaluated and identify the required degree of accuracy *(p. 447)*.

5. Describe how Sϕ and 3ϕ timer accuracy is evaluated, identify the appropriate tool for each, give examples of acceptable results, and identify the degree of accuracy required *(p. 447)*.

6. Explain what is meant by *reproducibility* and identify the degree of accuracy required *(p. 447)*.

7. Define *HVL* and list the three factors that influence it *(p. 447)*.

8. Explain how tube aging can result in increased HVL *(p. 447)*.

9. Identify *when* the focal spot size should be checked and the three *devices* that can be used to determine focal spot size *(pp. 447, 448)*.

10. Describe the conditions/faults/injuries that cassettes and intensifying screens should be visually checked for *(p. 448)*.

11. Explain the need for, and proper method of, periodic screen cleaning *(p. 448)*.

12. Describe the purpose and method of screen/film contact testing *(p. 448)*.

13. Explain how to check the condition of a grid *(p. 448)*.

14. Explain the necessity of QC checks on illumination *(p. 448)*.

15. Describe the proper care, storage, and checking of lead apparel *(p. 449)*.

A&U Chapter Review Questions

1. A quality control program includes checks on which of the following radiographic equipment conditions?
   1. reproducibility
   2. linearity
   3. positive beam limitation
   (A) 1 only
   (B) 1 and 2 only
   (C) 1 and 3 only
   (D) 1, 2, and 3

2. Which of the following contribute(s) to inherent filtration?
   1. x-ray tube glass envelope
   2. x-ray tube port window
   3. aluminum between tube housing and collimator
   (A) 1 only
   (B) 1 and 2 only
   (C) 1 and 3 only
   (D) 1, 2, and 3

3. Which of the following is used to evaluate focal spot size?
   (A) spinning top
   (B) wire-mesh
   (C) slit camera
   (D) penetrometer

4. Excessive anode heating can cause vaporized tungsten to be deposited on the port window. This can result in:
   1. decreased tube output
   2. tube failure
   3. electrical sparking
   (A) 1 only
   (B) 2 only
   (C) 1 and 2 only
   (D) 1, 2, and 3

5. Proper care of leaded apparel includes:
   1. periodic check for cracks
   2. careful folding following each use
   3. routine laundering with soap and water
   (A) 1 only
   (B) 1 and 2 only
   (C) 1 and 3 only
   (D) 1, 2, and 3

6. Periodic equipment calibration includes testing of the:
   1. focal spot
   2. mA
   3. kVp
   (A) 1 only
   (B) 1 and 3 only
   (C) 2 and 3 only
   (D) 1, 2, and 3

7. The spinning top test can be used to evaluate:
   1. timer accuracy
   2. rectifier failure
   3. effect of kVp on contrast
   (A) 1 only
   (B) 2 only
   (C) 1 and 2 only
   (D) 1, 2, and 3

8. Which of the following refers to a regular program of evaluation that ensures proper functioning of x-ray equipment, thereby protecting both patients and radiation workers?
   (A) sensitometry
   (B) densitometry
   (C) quality assurance
   (D) modulation transfer function

9. Poor screen–film contact can be caused by which of the following:
   1. damaged cassette frame
   2. foreign body in cassette
   3. warped cassette front
   (A) 1 only
   (B) 2 only
   (C) 1 and 3 only
   (D) 1, 2, and 3

10. Radiographs from a particular three phase, full wave rectified x-ray unit were underexposed, using known correct exposures. A synchronous spinning top test was performed using 100 mA, 1/20 second, and 70 kVp, and a 12-degree arc is observed on the test film. Which of the following is *most* likely the problem?
    (A) the 1/20 second time station is inaccurate
    (B) the 100 mA station is inaccurate
    (C) a rectifier is not functioning
    (D) the processor needs servicing

Answers and Explanations

1. (D) The accuracy of all three are important to ensure adequate patient protection. *Reproducibility* means that repeated exposures at a given technique must provide consistent intensity. *Linearity* means that a given mAs, using different mA stations with appropriate exposure time adjustments, will provide consistent intensity. *Positive beam limitation (PBL)* is automatic collimation and must be accurate to 2% of the source-to-image-receptor distance (SID). Light localized collimators must be available and must be accurate to within 2%.

2. (B) Inherent filtration is that which is "built into" the construction of the x-ray tube. Before exiting the x-ray tube, x-ray photons must pass through the tube's glass envelope and port window; the photons are filtered somewhat as they do so. This inherent filtration is usually the equivalent of 0.5 mm Al. Aluminum filtration *placed* between the x-ray tube housing and collimator is added in order to contribute to the total necessary requirement of 2.5 mm Al equivalent. The collimator itself is considered part of the added filtration (1.0 mm Al equivalent) because of the silver surface of the mirror within. It is important to remember that as aluminum filtration is added to the x-ray tube, the HVL increases.

3. (C) Focal spot size accuracy is directly related to the degree of *geometric blur;* that is, as focal spot size increases, blur increases. Manufacturer tolerance for new focal spots is 50% and focal spot size can increase in size as the x-ray tube ages; hence the importance of *testing* new focal spots and periodic testing to monitor any focal spot changes. Focal spot size can be measured with a *pinhole camera, slit camera,* or *star-pattern*–type *resolution device.* The pinhole camera and slit camera measure the physical size of the focal spot, while the star pattern measures focal spot size as a function of resolution/ geometric blur.

Perfect film–screen contact is essential to recorded detail and is evaluated with a *wire-mesh* test. A *spinning top* test is used to evaluate timer accuracy and rectifier operation. A *penetrometer* (aluminum step-wedge) is used to illustrate the effect of kVp on contrast.

4. (D) Vaporized tungsten may be deposited on the inner surface of the glass envelope at the tube (port) window. It acts as an *additional filter,* thereby *reducing tube output.* The tungsten deposit may also attract electrons from the filament, *creating sparking* and *causing puncture* of the glass envelope and subsequent tube failure.

5. (A) Protective lead aprons and gloves are made of lead impregnated vinyl or leather. They should be checked for cracks radiographically from time to time. Otherwise, minimal care is required. Lead aprons and gloves should always be hung on appropriate hangers. Glove supports permit air to circulate within the glove. Apron hangers provide convenient storage without folding. If lead aprons are folded (or just left in a heap!) cracks are more likely to form. If lead aprons or gloves become soiled, cleaning with a damp cloth and appropriate solution is all that is required. Excessive moisture should be avoided.

6. (D) Radiographic results should be consistent and predictable not only in positioning accuracy but with respect to exposure factors and image sharpness as well. X-ray equipment should be calibrated periodically as part of an ongoing QA program. The quantity (mAs) and quality (kVp) of the primary beam have a big impact on the quality of the finished radiograph. The focal spot should be tested periodically to evaluate its impact on image sharpness.

7. (C) The spinning top test is used to evaluate *timer accuracy* or *rectifier failure*. With single-phase, full-wave rectified equipment (120 pulses per second) for example, 12 dots should be visualized when using the 1/10 second station. A few more or less indicates timer inaccuracy. If the test demonstrated five dots, one might suspect rectifier failure. With three-phase equipment a special synchronous spinning top (or oscilloscope) is used and a solid black arc is obtained rather than dots. The length of this arc is measured and compared with the known correct arc.

8. (C) Sensitometry and densitometry are used in evaluation of the film processor, just one part of a complete quality assurance (QA) program. Modulation transfer function (MTF) is used to express spatial resolution, which is another component of the QA program. A complete QA program includes testing of all components of the imaging system: processors, focal spot, x-ray timers, filters, intensifying screens, beam alignment, and so on.

9. (D) Perfect contact between the intensifying screens and film is essential in order to maintain image sharpness. Any separation between them allows diffusion of fluorescent light and subsequent blurriness and loss of detail. Screen–film contact can be diminished if the cassette frame is damaged and misshapen, if the front is warped, or if there is a foreign body between the screens elevating them.

10. (A) A synchronous spinning top test is used to test timer accuracy or rectifier function in three phase equipment. Because three-phase, full-wave rectified current would expose a 360-degree arc per second, a 1/20 second exposure should expose an 18-degree arc. Anything more or less indicates timer inaccuracy. If exactly one-half the expected arc appears, one should suspect rectifier failure.

Practice Test

This practice test is intended to simulate the actual certification examination. Set aside special time for this test after your preparations for the actual exam are complete. Try to simulate the actual examination environment as much as possible. Choose a quiet place free from distractions and interruptions, gather the necessary materials, and arrange to be uninterrupted for up to 3 hours.

Each of the numbered items or incomplete statements in this section is followed by answers or by completions of the statement. Select the lettered answer or completion that is *best* in each case.

1. Required components of a digital fluoroscopy system include:
        1. computer
        2. video monitor
        3. image manipulation console
    (A) 1 only
    (B) 1 and 2 only
    (C) 2 and 3 only
    (D) 1, 2, and 3

2. Mammographic x-ray tube target materials include:
        1. molybdenum
        2. tungsten
        3. rhodium
    (A) 1 only
    (B) 1 and 2 only
    (C) 2 and 3 only
    (D) 1, 2, and 3

3. A blurry area seen on a radiographic image that also exhibits increased density and loss of contrast is probably caused by:
    (A) large effective focal spot
    (B) poor screen–film contact
    (C) fast screen–film system
    (D) chemical fog

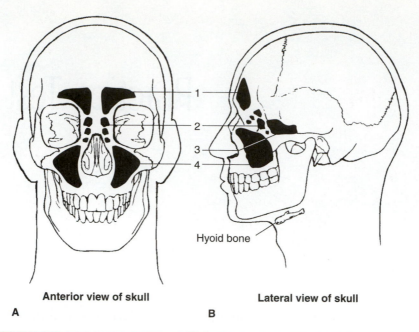

Anterior view of skull

A

Lateral view of skull

B

Hyoid bone

Figure 17–1.

4. Which position will best demonstrate the paranasal sinuses identified by the *number 4* in *Figure 17–1?*
   (A) PA axial (Caldwell)
   (B) parietoacanthial (Waters)
   (C) lateral
   (D) submentovertical

5. Which of the following structures is (are) located in the RLQ?
   1. gallbladder
   2. hepatic flexure
   3. cecum
   (A) 1 only
   (B) 1 and 2 only
   (C) 3 only
   (D) 1, 2, and 3

6. The *best* way to control voluntary motion is:
   (A) immobilization of the part
   (B) careful explanation of the procedure
   (C) short exposure time
   (D) physical restraint

7. Anaphylactic shock manifests early symptoms that include:
   1. dysphagia
   2. itching of palms and soles
   3. constriction of the throat
   (A) 1 only
   (B) 2 only
   (C) 2 and 3 only
   (D) 1, 2, and 3

8. Which of the following are well demonstrated in the lateral position of the cervical spine?
   1. intervertebral foramina
   2. apophyseal joints
   3. intervertebral joints
   (A) 1 only
   (B) 1 and 2 only
   (C) 2 and 3 only
   (D) 1, 2, and 3

9. Radiographers use monitoring devices to record their monthly exposure to radiation. The types of devices suited for this purpose include:
   1. pocket dosimeter
   2. TLD
   3. OSL
   (A) 1 only
   (B) 1 and 2 only
   (C) 2 and 3 only
   (D) 1, 2, and 3

10. Which ethical principle is related to the theory that patients have the right to de-
    cide what will not be done to them?
    (A) autonomy
    (B) beneficence
    (C) fidelity
    (D) veracity

11. *Somatic effects* of radiation refer to effects that are manifested:
    (A) in the descendants of the exposed individual
    (B) during the life of the exposed individual
    (C) in the exposed individual and their descendants
    (D) in the reproductive cells of the exposed individual

12. The junction of the transverse colon and descending colon forms the:
    (A) hepatic flexure
    (B) splenic flexure
    (C) transverse flexure
    (D) sigmoid flexure

13. Which of the following imaging procedures do *not* require the use of ionizing ra-
    diation to produce an image?
    1. ultrasonography
    2. computerized axial tomography
    3. magnetic resonance imaging
    (A) 1 and 2 only
    (B) 1 and 3 only
    (C) 2 and 3 only
    (D) 1, 2, and 3

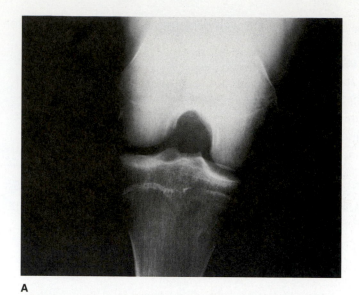

Figure 17–2.

14. A lesion with a stalk, projecting from the intestinal mucosa into the lumen is a/an:
    (A) fistula
    (B) polyp
    (C) diverticulum
    (D) abscess

15. The position seen in Figure 17–2 is used to demonstrate:
    (A) patellofemoral joint
    (B) femorotibial joint
    (C) intercondyloid fossa
    (D) tibiofibular articulation

16. The AP axial projection (Towne's method) of the skull *best* demonstrates the:
    (A) occipital bone
    (B) frontal bone
    (C) facial bones
    (D) sphenoid bone

17. Red blood cells are formed in:
    (A) liver
    (B) spleen
    (C) bone marrow
    (D) small intestine

18. Cervical spine positions performed to demonstrate the foramina closest to the image recorder are:
    (A) RAO and LAO
    (B) RPO and LPO
    (C) AP and lateral
    (D) flexion and extension laterals

19. With the body in the erect position, the diaphragm moves:
    (A) 2 to 4 inches higher than when recumbent
    (B) 2 to 4 inches lower than when recumbent
    (C) 2 to 4 inches superiorly
    (D) very slightly

20. With all other factors constant, as a digital image matrix size increases:
    1. pixel size decreases
    2. resolution increases
    3. pixel size increases
    (A) 1 only
    (B) 2 only
    (C) 1 and 2 only
    (D) 2 and 3 only

21. During a gastrointestinal examination, the AP recumbent projection of a stomach of average shape will usually demonstrate:
    1. barium-filled fundus
    2. double-contrast of distal stomach portions
    3. barium-filled duodenum and pylorus
    (A) 1 only
    (B) 1 and 2 only
    (C) 1 and 3 only
    (D) 1, 2, and 3

22. An ambulatory patient is one who:
    (A) is able to walk
    (B) is unable to walk
    (C) has difficulty breathing
    (D) arrives by ambulance

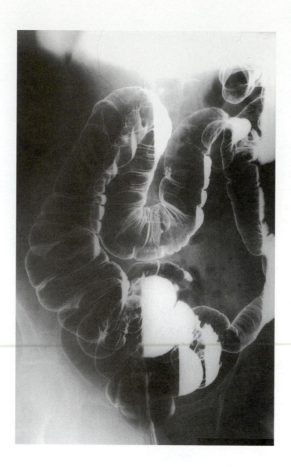

Figure 17–3. From the American College of Radiology Learning File. Courtesy of the American College of Radiology.

23. The radiograph seen in Figure 17–3 was made in which of the following positions?
    (A) AP erect
    (B) PA recumbent
    (C) right lateral decubitus
    (D) left lateral decubitus

24. Moving the image intensifier closer to the patient during fluoroscopy, while the x-ray tube remains stationary:
    1. decreases the SID
    2. decreases patient dose
    3. improves image quality
    (A) 1 only
    (B) 1 and 2 only
    (C) 1 and 3 only
    (D) 1, 2, and 3

25. The exposure factors used for a particular nongrid radiograph were 400 mA, 0.02 sec, and 90 kVp. Another radiograph using an 8:1 grid is requested. Which of the following groups of factors is *most* appropriate?
    (A) 400 mA, 0.02 sec, 110 kVp
    (B) 200 mA, 0.08 sec, 90 kVp
    (C) 300 mA, 0.05 sec, 100 kVp
    (D) 400 mA, 0.08 sec, 90 kVp

26. Radiographic contrast is a result of:
    1. differential tissue absorption
    2. emulsion characteristics
    3. proper regulation of mAs
    (A) 1 only
    (B) 1 and 2 only
    (C) 1 and 3 only
    (D) 1, 2, and 3

27. Which of the following conditions would require an increase in exposure factors?
    1. congestive heart failure
    2. pleural effusion
    3. emphysema
    (A) 1 only
    (B) 1 and 2 only
    (C) 1 and 3 only
    (D) 1, 2, and 3

28. An autoclave is used for:
    (A) dry heat sterilization
    (B) chemical sterilization
    (C) gas sterilization
    (D) steam sterilization

29. When examining the third through fifth fingers in the lateral position, which side of the forearm should be closest to the image recorder?
    (A) anterior
    (B) posterior
    (C) medial
    (D) lateral

30. The input phosphor of the image intensifier tube functions to convert:
    (A) kinetic energy to light
    (B) x-ray to light
    (C) electrons to light
    (D) fluorescent light to electrons

31. Recorded detail can be improved by decreasing:
    1. the SID
    2. the OID
    3. motion unsharpness
    (A) 1 only
    (B) 3 only
    (C) 2 and 3 only
    (D) 1, 2, and 3

32. Examples of secondary radiation barriers include:
    1. the control booth
    2. lead aprons
    3. x-ray tube housing
    (A) 2 only
    (B) 1 and 2 only
    (C) 2 and 3 only
    (D) 1, 2, and 3

33. Hysterosalpingography may be performed for demonstration of:
    1. uterine tubal patency
    2. mass lesions in the uterine cavity
    3. uterine position
    (A) 1 and 2 only
    (B) 1 and 3 only
    (C) 2 and 3 only
    (D) 1, 2, and 3

34. Diseases whose mode of transmission is through the air include:
    1. tuberculosis
    2. mumps
    3. rubella
    (A) 1 only
    (B) 1 and 2 only
    (C) 1 and 3 only
    (D) 1, 2 and 3

35. Which of the following image matrix sizes will provide the best spatial resolution?
    (A) 256×256
    (B) 512×512
    (C) 1024×1024
    (D) 2048×2048

36. The radiograph seen in *Figure 17–4* was made in which of the following positions?
    (A) AP erect
    (B) PA recumbent
    (C) right lateral decubitus
    (D) dorsal decubitus

37. The maximum base plus fog density consistent with diagnostic imaging is:
    (A) 0.04
    (B) 0.20
    (C) 0.40
    (D) 2.5

38. What do the developer, fixer, and wash all have in common?
    (A) water
    (B) acetic acid
    (C) potassium bromide
    (D) sodium sulfite

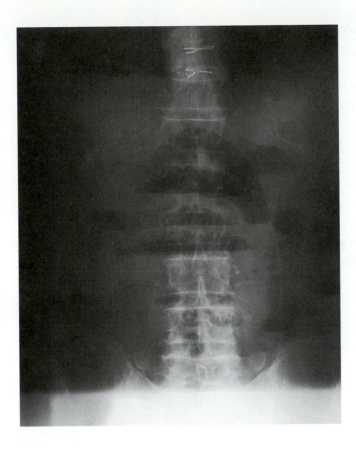

Figure 17–4. Courtesy of The Stamford Hospital, Department of Radiology.

39. With the OML perpendicular to the image recorder and the CR directed 25 degrees cephalad:
   1. the occipital bone is well demonstrated
   2. the dorsum sella is seen within the foramen magnum
   3. the petrous pyramids fill the orbits
   (A) 1 only
   (B) 1 and 2 only
   (C) 2 and 3 only
   (D) 1, 2, and 3

40. A profile view of the glenoid fossa can be obtained with the CR directed perpendicular to the glenoid fossa and the patient rotated:
   (A) 20 degrees affected side down
   (B) 20 degrees affected side up
   (C) 45 degrees affected side down
   (D) 45 degrees affected side up

41. Characteristics of nonstochastic effects of radiation include:
   1. they have predictability
   2. they have a threshold
   3. severity is directly related to dose
   (A) 1 only
   (B) 1 and 2 only
   (C) 2 and 3 only
   (D) 1, 2, and 3

42. Which of the following medical equipment is used to determine blood pressure?
    1. pulse oximeter
    2. stethoscope
    3. sphygmomanometer
(A) 1 and 2 only
(B) 1 and 3 only
(C) 2 and 3 only
(D) 1, 2 and 3

43. How is the thickness of the tomographic section related to the tomographic angle?
(A) The greater the tomographic angle, the thicker the section.
(B) The greater the tomographic angle, the thinner the section.
(C) The lesser the tomographic angle, the thinner the section.
(D) The tomographic angle is unrelated to section thickness.

44. In which of the following locations can the pulse be detected only by the use of a stethoscope?
(A) wrist
(B) apex of the heart
(C) groin
(D) neck

45. Mobile fluoroscopic equipment has all of the following features, *except*:
(A) an image intensifier
(B) a spot-film device
(C) a TV monitor
(D) a TV camera

46. The radiograph seen in *Figure 17–5 B* was made in which position?
(A) AP erect
(B) AP recumbent
(C) PA erect
(D) PA recumbent

47. The production of scattered radiation can be reduced by using the following methods:
    1. compression
    2. beam restriction
    3. a grid
(A) 1 and 2 only
(B) 1 and 3 only
(C) 2 and 3 only
(D) 1, 2, and 3

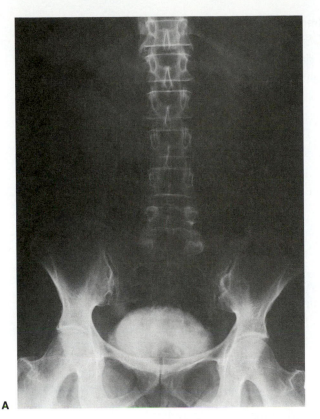 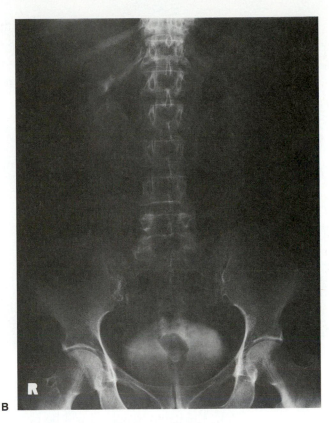

Figure 17–5. **(A)** and **(B)** Courtesy of The Stamford Hospital, Department of Radiology.

48. Chemical substances that inhibit growth of pathogenic microorganisms without necessarily killing them are called:
    1. antiseptics
    2. germicides
    3. disinfectants
    (A) 1 only
    (B) 1 and 2 only
    (C) 2 and 3 only
    (D) 1, 2 and 3

49. During GI radiography, the position of the stomach often varies depending on:
    1. respiratory phase
    2. body habitus
    3. patient position
    (A) 1 and 2 only
    (B) 1 and 3 only
    (C) 2 and 3 only
    (D) 1, 2, and 3

50. To better demonstrate ribs below the diaphragm:
     1. suspend respiration at the end of full exhalation
     2. suspend respiration at the end of deep inhalation
     3. perform the exam in the recumbent position
   (A) 1 only
   (B) 2 only
   (C) 1 and 3 only
   (D) 2 and 3 only

51. Any wall that the useful x-ray beam can be directed toward is called a:
   (A) secondary barrier
   (B) primary barrier
   (C) leakage barrier
   (D) scattered barrier

52. A "blowout fracture" usually occurs in which aspect of the orbital wall?
   (A) superior
   (B) inferior
   (C) medial
   (D) lateral

53. The carpal scaphoid will be best demonstrated in the following projection:
   (A) lateral wrist
   (B) radial flexion
   (C) semipronation oblique
   (D) carpal tunnel

54. Classify the following tissues in order according to *decreasing* radiosensitivity:
     1. liver cells
     2. intestinal crypt cells
     3. muscle cells
   (A) 1, 3, 2
   (B) 2, 3, 1
   (C) 2, 1, 3
   (D) 3, 1, 2

55. Which of the following can contribute to radiographic image distortion?
     1. tube angle
     2. the position of the organ or structure within the body
     3. radiographic positioning of the part
   (A) 1 only
   (B) 1 and 2 only
   (C) 2 and 3 only
   (D) 1, 2, and 3

56. Glenohumeral joint dislocation can be evaluated with which of the following?
     1. inferosuperior axial
     2. transthoracic lateral
     3. scapular Y projection
   (A) 1 only
   (B) 1 and 2 only
   (C) 2 and 3 only
   (D) 1, 2, and 3

57. Characteristics of a 16:1 grid include:
     1. absorbs more primary radiation than an 8:1 grid
     2. has more centering latitude than an 8:1 grid
     3. used with higher kVp exposures than an 8:1 grid
   (A) 1 only
   (B) 1 and 3 only
   (C) 2 and 3 only
   (D) 1, 2, and 3

58. Under which of the following conditions is biologic material most sensitive to radiation exposure?
   (A) anoxic
   (B) hypoxic
   (C) oxygenated
   (D) deoxygenated

59. Which of the following is a fast acting vasodilator used to lower blood pressure and relieve the pain of angina pectoris?
   (A) digitalis
   (B) Dilantin
   (C) nitroglycerin
   (D) cimetidine (Tagamet)

60. The image intensifier's input phosphor is generally composed of:
   (A) cesium iodide
   (B) zinc cadmium sulfide
   (C) gadolinium oxysulfide
   (D) calcium tungstate

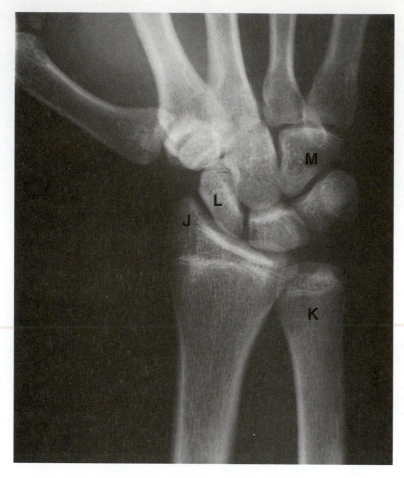

Figure 17–6. Courtesy of Bob Wong.

61. What does the letter *M* represent in *Figure 17–6?*
    (A) scaphoid
    (B) pisiform
    (C) trapezium
    (D) hamate

62. Which of the following formulas would the radiographer use to determine the total number of heat units produced with a given exposure using 3-phase, 12-pulse equipment?
    (A) mA × time × kVp
    (B) mA × time × kVp × 3.0
    (C) mA × time × kVp × 1.35
    (D) mA × time × kVp × 1.41

63. Double-contrast examinations of the stomach or large bowel are performed for better visualization of:
    (A) position of the organ
    (B) size and shape of the organ
    (C) diverticula
    (D) gastric or bowel mucosa

64. If the exposure rate at 3 feet from the fluoroscopic table is 40 mR/hr, what will be the exposure rate for 30 minutes at a distance of 5 feet from the table?
    (A) 7 mR
    (B) 12 mR
    (C) 14 mR
    (D) 24 mR

65. The medical abbreviation meaning *every hour* is:
    (A) tid
    (B) qid
    (C) qh
    (D) pc

66. Symptoms of shock include:
    1. Pallor and weakness
    2. increased pulse rate
    3. fever
    (A) 1 only
    (B) 1 and 2 only
    (C) 1 and 3 only
    (D) 1, 2 and 3

67. Structures found within the mediastinum include all of the following, *except* the:
    (A) esophagus
    (B) thymus
    (C) heart
    (D) terminal bronchiole

68. A student radiographer who is younger than 18 years of age must not receive an annual occupational dose greater than:
    (A) 0.1 rem (1 mSv)
    (B) 0.5 rem (5 mSv)
    (C) 5 rem (50 mSv)
    (D) 10 rem (100 mSv)

69. Proper body mechanics includes a wide base of support. The base of support is the portion of the body:
    (A) in contact with the floor or other horizontal surface
    (B) in the midportion of the pelvis or lower abdomen
    (C) passing through the center of gravity
    (D) none of the above

70. The most important scattering object in both radiography and fluoroscopy is the:
    (A) x-ray table
    (B) x-ray tube
    (C) patient
    (D) film

71. Accurate operation of the AEC device is dependent on:
    1. thickness and density of the object
    2. positioning of the object with respect to the ionization chamber
    3. beam restriction
    (A) 1 only
    (B) 1 and 2 only
    (C) 2 and 3 only
    (D) 1, 2, and 3

72. Major effect(s) of deoxyribonucleic acid (DNA) irradiation include:
    1. malignant disease
    2. chromosome aberration
    3. cell death
    (A) 1 only
    (B) 1 and 2 only
    (C) 2 and 3 only
    (D) 1, 2, and 3

73. Inspiration and expiration projections of the chest may be performed to demonstrate
    1. pneumothorax
    2. foreign body
    3. atelectasis
    (A) 1 only
    (B) 1 and 2 only
    (C) 1 and 3 only
    (D) 1, 2, and 3

74. When a radiographer is obtaining patient history, both subjective and objective data should be obtained. An example of *subjective* data is:
    (A) the patient appears to have a productive cough
    (B) the patient has a blood pressure of 130/95
    (C) the patient states he experiences extreme pain in the upright position
    (D) the patient has a palpable mass in the right upper quadrant of the left breast

75. Compression of breast tissue during mammographic imaging improves image quality because:
    1. geometric blurring is decreased
    2. less scatter radiation is produced
    3. patient motion is reduced
    (A) 1 only
    (B) 3 only
    (C) 2 and 3 only
    (D) 1, 2, and 3

76. All of the following statements regarding breast cancer management are true, *except*:
    (A) early stages of disease respond well to surgical treatment
    (B) BSE helps provide an early diagnosis
    (C) survival improves with early diagnosis
    (D) a baseline mammogram should be made once menopause begins

77. Which of the following medical abbreviations means *three times a day*?
    (A) tid
    (B) qid
    (C) qh
    (D) pc

78. The energy of x-ray photons has an inverse relationship with:
    1. photon wavelength
    2. applied mA
    3. applied kVp
    (A) 1 only
    (B) 1 and 2 only
    (C) 1 and 3 only
    (D) 1, 2, and 3

79. The term "effective dose" refers to:
    (A) whole-body dose
    (B) localized organ dose
    (C) genetic effects
    (D) somatic and genetic effects

80. A patient was positioned for a radiographic projection with the x-ray tube, grid, and image recorder properly aligned but the body part angled. Which of the following will result?
    (A) grid cutoff at the periphery of the image
    (B) grid cutoff along the center of the image
    (C) increased density at the periphery
    (D) image distortion

81. The advantages of 100-mm spot-film cameras over 90-mm spot-film cameras, include:
    1. improved image quality
    2. decreased patient dose
    3. decreased x-ray tube heat load
    (A) 1 only
    (B) 1 and 2 only
    (C) 2 and 3 only
    (D) 1, 2, and 3

82. What does the letter *D* represent in *Figure 17–7*?
    (A) fundus
    (B) pylorus
    (C) body of stomach
    (D) bulb of duodenum

83. What does the letter *H* represent in *Figure 17–7*?
    (A) jejunum
    (B) ascending duodenum
    (C) descending duodenum
    (D) bulb of duodenum

84. What structure occupies the area represented by the letter *G* in *Figure 17–7*?
    (A) gallbladder
    (B) right lobe of the liver
    (C) head of the pancreas
    (D) hepatic flexure of the colon

85. In what position was the radiograph seen in *Figure 17–7* made?
    (A) AP
    (B) LPO
    (C) RAO
    (D) Lateral

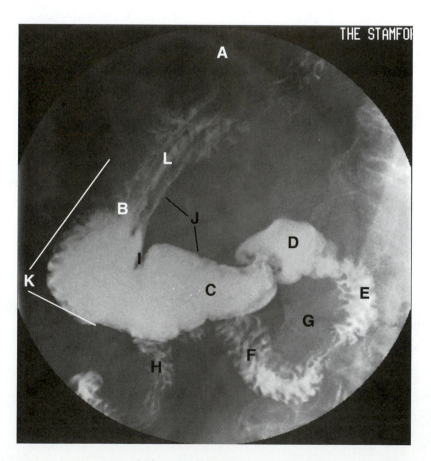

Figure 17–7. Courtesy of The Stamford Hospital, Department of Radiology.

86. The four major arteries supplying the brain include the:
    1. brachiocephalic artery
    2. common carotid arteries
    3. vertebral arteries
    (A) 1 and 2 only
    (B) 1 and 3 only
    (C) 2 and 3 only
    (D) 1, 2, and 3

87. Most laser film must be handled:
    (A) under a Wratten 6B safelight
    (B) in total darkness
    (C) under a GBX safelight
    (D) with high-temperature processors

88. Which of the following will have an effect on radiographic contrast?
    1. beam restriction
    2. grids
    3. focal spot size
    (A) 1 only
    (B) 1 and 2 only
    (C) 2 and 3 only
    (D) 1, 2, and 3

89. Chemical substances that are used to kill pathogenic bacteria are called:
    1. antiseptics
    2. germicides
    3. disinfectants
    (A) 1 only
    (B) 1 and 2 only
    (C) 2 and 3 only
    (D) 1, 2 and 3

90. Which of the following statements regarding human gonadal cells is/are accurate?
    1. The female oogonia reproduce only during fetal life.
    2. The male spermatogonia reproduce continuously.
    3. Both male and female stem cells reproduce only during fetal life.
    (A) 1 only
    (B) 2 only
    (C) 1 and 2 only
    (D) 3 only

91. Lateral deviation of the nasal septum may be *best* demonstrated in the:
    (A) lateral projection
    (B) PA axial (Caldwell method) projection
    (C) parietoacanthial (Water's method) projection
    (D) AP axial (Grashey/Towne method) projection

92. Exposure rate increases with an increase in:
     1. mA
     2. kVp
     3. SID
   (A)   1 only
   (B)   1 and 2 only
   (C)   2 and 3 only
   (D)   1, 2, and 3

93. Characteristic of anemia include:
     1. decreased number of circulating red blood cells
     2. decreased hemoglobin
     3. hematuria
   (A)   1 only
   (B)   1 and 2 only
   (C)   1 and 3 only
   (D)   1, 2, and 3

94. Developer solution is prevented from entering the fixer tank in automatic processing by the:
   (A)   guide shoes
   (B)   rollers
   (C)   switch
   (D)   timer

95. The artifacts seen in *Figure 17–8* are representative of:
   (A)   safelight fog
   (B)   inadequate developer replenishment
   (C)   guide shoe marks
   (D)   hair braids

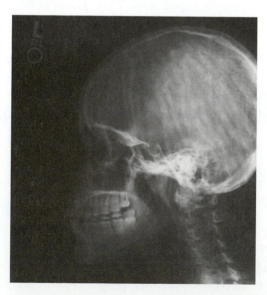

Figure 17–8. Courtesy of The Stamford Hospital, Department of Radiology.

96. Which of these radiation exposure situations is likely to be the most harmful?
    (A) a large dose to a specific area all at once
    (B) a small dose to the whole body over a period of time
    (C) a large dose to the whole body all at one time
    (D) a small dose to a specific area over a period of time

97. Which of the following positions would best demonstrate the proximal tibiofibular articulation?
    (A) AP
    (B) 90 degrees mediolateral
    (C) 45 degrees internal rotation
    (D) 45 degrees external rotation

98. The following bones participate in the formation of the knee joint:
        1. femur
        2. tibia
        3. patella
    (A) 1 and 2 only
    (B) 1 and 3 only
    (C) 2 and 3 only
    (D) 1, 2, and 3

99. Which of the following is a vasopressor and may be used for an anaphylactic reaction or cardiac arrest?
    (A) nitroglycerin
    (B) epinephrine
    (C) hydrocortisone
    (D) digitoxin

100. The absorption of excessive primary radiation by a grid is called:
    (A) grid selectivity
    (B) contrast improvement factor
    (C) grid cutoff
    (D) latitude

101. Hormonal factors that increase the risk of a woman developing breast cancer include:
        1. family history
        2. early menses
        3. nulliparity
    (A) 1 only
    (B) 1 and 2 only
    (C) 2 and 3 only
    (D) 1, 2, and 3

102. In which of the following positions should you place a patient who is experiencing syncope?
    (A) dorsal recumbent with head elevated
    (B) dorsal recumbent with feet elevated
    (C) lateral recumbent
    (D) seated with feet supported

103. What is the usual developer temperature in a 90-second automatic processor?
    (A) 75° to 80°F
    (B) 80° to 85°F
    (C) 85° to 90°F
    (D) 90° to 95°F

104. What is the device that is used to give a predetermined exposure to a film in order to test its response to processing?
    (A) sensitometer
    (B) densitometer
    (C) step-wedge
    (D) spinning top

105. Late or long term effects of radiation exposure are generally represented by which of the following dose-response curves?
    (A) linear threshold
    (B) linear nonthreshold
    (C) nonlinear threshold
    (D) nonlinear nonthreshold

106. Subacromial or subcoracoid dislocation will be best demonstrated in which of the following projections or positions?
    (A) tangential
    (B) AP axial
    (C) transthoracic lateral
    (D) PA oblique scapular Y

107. Typical examples of digital imaging include:
        1. magnetic resonance imaging (MRI)
        2. computed tomography (CT)
        3. pluridirectional tomography
    (A) 1 only
    (B) 1 and 2 only
    (C) 1 and 3 only
    (D) 1, 2, and 3

108. The function of the developer solution chemicals is to:
    (A)   reduce the manifest image to a latent image
    (B)   increase production of silver halide crystals
    (C)   reduce the latent image to a manifest image
    (D)   remove the unexposed crystals from the film

109. Which of the following conditions will demonstrate least x-ray penetrability?
    (A)   fibrosarcoma
    (B)   osteomalacia
    (C)   paralytic ileus
    (D)   ascites

110. In the parieto-orbital projection (Rhese method) of the optic canal, the median sagittal plane and central ray form what angle?
    (A)   90 degrees
    (B)   37 degrees
    (C)   53 degrees
    (D)   45 degrees

111. A radiographic image exhibiting few shades of gray between black and white is said to possess:
    (A)   no contrast
    (B)   high contrast
    (C)   low contrast
    (D)   little contrast

112. A small bottle containing a single dose of medication is termed:
    (A)   an ampule
    (B)   a vial
    (C)   a bolus
    (D)   a carafe

113. A patient suffering from orthopnea would experience the *least* discomfort in which body position?
    (A)   Fowler's
    (B)   Trendelenburg
    (C)   recumbent
    (D)   erect

114. Which of the following is the most proximal structure on the adult ulna?
    (A)   capitulum
    (B)   styloid process
    (C)   coronoid process
    (D)   olecranon process

115. In *Figure 17–9*, the letter *E* represents the:
    (A) trochlea
    (B) capitulum
    (C) lateral epicondyle
    (D) medial epicondyle

116. In *Figure 17–9*, the letter *D* represents the:
    (A) trochlea
    (B) capitulum
    (C) lateral epicondyle
    (D) medial epicondyle

117. What is the intensity of scattered radiation perpendicular to and 1 meter from the patient, compared to the useful beam at the patient's surface?
    (A) 0.01%
    (B) 0.1%
    (C) 1.0%
    (D) 10.0%

118. Proper care of leaded apparel includes:
    1. periodic check for cracks
    2. careful folding following each use
    3. routine laundering with soap and water
    (A) 1 only
    (B) 1 and 2 only
    (C) 2 and 3 only
    (D) 1, 2, and 3

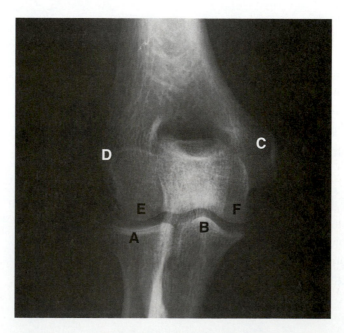

Figure 17–9. Courtesy of The Stamford Hospital, Department of Radiology.

119. A 3-inch object to be radiographed at 36 inches SID lies 4 inches from the image recorder. What will be the image width?
    (A) 2.6 inches
    (B) 3.3 inches
    (C) 26 inches
    (D) 33 inches

120. The sternoclavicular joints are best demonstrated with the patient PA and:
    (A) in a slight oblique, affected side adjacent to image recorder
    (B) in a slight oblique, affected side away from image recorder
    (C) erect, weight bearing
    (D) erect, with and without weights

121. Which of the following criteria is (are) required for accurate visualization of the greater tubercle in profile?
        1. epicondyles parallel to the image receptor
        2. arm in external rotation
        3. humerus in AP position
    (A) 1 only
    (B) 1 and 3 only
    (C) 2 and 3 only
    (D) 1, 2, and 3

122. All of the following positions are likely to be employed for both single-contrast and double-contrast examinations of the large bowel *except*:
    (A) lateral rectum
    (B) AP axial rectosigmoid
    (C) right and left lateral decubitus abdomen
    (D) RAO and LAO abdomen

123. Protective or "reverse" isolation is required in which of the following conditions?
        1. tuberculosis
        2. burns
        3. leukemia
    (A) 1 only
    (B) 1 and 2 only
    (C) 2 and 3 only
    (D) 1, 2 and 3

124. The amount and type of filtration most likely to be used in mammography is:
    (A) 0.5 mm Mo
    (B) 1.5 mm Al
    (C) 1.5 mm Cu
    (D) 2.0 mm Cu

125. A radiograph made with a parallel grid demonstrates decreased density on its lateral edges. This is most likely caused by:
    (A) static electrical discharge
    (B) the grid off-centered
    (C) improper tube angle
    (D) decreased SID

126. When reviewing patient blood chemistry levels, what is considered the normal creatinine range?
    (A) 0.6 to 1.5 mg /100 mL
    (B) 4.5 to 6 mg /100 mL
    (C) 8 to 25 mg/100 mL
    (D) up to 50 mg/100 mL

127. The manubrial notch, a bony landmark used in radiography of the sternoclavicular joints, is located at the same level as the:
    (A) vertebra prominens
    (B) first thoracic vertebra
    (C) third thoracic vertebra
    (D) ninth thoracic vertebra

128. Which of the following functions to protect the x-ray tube and patient from overexposure in the event the automatic exposure control fails to terminate an exposure?
    (A) circuit breaker
    (B) backup timer
    (C) rheostat
    (D) fuse

129. Which of the following would be appropriate cassette front material?
        1. tungsten
        2. magnesium
        3. Bakelite
    (A) 1 only
    (B) 1 and 2 only
    (C) 2 and 3 only
    (D) 1, 2, and 3

130. What type of precaution prevents the spread of infectious agents in aerosol form?
    (A) strict isolation
    (B) protective isolation
    (C) airborne precautions
    (D) contact precautions

131. In the lateral projection of the foot, the:
        1. plantar surface should be perpendicular to the image receptor
        2. metatarsals are superimposed
        3. talofibular joint should be visualized
    (A) 1 only
    (B) 1 and 2 only
    (C) 2 and 3 only
    (D) 1, 2, and 3

132. The artifact seen in *Figure 17–10* is representative of:
    (A) processor artifact
    (B) exposure artifact
    (C) handling artifact
    (D) chemical fog

133. Factor(s) that can be used to regulate radiographic density is (are):
    1. milliamperage
    2. exposure time
    3. kilovoltage
    (A) 1 only
    (B) 2 only
    (C) 1 and 2 only
    (D) 1, 2, and 3

134. Screen contact is evaluated by which of the following tests?
    (A) spinning top test
    (B) wire-mesh test
    (C) penetrometer test
    (D) star-pattern test

135. The mechanical device used to correct an ineffectual cardiac rhythm is a(n):
    (A) defibrillator
    (B) cardiac monitor
    (C) crash cart
    (D) resuscitation bag

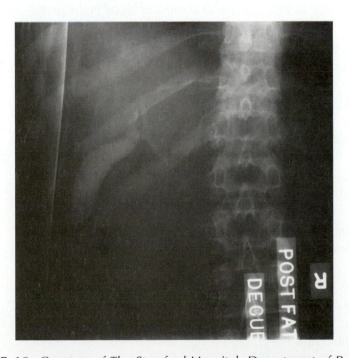

Figure 17–10. Courtesy of The Stamford Hospital, Department of Radiology.

136. The term that refers to parts closer to the source or beginning is:
    (A)   cephalad
    (B)   caudad
    (C)   proximal
    (D)   medial

137. The photoelectric process is an interaction between an x-ray photon and:
    (A)   an inner shell electron
    (B)   an outer shell electron
    (C)   a nucleus
    (D)   another photon

138. As a result of the anode heel effect, the intensity of the x-ray beam is greatest along the:
    (A)   path of the central ray
    (B)   anode end of the beam
    (C)   cathode end of the beam
    (D)   transverse axis of the image receptor

139. The total brightness gain of an image intensifier is a result of:
       1. flux gain
       2. minification gain
       3. focusing gain
    (A)   1 only
    (B)   2 only
    (C)   1 and 2 only
    (D)   1 and 3 only

140. The type of shock associated with pooling of blood in the peripheral vessels is classified as:
    (A)   neurogenic
    (B)   cardiogenic
    (C)   hypovolemic
    (D)   septic

141. What projection of the calcaneus is obtained with the leg extended, plantar surface vertical and perpendicular to the image receptor, and central ray directed 40 degrees caudad?
    (A)   axial plantodorsal projection
    (B)   axial dorsoplantar projection
    (C)   lateral projection
    (D)   weight-bearing lateral

142. The uppermost portion of the iliac crest is approximately at the same level as the:
    (A)   costal margin
    (B)   umbilicus
    (C)   xiphoid tip
    (D)   fourth lumbar vertebra

143. Which of the following factors impacts radiation damage to biologic tissue?
    1. radiation quality
    2. absorbed dose
    3. size of irradiated area
    (A)   1 only
    (B)   2 only
    (C)   1 and 2 only
    (D)   1, 2, and 3

144. What apparatus is needed for the construction of a characteristic curve?
    1. penetrometer
    2. densitometer
    3. electrolytic canister
    (A)   1 and 2 only
    (B)   1 and 3 only
    (C)   2 and 3 only
    (D)   1, 2, and 3

145. The type(s) of radiation produced at the tungsten target is/are:
    1. photoelectric
    2. characteristic
    3. Bremsstrahlung
    (A)   1 only
    (B)   1 and 2 only
    (C)   2 and 3 only
    (D)   1, 2, and 3

146. To produce just a perceptible increase in radiographic density, the radiographer must increase the:
    (A)   mAs by 30%
    (B)   mAs by 15%
    (C)   kVp by 15%
    (D)   kVp by 30%

147. Characteristics of the typical diagnostic x-ray tube and its construction include:
    1. The target material should have a high atomic number and melting point.
    2. The useful beam emerges from the port window.
    3. The cathode assembly receives both low and high voltages.
    (A)   1 only
    (B)   2 only
    (C)   1 and 2 only
    (D)   1, 2, and 3

148. During chest radiography, the act of inspiration:
    1. elevates the diaphragm
    2. raises the ribs
    3. depresses the abdominal viscera
    (A)   1 only
    (B)   1 and 2 only
    (C)   2 and 3 only
    (D)   1, 2, and 3

149. The stomach of an asthenic patient is *most* likely to be located:
    (A) high, transverse, and lateral
    (B) low, transverse, and lateral
    (C) high, vertical, and toward the midline
    (D) low, vertical, and toward the midline

150. The microswitch for controlling the amount of replenishment used in an automatic processor is located at the:
    (A) receiving bin
    (B) crossover roller
    (C) entrance roller
    (D) replenishment pump

151. An increase in kVp will have which of the following effects?
    1. More scatter radiation will be produced.
    2. The exposure rate will increase.
    3. Radiographic contrast will increase.
    (A) 1 only
    (B) 1 and 2 only
    (C) 2 and 3 only
    (D) 1, 2, and 3

152. The position illustrated in *Figure 17–11* can be improved by:
    (A) bringing the chin up more
    (B) bringing the chin down more
    (C) angling the CR caudad
    (D) opening the mouth more

153. The medical term referring to *nosebleed* is:
    (A) vertigo
    (B) urticaria
    (C) epistaxis
    (D) aura

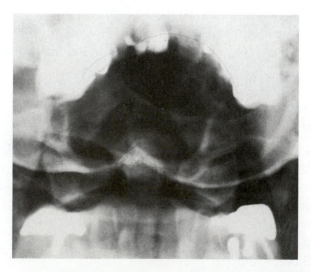

Figure 17–11. Courtesy of The Stamford Hospital, Department of Radiology.

CHAPTER 17. PRACTICE TEST   **485**

154. The most significant risk factor for breast cancer is:
    (A) age
    (B) gender
    (C) family history
    (D) personal history

155. Which of the following are methods used to help reduce colonic spasms during fluoroscopic filling of the large bowel?
    1. placing the patient in the Trendelenburg position
    2. administration of glucagon prior to the exam
    3. temporarily slowing or stopping the flow of barium
    (A) 1 and 2 only
    (B) 1 and 3 only
    (C) 2 and 3 only
    (D) 1, 2, and 3

156. Radiation exposure to the developing fetus can cause:
    1. mental retardation
    2. growth retardation
    3. organ damage
    (A) 1 only
    (B) 1 and 2 only
    (C) 2 and 3 only
    (D) 1, 2, and 3

157. A patient is usually required to drink barium sulfate suspension in order to demonstrate which of the following structure(s)?
    1. pylorus
    2. sigmoid
    3. duodenum
    (A) 1 and 2 only
    (B) 1 and 3 only
    (C) 2 and 3 only
    (D) 3 only

158. OID is related to recorded detail in which of the following ways?
    (A) Radiographic detail is directly related to OID.
    (B) Radiographic detail is inversely related to OID.
    (C) As OID increases, so does radiographic detail.
    (D) OID is unrelated to radiographic detail.

159. Which of the following devices is used to overcome severe variation in patient anatomy or tissue density, providing more uniform radiographic density?
    (A) compensating filter
    (B) grid
    (C) collimator
    (D) intensifying screen

160. A radiograph demonstrating a long scale of contrast is most likely to be produced by increasing:
(A) photon energy
(B) screen speed
(C) mAs
(D) SID

161. Glossitis refers to inflammation of the:
(A) epiglottis
(B) ossicles
(C) tongue
(D) salivary glands

162. Of the following groups of technical factors, which will produce the greatest radiographic density?
(A) 10 mAs, 74 kVp, 44 inches SID
(B) 10 mAs, 74 kVp, 36 inches SID
(C) 5 mAs, 85 kVp, 48 inches SID
(D) 5 mAs, 85 kVp, 40 inches SID

163. What is the best way to reduce magnification distortion?
(A) Use a small focal spot.
(B) Increase the SID.
(C) Decrease the OID.
(D) Use a slow screen–film combination.

164. *Somatic effects* of radiation refer to effects that are manifested:
(A) in the descendants of the exposed individual
(B) during the life of the exposed individual
(C) in the exposed individual and their descendants
(D) in the reproductive cells of the exposed individual

165. The energy of ionizing electromagnetic radiations is measured in:
(A) mA
(B) mAs
(C) keV
(D) kVp

166. The total number of x-ray photons produced at the target is contingent on:
    1. tube current
    2. target material
    3. square of the kilovoltage
(A) 1 only
(B) 1 and 2 only
(C) 2 and 3 only
(D) 1, 2, and 3

167. With the patient positioned as for a parietoacanthial projection (Water's method), and the central ray directed through the patient's open mouth, which of the following sinus groups is demonstrated through the open mouth?
    (A) frontal
    (B) ethmoid
    (C) maxillary
    (D) sphenoid

168. Involuntary patient motion can be caused by:
    1. posttraumatic shock
    2. medication
    3. room temperature
    (A) 1 only
    (B) 1 and 2 only
    (C) 1 and 3 only
    (D) 1, 2, and 3

169. What is the fetal dose-limit for pregnant radiographers for the entire gestation period?
    (A) 0.1 rem
    (B) 0.5 rem
    (C) 5.0 rem
    (D) 10 rem

170. The following statement(s) is (are) accurate with respect to the differences between the male and female bony pelvis:
    1. The female pelvic outlet is wider.
    2. The pubic angle is 90 degrees or less in the male.
    3. The male pelvis is more shallow.
    (A) 1 only
    (B) 1 and 2 only
    (C) 2 and 3 only
    (D) 1, 2, and 3

171. Which of the following is a condition in which an occluded blood vessel stops blood flow to a portion of the lungs?
    (A) pneumothorax
    (B) atelectasis
    (C) pulmonary embolism
    (D) hypoxia

172. An accurately positioned oblique projection of the first through fourth lumbar vertebrae will demonstrate the classic "scotty dog." What bony structure does the scotty dog's "ear" represent?
    (A) superior articular process
    (B) pedicle
    (C) transverse process
    (D) pars interarticularis

173. The voltage ripple associated with a 3-phase, 12-pulse rectified generator is approximately:
     (A) 100%
     (B) 32%
     (C) 13%
     (D) 3%

174. What minimum total amount of filtration (inherent plus added) is required in x-ray equipment operated above 70 kVp?
     (A) 2.5 mm Al equivalent
     (B) 3.5 mm Al equivalent
     (C) 2.5 mm Cu equivalent
     (D) 3.5 mm Cu equivalent

175. The automatic exposure device that is located immediately under the x-ray table is the:
     (A) ionization chamber
     (B) scintillation camera
     (C) photomultiplier
     (D) photocathode

176. Which of the following is demonstrated in a 25-degree LPO position with the central ray entering 1-inch medial to the elevated anterior superior iliac spine (ASIS)?
     (A) left sacroiliac joint
     (B) right sacroiliac joint
     (C) left ilium
     (D) right ilium

177. The image seen in *Figure 17–12* was made using the following type x-ray equipment:
     (A) single phase
     (B) 3-phase, 6-pulse
     (C) 3-phase, 12-pulse
     (D) high frequency

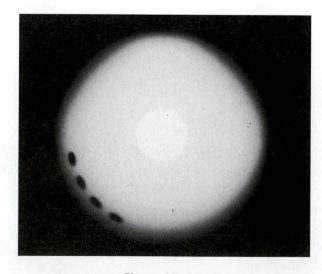

Figure 17–12.

178. If the test image seen in *Figure 17–12* is known to represent correctly operating equipment, then at what exposure time was it made?
     (A)   1/15 second
     (B)   1/30 second
     (C)   1/60 second
     (D)   1/120 second

179. What is meant by the term "controlled area"?
     1. one that is occupied by people trained in radiation safety
     2. one that is occupied by people who wear radiation monitors
     3. one whose occupancy factor is one
     (A)   1 and 2 only
     (B)   2 only
     (C)   1 and 3 only
     (D)   1, 2, and 3

180. With all other factors remaining the same, as grid ratio is increased:
     (A)   recorded detail decreases
     (B)   optical density decreases
     (C)   focal spot distortion decreases
     (D)   the scale of contrast becomes longer

181. All of the following statements concerning respiratory structures are true *except:*
     (A)   the right lung has two lobes
     (B)   the uppermost portion of the lung is the apex
     (C)   each lung is enclosed in pleura
     (D)   the trachea bifurcates into mainstem bronchi

182. To demonstrate the pulmonary apices in the AP position, the:
     (A)   central ray is directed 15 to 20 degrees cephalad
     (B)   central ray is directed 15 to 20 degrees caudad
     (C)   exposure is made on full exhalation
     (D)   patient's shoulders are rolled forward

183. If a particular radiograph allows 10% of the illuminator light to pass through the film, that radiograph has a density of:
     (A)   0.01
     (B)   0.1
     (C)   1.0
     (D)   2.0

184. The sigmoid colon is located in the:
     (A)   left lower quadrant (LLQ)
     (B)   left upper quadrant (LUQ)
     (C)   right lower quadrant (RLQ)
     (D)   right upper quadrant (RUQ)

185. A 15% increase in kVp accompanied by a 50% decrease in mAs will result in a(an):
    (A) shorter scale contrast
    (B) increase in exposure latitude
    (C) increase in radiographic density
    (D) decrease in recorded detail

186. What will result from using double-emulsion film in a cassette having a single intensifying screen?
    (A) double exposure
    (B) decreased density
    (C) increased recorded detail
    (D) greater latitude

187. The AP projection of the scapula requires that the:
        1. patient's arm be abducted at right angles to the body
        2. patient's elbow be flexed with hand supinated
        3. exposure be made during quiet breathing
    (A) 1 and 2 only
    (B) 1 and 3 only
    (C) 3 only
    (D) 1, 2, and 3

188. The effects of radiation to biologic material are dependent on several factors. If a quantity of radiation is delivered to a body over a long period of time, the effect
    (A) will be greater than if it were delivered all at one time
    (B) will be less than if it were delivered all at one time
    (C) has no relation to how it is delivered in time
    (D) is solely dependent on the radiation quality

189. Which of the following types of adult tissues is (are) relatively insensitive to radiation exposure?
        1. muscle tissue
        2. nerve tissue
        3. epithelial tissue
    (A) 1 only
    (B) 1 and 2 only
    (C) 2 and 3 only
    (D) 1, 2, and 3

190. The radiograph seen in *Figure 17–13* illustrates the joint space obscured by the:
    (A) medial femoral condyle
    (B) lateral femoral condyle
    (C) intercondylar eminences
    (D) tibial tuberosity

191. Underexposure of a radiograph can be caused by all of the following *except:*
    (A) insufficient mA
    (B) insufficient exposure time
    (C) insufficient kVp
    (D) insufficient SID

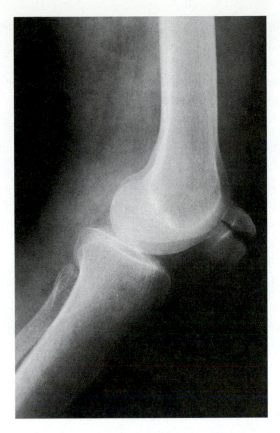

Figure 17–13.

192. When a patient is received in the radiology department with a urinary Foley cath-
     eter bag, it is important to:
     (A) place the drainage bag above the level of the bladder
     (B) place the drainage bag at the same level as the bladder
     (C) place the drainage bag below the level of the bladder
     (D) clamp the Foley catheter

193. A slit camera is used to measure:
         1. focal spot size
         2. intensifying screen resolution
         3. source-to-image-receptor distance (SID) resolution
     (A) 1 only
     (B) 1 and 2 only
     (C) 1 and 3 only
     (D) 1, 2, and 3

194. The *most* effective method of sterilization is:
     (A) dry heat
     (B) moist heat
     (C) pasteurization
     (D) freezing

195. What should be the radiographer's main objective regarding personal radiation safety?
    (A)   not to exceed his or her dose limit
    (B)   to keep personal exposure as far below the dose limit as possible
    (C)   to avoid whole-body exposure
    (D)   to wear protective apparel when "holding" patients for exposures

196. Which of the following factor(s) is(are) important in determining thickness of protective barriers?
    1. distance between x-ray source and barrier
    2. occupancy factor time
    3. workload (mA-min/wk)
    (A)   1 only
    (B)   1 and 2 only
    (C)   2 and 3 only
    (D)   1, 2, and 3

197. Conditions contributing to poor radiographic film archival quality include:
    1. fixer retention
    2. insufficient developer replenishment
    3. poor storage conditions
    (A)   1 only
    (B)   3 only
    (C)   2 and 3 only
    (D)   1, 2, and 3

198. An exposure was made at 38 inches SID using 300 mA, 0.03 second exposure, and 80 kVp with a 400 film–screen combination and an 8:1 grid. It is desired to repeat the radiograph and, in order to improve recorded detail, use 42 inches SID and 200 film–screen combination. With all other factors remaining constant, what exposure time will be required to maintain the original radiographic density?
    (A)   0.03 second
    (B)   0.07 second
    (C)   0.14 second
    (D)   0.36 second

199. The dose of radiation that will cause a noticeable skin reaction is referred to as the:
    (A)   LET
    (B)   SSD
    (C)   SED
    (D)   SID

200. You encounter a person who is apparently unconscious. Although his airway is open, there is no rise and fall of his chest and you can hear no breath sounds. You should:
    (A)   begin mouth-to-mouth rescue breathing, giving two full breaths
    (B)   proceed with the Heimlich maneuver
    (C)   begin external chest compressions at a rate of 80 to 100 per minute
    (D)   begin external chest compressions at a rate of at least 100 per minute

Answers and Explanations

1. (D) The advantages of digital fluoroscopy (DF) over conventional fluoroscopy (CF) include higher speed acquisition and availability of post processing for image/contrast enhancement. Although DF appears fundamentally the same as CF, DF has special requirements: a computer, two video monitors, and an operating console that is far more complex than the conventional console. A computer is located between the TV camera and the TV monitor, and serves to convert the analog image to a digital image. The operating console has many special function keys for patient data entry, for data acquisition, image display, and image post processing manipulation. Two video monitors are required—the second monitor is for display of the subtracted image. *(Bushong, pp. 372, 380)*

2. (D) Target materials for mammographic x-ray tubes are often quite different than materials used for conventional radiography. *Tungsten targets* (Z = 74) will produce 17 to 24 keV x-rays, but also produces many x-rays above and below those values. Tungsten mammographic x-ray tubes often use a molybdenum or rhodium filter to reduce the (higher energy) Bremsstrahlung x-rays. *Molybdenum targets* (Z = 42) are widely used and produce about 19 keV K characteristic x-rays with almost no Bremsstrahlung x-rays. *Rhodium targets* (Z = 45) produce slightly higher energy x-ray (because of its higher Z number) of approximately 23 keV. The molybdenum and rhodium target tubes are *filtered* by either molybdenum or rhodium. *(Bushong, pp. 310–312)*

3. (B) Overall blurriness represents loss of recorded detail, and that might be attributed to a large focal spot, fast intensifying screens, or poor screen/film contact. However, when the blurriness is *localized* and *accompanied by increased density and loss of contrast*, the cause can only be poor screen/film contact. When intensifying screens have even a slight buckle or separation, fluorescent light is allowed greater diffusion and it is this diffusion that is responsible for loss of recorded detail. The diffusion of light over a larger area also causes the film emulsion to receive more exposure, resulting in increased density and loss of contrast. *(Carlton & Adler, pp. 332–333)*

4. (B) There are four paired paranasal sinuses: *frontal, ethmoidal, maxillary,* and *sphenoidal* (Fig. 7–1). The left and right *frontal* sinuses are usually asymmetrical and are located behind the glabella and superciliary arches of the frontal bone. The *ethmoidal* sinuses are composed of 6 to 18 thin-walled air cells occupying the bony labyrinth of the ethmoid bone. The *frontal and ethmoidal sinuses* are demonstrated in the posteroanterior (PA) axial projection (Caldwell position). The *maxillary* sinuses (antra of Highmore) are the largest of the paranasal sinuses and are located in the body of the maxillae. They are particularly prone to infection and collections of stagnant mucus. The maxillary sinuses are well demonstrated in the *parietoacanthial* projection (Waters position). The *sphenoidal* sinuses are located in the body of the sphenoid bone and are usually asymmetrical. They are well demonstrated in the *SMV* projection. All sinuses are seen in the *lateral* projection, although the left and right of each group are superimposed. Radiography of the paranasal sinuses must be performed in the erect position so that any *fluid levels* may be demonstrated and to distinguish between fluid and other pathology such as *polyps*.

5. (C) The gallbladder is located on the posterior surface of the liver in the right upper quadrant (RUQ). The hepatic flexure, named because of its close proximity to the liver, is also in the RUQ. The vermiform appendix projects from the first portion of the large bowel, the cecum, located in the right lower quadrant (RLQ). *(Saia, p. 173)*

6. (B) Patients who are able to cooperate are usually able to control *voluntary* motion if they are provided with an adequate explanation of the procedure. Once patients understand what is needed, most will cooperate to the best of their ability (by suspending respiration and holding still for the exposure). Certain body functions and responses, such as heart action, peristalsis, pain, and muscle spasm, cause *involuntary* motion uncontrollable by the patient. The best way to control involuntary and voluntary motion is by always selecting the shortest possible exposure time. Voluntary motion may also be minimized by careful explanation, immobilization, and (as a last resort and only in certain cases) restraint. *(Ballinger & Frank, vol 1, pp. 12–13)*

7. (D) Adverse reactions to the intravascular administration of iodinated contrast are not uncommon, and although the risk of a life-threatening reaction is relatively rare, the radiographer must be alert to recognize and deal effectively should a serious reaction occur. Minor reaction is characterized by flushed appearance and nausea, occasionally vomiting and a few hives. *Early* symptoms of a possible anaphylactic reaction include constriction of the throat, possibly caused by laryngeal edema, dysphagia, (difficulty swallowing) and itching of the palms and soles. The radiographer must maintain the patient's airway, summon the radiologist and call a "code" *(Ehrlich et al, p. 176)*

8. (C) *Intervertebral joints* are well visualized in the *lateral* projection of all the vertebral groups. Cervical articular facets (forming *apophyseal joints*) are 90 degrees to the midsagittal plane and therefore are also well demonstrated in the *lateral* projection. The cervical *intervertebral foramina* lie 45 degrees to the midsagittal plane (and 15 to 20 degrees to a transverse plane) and are therefore demonstrated in the *oblique* position. *(Ballinger & Frank, vol 1, p. 401)*

9. (C) The OSL (optically stimulated luminescence) is rapidly becoming the most commonly used personnel monitor today. Film badges and TLDs (thermoluminescent dosimeters) have been successfully used for years. A pocket dosimeter is used primarily when working with large amounts of radiation and when a daily reading is desired. *(Sherer et al, pp. 222–223)*

10. (A) *Autonomy* is the ethical principle related to the theory that patients have the right to decide what will or will not be done to them. *Beneficence* is related to the idea of doing good and being kind. *Fidelity* is faithfulness and loyalty. *Veracity* is not only telling the truth, but also not practicing deception. *(Adler & Carlton, p. 324)*

11. (B) *Somatic effects* of radiation refer to those effects experienced directly by the exposed individual such as erythema, epilation, and cataracts. *Genetic effects* of radiation exposure are caused by irradiation of the reproductive cells of the exposed individual and transmitted from one generation to the next. *(Sherer et al, pp. 115, 131)*

12. (B) The approximately 5-foot-long large intestine (colon) functions in the formation, transport, and evacuation of feces. The colon (see Fig. 2–60) commences at the terminus of the small intestine; its first portion is the sac-like *cecum* in the RLQ, located inferior to the ileocecal valve. The ascending colon is continuous with the cecum and is located along the right side of the abdominal cavity. It bends medially and anteriorly forming the right colic *(hepatic)* flexure. The colon traverses the abdomen as the transverse colon and bends posteriorly and inferiorly to form the left colic *(splenic)* flexure. The descending colon continues down the left side of the abdominal cavity and at about the level of the pelvic brim, in the *left lower quadrant (LLQ),* the colon moves medially to form the S-shaped *sigmoid* colon. The rectum, approximately 5 inches in length, lies between the sigmoid and anal canal. *(Ballinger & Frank, vol 2, p. 89)*

13. (B) Neither ultrasonography nor magnetic resonance imaging requires the use of ionizing radiation to produce an image. Computerized axial tomography does require ionizing radiation to produce an image. Ultrasonography requires the use of high-frequency sound waves (ultrasound) to produce images of soft-tissue structures and certain blood vessels within the body. Magnetic resonance imaging relies on the use of a very powerful magnet and specially designed coils that send and receive radio wave signals to produce the image. *(Torres, pp. 244, 245)*

14. (B) A *polyp* is a tumor with either a pedicle (pedunculated, or having a stalk) or a braod base (sessile), commonly found in vascular organs projecting inward from its mucosal wall. They are usually removed surgically because, although usually benign, they can become malignant. A *diverticulum* is an *out*pouching from the wall of an organ, such as the colon. A *fistula* is an abnormal tubelike passageway between organs or an organ and the surface. An *abscess* is a localized collection of pus as a result of inflammation. *(Tortora & Grabowski, p. 899)*

15. (C) The knee is formed by the proximal tibia, the patella, and the distal femur, which articulate to form the *femorotibial* and *patellofemoral* joints. The distal posterior femur presents two large *medial and lateral condyles* separated by the deep *intercondyloid fossa.* Two small prominences, the medial and lateral epicondyles, are just superior to the condyles. The femoral and tibial condyles articulate to form the femorotibial joint. Figure 17–2 illustrates positioning for the *intercondyloid fossa* (Camp–Coventry method). The patient is posteroanterior (PA) recumbent with knee flexed so tibia forms 40 degrees angle with the tabletop and with foot rested on support. The CR is directed 40 degrees caudad (perpendicular to the long axis of the tibia) to the knee joint. This results in a *PA axial* (superoinferior) projection of the intercondyloid fossa, tibial plateau, and eminences. It is referred to as the *"tunnel view";* see Figure 7–34B. *(Ballinger & Frank, vol 1, p. 302)*

16. (A) The *anteroposterior (AP) axial* projection (Towne's method) of the skull is used to demonstrate the *occipital* bone. The skull is positioned AP and the CR is directed caudally. This serves to project the anterior structures inferiorly and away from superimposition on the occipital bone. The frontal bone is best demonstrated in the PA projection; the facial bones in the parietoacanthial (Water's) position. The sphenoid bone can be seen in the lateral and basal projections. *(Ballinger & Frank, vol 2, p. 268)*

17. (C) The production of red blood cells is called erythropoiesis. This process takes place in the bone marrow of the extremities of long bone, pelvis, ribs, sternum, and vertebrae. Red blood cells have no nucleus and a life span of about 120 days. After red blood cells die, they are removed from circulation by phagocytic action in the liver and spleen. *(Tortora & Grabowski, p. 642)*

18. (A) The cervical intervertebral foramina lie 45 degrees to the midsagittal plane and 15 to 20 degrees to a transverse plane. When the *posterior oblique* position (LPO, RPO) is used, the cervical intervertebral foramina demonstrated are those *further* from the image receptor. There is therefore some magnification of the foramina. In the *anterior oblique* position (LAO, RAO), the foramina disclosed are those *closer* to the image receptor. *(Ballinger & Frank, vol 1, p. 402)*

19. (B) When the body is erect the diaphragm is more easily moved to a lower position during inspiration. For this reason, chest radiography is performed erect to allow maximum lung expansion. With the body in the supine position, the abdominal viscera exert greater pressure on the diaphragm and it usually assumes a position 2 to 4 inches higher than when erect. *(Ballinger & Frank, vol 1, p. 516)*

20. (C) A digital image is formed by a *matrix* of *pixels* (picture elements) in rows and columns. A matrix having 512 pixels in each row and column is a 512 × 512 matrix. The term *field of view* is used to describe how much of the patient (eg, 150-mm diameter) is included in the matrix. The matrix and/or field of view can be changed without affecting the other, but changes in either will change pixel size. As in traditional radiography, *spatial resolution* is measured in line pairs per mm (*lp/mm*). As matrix size is increased, there are more and smaller pixels in the matrix, therefore improved resolution. Fewer and larger pixels results in a poor resolution "pixelly" image, that is, one that you can actually see the individual pixel boxes. *(Fosbinder & Kelsey, p. 286)*

21. (B) With the body in the anteroposterior (AP) recumbent position, barium flows easily into the fundus of the stomach, displacing it somewhat superiorly. The fundus, then, is filled with barium, while the air that had been in the fundus is displaced into the gastric body, pylorus, and duodenum, illustrating them in double-contrast fashion. Air contrast delineation of these structures allows us to see through the stomach, to retrogastric areas and structures. Barium-filled duodenum and pylorus is best demonstrated in the right anterior oblique (RAO) position. *(Ballinger & Frank, vol 2, pp. 116–117)*

22. (A) An *ambulatory* patient is one who is able to walk with minimal or no assistance. Outpatients are usually ambulatory as well as many inpatients. Patients that are not ambulatory are usually transported to the radiology department via stretcher. *(Adler & Carlton, p. 158)*

23. (D) The pictured radiograph was made in the *left lateral decubitus* position. It is part of a series of radiographs made during an air contrast (double-contrast) barium enema (BE) examination. A *double-contrast examination* of the large bowel is performed in order to see *through* the bowel to is posterior wall and to visualize any *intraluminal* (eg, polypoid) *lesions* or *masses*. Various body positions are used to redistribute the barium and air. To demonstrate the medial and lateral walls of the bowel, decubitus positions are performed. The radiograph presents a left lateral decubitus position, because the *barium has gravitated* to the left side (the side of the splenic flexure). The *air rises* and delineates the medial side of the descending colon and the lateral side of the ascending colon. *(Ballinger & Frank, vol 2, pp. 150–151)*

24. (D) Moving the image intensifier *closer to the patient* during fluoroscopy *reduces* the distance between the x-ray tube (source) and the image intensifier (image receptor), that is, the *SID (source-to-image-receptor distance)*. It follows that the distance between the part being imaged (object) and the image intensifier (image receptor) is also reduced, that is, the *OID (object-to-image-receptor distance)*. The shorter OID produces *less magnification* and *better image quality*. As SID is reduced, the intensity of the x-ray photons at the image intensifier's input phosphor increases, stimulating the automatic brightness control (ABC) to decrease the mA (milliamperage), thereby *decreasing patient dose*. *(Fosbinder & Kelsey, pp. 265–267)*

25. (D) The addition of a grid will help clean up the scatter radiation produced by higher kVp, but it requires an *mAs adjustment*. According to the grid conversion factors listed below, the addition of an 8:1 grid requires that the original mAs be multiplied by a factor of four:

$$\text{No grid} = 1 \times \text{original mAs}$$

$$5:1 \text{ grid} = 2 \times \text{original mAs}$$

$$6:1 \text{ grid} = 3 \times \text{original mAs}$$

$$8:1 \text{ grid} = 4 \times \text{original mAs}$$

$$12:1 \text{ grid} = 5 \times \text{original mAs}$$

$$16:1 \text{ grid} = 6 \times \text{original mAs}$$

The adjustment therefore requires 32 mAs at 90 kVp. *(Saia, p. 328)*

26. (B) Radiographic contrast is defined as the degree of *difference between adjacent densities*. These density differences represent sometimes very subtle differences in absorbing properties of adjacent body tissues. The type of *film emulsion* used also brings with it its own contrast characteristics. Different types of film emulsions have different degrees of contrast "built into" them chemically. The technical factor used to regulate contrast is kilovoltage. Radiographic contrast is unrelated to mAs. *(Bushong, p. 265)*

27. (B) *Emphysema* is abnormal distention of alveoli (or tissue spaces) with air. The presence of abnormal amounts of air makes it necessary to decrease from normal exposure factors. *Congestive heart failure* and *pleural effusion* involve abnormal amounts of fluid in the chest and thus require an *increase* in exposure factors. *(Saia, p. 333)*

28. (D) Sterilization is the complete elimination of all living microorganisms, and can be accomplished by several methods. *Pressurized steam*, in an *autoclave*, is probably the most familiar means of sterilization; the pressure allows higher temperatures to be achieved. *Gas* or *chemical* sterilization is used for items unable to withstand moisture and/or high temperatures. Other methods of sterilization include *dry heat*, ionizing *radiation*, and microwaves (*nonionizing radiation*). *(Torres, pp. 106–107)*

29. (C) When examining the third through fifth fingers in the lateral position, the *medial* side of the forearm (*ulnar side*) should be closest to the image recorder. This *minimizes magnification* by achieving the shortest possible OID (object-to-image-receptor distance). The terms medial and lateral are identified while viewing the part in the anatomic position. *(Ballinger & Frank, vol 1, p. 95)*

30. (B) The image intensifier's input phosphor receives the remnant radiation emerging from the patient and converts it into a fluorescent light image. Very close to the input phosphor, separated by a thin, transparent layer, is the photocathode. The photocathode is made of a photoemissive alloy, usually an antimony and cesium compound. The fluorescent light image strikes the photocathode and is converted to an electron image that is focused by the electrostatic lenses to the output phosphor. *(Fosbinder & Kelsey, p. 260)*

31. (C) *Motion*, voluntary or involuntary, is most detrimental to good recorded detail. Though all other detail factors may be adjusted to maximize detail, if motion occurs during exposure, detail is lost. The most important ways to reduce the possibility of motion are by using the shortest possible exposure time, by careful patient instruction (for suspended respiration), and by adequate immobilization when necessary. Minimizing magnification through the use of *increased* SID (source-to-image-receptor distance) and *decreased* OID (object-to-image-receptor distance) functions to improve recorded detail. *(Selman, pp. 319–320, 327)*

32. (D) *Secondary* radiation includes *leakage and scattered* radiation. The control booth wall is a secondary barrier; therefore the primary beam must never be directed toward it. The x-ray tube housing must reduce leakage radiation to less than 100 mR/h at a distance of 1 m from the housing. Lead aprons, lead gloves, portable x-ray barriers, and the like are also designed to protect the user from exposure to *scattered* radiation, and will not protect from the primary beam. *(Sherer et al, pp. 193–194)*

33. (D) Hysterosalpingography may be performed for demonstration of uterine tubal patency, mass lesions in the uterine cavity, and uterine position. Although hysterosalpingography is often performed to check tubal patency, the uterine anatomy, position, and morphology are exhibited. Additionally, polyps, fibroids, or space occupying lesions within the uterus are well demonstrated. *(Ballinger & Frank, vol 2, p. 218)*

34. (D) *Indirect contact* involves transmission of microorganisms via *airborne* contamination, *fomites*, and *vectors*. Airborne precaution *requires the patient to wear a mask* to avoid the spread of acid-fast bacilli (in bronchial secretions of TB patients) or other pathogens during coughing. If the patient is unable or unwilling to wear a mask, the radiographer must wear one. The radiographer should wear gloves, but a gown is required only if flagrant contamination is likely. Patients infected with *airborne precaution* require a *private, specially ventilated (negative pressure) room*. A private room is indicated for all patients on *droplet precaution*, that is, diseases transmitted via large droplets expelled from the patient while speaking, sneezing, or coughing. The pathogenic droplets can infect others when they come in contact with mouth or nasal mucosa or conjunctiva. *Rubella* ("German measles"), *mumps*, and *influenza* are among the diseases spread by droplet contact; *a private room is required* for the patient, and health care practitioners must use gown and gloves. *(Adler & Carlton, p. 115)*

35. (D) Image storage is located in a *pixel*, which is a two dimensional "picture element" (see Fig. 15–15) measured in the "XY" direction. The third dimension in the matrix of pixels is the *depth* which together with the pixel is referred to as the *voxel* (see Fig. 15–16), measured in the "Z" direction.

A digital image is formed by a *matrix* of *pixels* in rows and columns. The *matrix* is the number of pixels in the XY direction. *The larger the matrix size, the better the image resolution* (see Fig. 15–17).

A matrix having 512 pixels in each row and column is a 512 × 512 matrix. The term *field of view* is used to describe how much of the patient (eg, 150-mm diameter) is included in the matrix. The matrix and/or field of view can be changed without one affecting the other, but changes in either will change pixel size. *As in traditional radiography, spatial resolution is measured in line pairs per mm (lp/mm). As matrix size is increased, there are more and smaller pixels in the matrix, therefore improved resolution.* Fewer and larger pixels results in a poor resolution "pixelly" image, that is, one that you can actually see the individual pixel boxes (see Fig. 15–17).

Typical image matrix sizes used in radiography are:

- Nuclear medicine   128 × 128
- Digital subtraction angiography (DSA) (Fig. 15–23)   512 × 512
- Computed tomography (CT)   512 × 512
- Chest radiography   2048 × 2048

(Fosbinder & Kelsey, p. 284)

36. (A) The anteroposterior (AP) projection provides a general survey of the abdomen, showing the size and shape of the liver, spleen, and kidneys. When performed *erect*, it should demonstrate both hemidiaphragms. The *erect* position is used to demonstrate air/fluid levels (as seen in the radiograph, Fig. 17–4). Air or fluid levels will be clearly demonstrated only if the central ray is directed *parallel* to them. The manner (direction) in which the levels are seen indicates the position in which the image was made. *(Ballinger & Frank, vol 1, p. 38)*

37. (B) Film base material is a durable *polyester* plastic that will not tear, and with a dimensional stability that will be unaffected as it travels through the processor roller system and various chemical temperatures. Film base is not absolutely clear; it has a mea-surable density, referred to as the *base density*. Base density is the sum of environmental exposure received during production and storage as well as the density resulting from the base material tint and dye. An additional, approximately equal, amount of fog density results from processing. It is recommended that the total *base plus fog* density should not exceed 0.2 as measured by a densitometer. *(Bushong, p. 258)*

38. (A) Processing chemicals in concentrated form require dilution. Water is used for dilution of developer and fixer to usable concentration. And, of course, water is used for the wash. Sodium sulfite is common to the developer and fixer (but not wash) as the preservative. Potassium bromide is the restrainer found only in the developer. *(Bushong, p. 195)*

39. (B) The posteroanterior (PA) axial projection (Haas method/nuchofrontal projection) of the skull requires that the central ray be angled 25 degrees cephalad to the perpendicular orbitomeatal line (OML). This position is used to demonstrate the *occipital bone* in kyphotic patients and other patients who are unable to assume the AP recumbent position. If positioned accurately, the *dorsum sella and posterior clinoid processes* will be demonstrated within the foramen magnum. If the central ray is angled excessively, the *posterior aspect of the arch of C1* will appear in the foramen magnum. *(Ballinger & Frank, vol 2, p. 274)*

40. (C) A profile view of the glenoid fossa can be obtained in the anteroposterior (AP) oblique projection (*left posterior oblique [LPO]* or *right posterior oblique [RPO]*, Grashey method). In the anatomic position, the bony glenoid fossa is seen to project *posteriorly and laterally* about 40 degrees. Therefore, if the shoulder is positioned with the body rotated *35 to 45 degrees toward the affected side*, the glenoid fossa will be placed parallel with the CR (*perpendicular to the image recorder*) and a profile view of the fossa is obtained. *(Ballinger & Frank, vol 1, pp. 182, 183)*

41. (D) *Nonstochastic* effects are somatic effects that are predictable, threshold responses; that is, a certain quantity of radiation must be received before the effect will occur, and the greater the dose the more severe the effect. Examples of nonstochastic effects are erythema, blood changes, cataract formation, and epilation. *Stochastic* effects of radiation are nonthreshold and randomly occurring. Examples of stochastic effects include carcinogenesis and genetic effects. The chance of occurrence of stochastic effects is directly related to the radiation dose; that is, as radiation dose increases there is a greater likelihood of genetic alterations or development of cancer. *(Sherer et al, pp. 60–61)*

42. (C) A *pulse oximeter* is used to measure a patient's pulse rate and oxygen saturation level. A *stethoscope and a sphygmomanometer* are used together to measure blood pressure. The first sound heard is the systolic pressure and the normal range is 110 to 140 mm Hg. When no more sound is heard, the diastolic pressure is recorded. The normal diastolic range is 60 to 90 mm Hg. Elevated blood pressure is called *hypertension*. *Hypotension*, low blood pressure, is not of concern unless it is caused by injury or disease; in that case, it results in shock. *(Adler & Carlton, pp. 185–187)*

43. (B) Tomography is a procedure that uses reciprocal motion between x-ray tube and image receptor-to-image structures at a particular level in the body, while blurring everything above and below that level. The thickness of the level visualized can be varied by changing the tube angle (amplitude). In general, the greater the tube angle, the thinner the section imaged. Thinner sections may be used for imaging small or intricate structures. *(Bushong, p. 282)*

44. (B) As blood pulsates through the arteries, a throb can be detected. This throb or *pulse* can be readily palpated where the arteries are superficial (examples are *wrist, groin, neck*, and posterior surface of the *knee*). The apical pulse can be detected with a stethoscope. *(Torres, p. 63)*

45. (B) The *image intensifier* in mobile fluoroscopic ("C" arm) equipment has the same function as the image intensifier in fixed equipment; that is, it brightens the x-ray image so that it can be viewed in a room having normal lighting. The *TV camera* transmits the fluoroscopic image from the output phosphor of the image intensifier to the *TV monitor* for viewing. Mobile fluoroscopes/"C" arms have no *spot-film device*, although they frequently have features such as "last image hold" and capacity for digital recording. *(Fosbinder & Kelsey, pp. 266–268)*

46. (B) Radiograph *A* was performed *posteroanterior (PA)* and radiograph *B* performed *anteroposterior (AP)* as evidenced by the bony pelvis anatomy. The PA projection (image A) shows the ilia more foreshortened, giving the pelvis a "closed" appearance, while in the AP projection the ilia and bladder area appears more "open." There was an appropriate selection of exposure factors, for the required anatomic structures are well visualized: renal shadows, psoas muscle, lumbar transverse processes, and inferior margin of the liver. There is no evidence of the radiographs having been done erect, as the hemidiaphragms are not included and the gas patterns appear without leveling. *(Bontrager, pp. 109, 110)*

47. (A) Limiting the *size of the irradiated field* is a most effective method of decreasing the production of scattered radiation. The smaller the *volume of tissue* irradiated, the smaller the amount of scattered radiation generated; this can be accomplished using *compression* (prone position instead of supine or compression band). Use of a grid does not affect the *production* of scatter radiation, but rather *removes it* once it has been produced *(Fosbinder & Kelsey, p. 289)*

48. (A) Some chemical agents used in health care facilities function to *kill* pathogenic microorganisms, while others function to *inhibit the growth*/spread of pathogenic microorganisms. Germicides and disinfectants are used to kill pathogenic microorganisms and antiseptics (like alcohol) are used to stop their growth/spread. Sterilization is another associated term and refers to killing of all microorganisms and their spores. *(Ballinger & Frank, vol 1, p. 15)*

49. (D) When performing gastrointestinal (GI) radiography, the position of the stomach may vary depending on the respiratory phase, the body habitus, and the patient position. *Inspiration* causes the lungs to fill with air and the diaphragm to descend, thereby pushing the abdominal contents downward. On *expiration*, the diaphragm will rise, allowing the abdominal organs to ascend. Body *habitus* is an important factor in determining the size and shape of the stomach. An asthenic patient may have a long, J-shaped stomach, while the stomach may be transverse on a hypersthenic patient. The body habitus in an important consideration in determining the positioning and placement of the image receptor. The patient *position* can also alter the position of the stomach. If a patient turns from the right anterior oblique (RAO) position, into the anteroposterior (AP) position, the stomach will move into a more horizontal position. Although the cardiac sphincter and the pyloric sphincter are relatively fixed, the fundus is quite mobile, and will vary in position. *(Dowd & Wilson, vol 2, p. 778)*

50. (C) Ribs below the diaphragm are best demonstrated with the diaphragm elevated. This is accomplished by placing the patient in a recumbent position and by taking the exposure at the end of exhalation. Conversely, the ribs above the diaphragm are best demonstrated with the diaphragm depressed. Placing the patient in the erect position and taking the exposure at the end of deep inspiration accomplishes this. *(Ballinger & Frank, vol 1, p. 428)*

51. (B) Protective barriers are classified as either primary or secondary. Primary barriers protect from the useful, or primary, x-ray beam and consist of a certain thickness of lead. They are located anywhere the primary beam can possibly be directed, eg, the walls of the x-ray room. The walls of the x-ray room usually require 1/16 inch (1.5 mm) thickness of lead 7 feet high. Secondary barriers protect from secondary (scattered and leakage) radiation. Secondary barriers are control booths, lead aprons and gloves, the wall of the x-ray room *above 7 feet*. Secondary barriers require much less lead than primary barriers. *(Bushong, p. 512)*

52. (B) The bony walls of the orbit are thin, fragile, and subject to fracture. A direct blow to the eye results in a pressure that can cause fracture. That fracture is usually to the *orbital floor* (inferior aspect of the bony orbit). Because the fracture results from increased pressure within the eye, it is referred to as a "blowout" fracture. *(Ballinger & Frank, vol 2, p. 289)*

53. (C) The carpal scaphoid is somewhat curved, and consequently, is foreshortened radiographically in the posteroanterior (PA) projection. To better separate it from the adjacent lateral carpals, the semipronation oblique is frequently employed. Radial flexion is used to better demonstrate the medial carpals; ulnar flexion can also be used to better demonstrate the carpal scaphoid. The scaphoid is superimposed on adjacent carpals in the lateral projection. The carpal tunnel/canal does not demonstrate the carpal scaphoid. *(Saia, p. 96)*

54. (C) According to Bergonié and Tribondeau, the most radiosensitive cells are undifferentiated, rapidly dividing cells such as lymphocytes, intestinal crypt (of Lieberkühn) cells, and spermatogonia. Liver cells are among the types of cells that are somewhat differentiated and capable of mitosis. These characteristics render them somewhat radiosensitive. Muscle cells, as well as nerve cells and red blood cells, are highly differentiated and do not divide. Therefore, in order of *decreasing* sensitivity (from least to greatest sensitivity), the cells are intestinal crypt cells, liver cells, and muscle cells. *(Bushong, p. 460)*

55. (D) Distortion is caused by *improper alignment of the tube, body part, and image recorder*. Anatomic structures within the body are rarely parallel to the image receptor in a simple recumbent position. In an attempt to overcome this distortion, we position the part to be parallel with the image receptor, or angle the central ray to "open up" the part. Examples of this technique are obliquing the pelvis to place the ilium parallel to the image receptor, or angling the central ray cephalad in order to "open up" the sigmoid colon. *(Shephard, pp. 231–234)*

56. (C) Although the *inferosuperior axial* projection can be used to evaluate the glenohumeral joint, the required abduction of the arm would be contraindicated when evaluating a shoulder for possible dislocation. The *transthoracic* lateral projection is used to evaluate the glenohumeral joint and upper humerus when the patient is unable to abduct the arm (as in dislocation). The *scapular Y* projection is an oblique projection of the shoulder and is used in demonstrating anterior or posterior dislocation. *(Ballinger & Frank, vol 1, pp. 132, 142)*

57. (B) High kilovoltage exposures produce large amounts of scattered radiation, and high ratio grids are often used with high kV techniques in an effort to absorb more of this scattered radiation. However, as more scattered radiation is absorbed, *more primary radiation is absorbed* as well. This accounts for the *increase in mAs required* when changing from 8:1 to 16:1 grid. Additionally, precise *centering and positioning become more critical*; a small degree of inaccuracy is *more likely to cause grid cutoff* in a high ratio grid. *(Selman, pp. 362–363)*

58. (C) Tissue is most sensitive to radiation exposure when in an *oxygenated* condition. Anoxic refers to a general lack of oxygen in tissue; hypoxic refers to tissue with little oxygen. Anoxic and hypoxic tumors are typically avascular (with little or no blood supply) and therefore more radioresistant. *(Sherer et al, p. 109)*

59. (C) Angina pectoris is a spasmodic chest pain frequently caused by oxygen deficiency in the myocardium. The pain often radiates down the left arm and up to the left jaw. Angina pectoris attacks are frequently associated with exertion or emotional stress in individuals with coronary artery disease. Pain may be relieved with a vasodilator such as *nitroglycerin* given sublingually or transdermally. *Digitalis* is used to treat congestive heart failure. *Dilantin* is used in the control of seizure disorders, and *Tagamet* is used to treat duodenal ulcers. *(Torres, p. 257)*

60. (A) The image intensifier's input phosphor receives the remnant beam from the patient and converts it to a fluorescent light image. To maintain resolution, the input phosphor is made of cesium iodide crystals. *Cesium iodide* is much more efficient in this conversion process than was the phosphor previously used, zinc cadmium sulfide. Calcium tungstate was the phosphor used in cassette intensifying screens for many years prior to the development of rare earth phosphors such as gadolinium oxysulfide. *(Bushong, p. 324)*

61. (D) The wrist is composed of eight carpal bones arranged in two rows (proximal and distal). The proximal row consists of (from lateral to medial) the scaphoid, the lunate, the triquetrum, and the pisiform. The distal row (from lateral to medial) includes the trapezium, the trapezoid, the capitate, and the hamate. The radiograph seen in *Figure 17–6* is a *posteroanterior (PA) projection of the wrist*. The letter *L* represents the *scaphoid,* which is the most *lateral* carpal of the *proximal* row. Letter *M* points out the most *medial* carpal of the *distal* row, the *hamate*. The joints of the wrist include the *intercarpal joints* and the *radiocarpal joint.*

62. (D) The number of *heat units* produced during a given exposure with single phase equipment is determined by multiplying mA × sec × kVp. Correction factors are required with three phase equipment. Unless the equipment manufacturer specifies otherwise, three phase, *six* pulse heat units are determined by multiplying mA × sec × kVp × 1.35. Three-phase, *12*-pulse heat units are determined by multiplying mA × sec × kVp × 1.41. *(Selman, p. 220)*

63. (D) Double-contrast studies of the stomach or large intestine involve coating the organ with a thin layer of barium sulfate, and then introducing air. This permits seeing through the organ to structures behind it, and most especially allows visualization of the mucosal lining of the organ. A barium-filled stomach or large bowel demonstrates position, size, and shape of the organ, and any lesion that projects out from its walls, such as diverticula. Polypoid lesions, which project inward from the wall of an organ, may go unnoticed unless a double-contrast exam is performed. *(Ehrlich et al, p. 200)*

64. (A) The intensity or exposure rate of radiation at a given distance from a point source is inversely proportional to the square of the distance. This is the Inverse Square Law of Radiation and is expressed in the following equation:

$$\frac{I_1}{I_2} = \frac{D_2^2}{D_1^2}$$

Substituting known values:

$$\frac{40 \text{ mR/hr}}{x \text{ mR/hr}} = \frac{25}{9}$$

$$25x = 360$$

$$x = 14.4 \text{ mR/hr, therefore 7.2 mR in 30 minutes}$$

(Bushong, p. 47)

65. (C) Every hour is indicated by the abbreviation *qh*. The abbreviation *tid* means three times a day, and *qid* means four times a day. After meals is abbreviated *pc*. *(Torres, p. 192)*

66. (B) A patient going into shock may exhibit *pallor and weakness*, a significant *drop in blood pressure*, and an *increase in pulse rate*. The patient may also experience *apprehension and restlessness*, and have *cool, clammy skin*. A radiographer recognizing these symptoms should call them to the physician's attention immediately. Fever is not associated with shock. *(Ehrlich et al, pp. 176, 177)*

67. (D) The mediastinum is the space between the lungs that contains the heart, great vessels, trachea, esophagus, and thymus gland. It is bound anteriorly by the sternum and posteriorly by the vertebral column, and extends from the upper thorax to the diaphragm. *(Tortora & Grabowski, p. 18)*

68. (A) Because the established dose-limit formula guideline is used for occupationally exposed persons 18 years of age and older, guidelines had to be established in the event a student entered the clinical component of a radiography educational program prior to age 18 years. The guideline states that the occupational dose limit for students *younger than age 18 years* is *0.1 rem* (100 mrem or 1 mSv) in any given year. It is important to note that this 0.1 rem *is included* in the 0.5 rem dose limit allowed the student as a member of the general public. *(Bushong, p. 500)*

69. (A) Proper body mechanics includes a wide base of support. The *base of support* is the part of the body in touch with the floor or other horizontal plane. The *center of gravity* is the midpoint of the pelvis or lower abdomen, depending on body build. The *line of gravity* is the abstract line passing through the center of gravity, vertically. Proper body mechanics can help prevent painful back injuries by making proficient use of the muscles in the arms and legs. *(Ehrlich et al, p. 61)*

70. (C) The patient, as the first scatterer, is the most important scatterer. At 1 m from the patient, the intensity of the scattered beam is 0.1% of the intensity of the primary beam. Compton scatter emerging from the patient is almost as energetic as the primary beam entering the patient. *(Selman, p. 520)*

71. (C) The automatic exposure control (AEC) automatically terminates the exposure when the proper density has been recorded on the image receptor. The important advantage of the phototimer, then, is that it can accurately duplicate radiographic densities. It is very useful in providing accurate comparison in follow-up examinations, and in decreasing patient exposure dose by decreasing the number of "retakes" because of improper exposure. The AEC automatically adjusts the exposure required for body parts having different *thicknesses and densities.* Remember that proper functioning of the AEC depends on accurate positioning by the radiographer. The correct *ionization chamber*(s) must be selected and the anatomic part of interest must completely cover the ionization chamber in order to achieve the desired density. If *collimation* is inadequate, and a field size larger than the part is used, excessive scatter radiation from the body or tabletop can cause the AEC to terminate the exposure prematurely, resulting in an underexposed radiograph. *(Shephard, pp. 289–291)*

72. (D) *Chromosome aberration, cell death, and malignant disease* are major effects of deoxyribonucleic acid (DNA) irradiation, often as a result of abnormal metabolic activity. If the damage happens to the DNA of a germ cell, the radiation response may not occur until one or more generations later. *(Bushong, p. 472)*

73. (D) Phase of respiration is exceedingly important in thoracic radiography; lung expansion and the position of the diaphragm strongly influence the appearance of the finished radiograph. Inspiration and expiration radiographs of the chest are taken to demonstrate air in the pleural cavity *(pneumothorax),* to demonstrate *atelectasis* (partial or complete collapse of one or more pulmonary lobes) degree of *diaphragm excursion,* or to detect the presence of a *foreign body.* The expiration image will require a somewhat greater exposure (6 to 8 kV more) to compensate for the diminished quantity of air in the lungs. *(Ballinger & Frank, vol 1, p. 444)*

74. (C) Obtaining a complete and accurate history from the patient for the radiologist is an important aspect of a radiographer's job. Both subjective and objective data should be collected. *Objective* data include signs and symptoms that can be observed, such as a cough, a lump, or elevated blood pressure. *Subjective* data relates to what the patient feels, and to what extent. A patient may experience pain, but is it mild or severe? Is it localized or general? Does the pain increase or decrease under different circumstances? A radiographer should explore this with a patient and document additional information on the requisition for the radiologist. *(Adler & Carlton, p. 137)*

75. (D) Compression of the breast tissue during mammographic imaging improves the technical quality of the image for several reasons. Compression brings breast structures in *closer contact* with the image recorder, thus reducing geometric blur and improving detail. As the breast tissue is compressed and essentially becomes thinner, less *scatter radiation* is produced. Compression serves as excellent *immobilization* as well. *(Bushong, pp. 295–296)*

76. (D) Breast cancer is very successfully treated the earlier it is diagnosed. Every effort is made to detect breast cancer before it is palpable. Early detection, diagnosis, and treatment (eg: radiation therapy, surgery) has steadily increased breast cancer survival rates. Regular BSE (breast self examination), along with appropriate and regular mammography contribute to early detection and treatment. A baseline mammogram is recommended before the onset of menopause. *(Ballinger & Frank, vol 2, pp. 425, 428)*

77. (A) Three times a day is indicated by the abbreviation *tid.* The abbreviation *qid* means four times a day. Every hour is represented by *qh,* and *pc* means after meals. *(Ehrlich et al, p. 277)*

78. (A) As kVp is increased, more *high energy* photons are produced and the overall energy of the primary beam is increased. *Photon energy is inversely related to wavelength;* that is, as photon energy increases, wavelength decreases. An increase in milliamperage serves to increase the number of photons produced at the target, but is unrelated to their energy. *(Selman, p. 177)*

79. (A) Every radiographic examination involves an *entrance skin exposure* (ESE) which can be determined fairly easily. It also involves a gonadal dose and marrow dose that, if needed, can be calculated by the radiation physicist. If the ESE of a particular exam was calculated to determine the *equivalent whole-body dose*, this is termed *effective dose*. For example, the ESE of a posteroanterior (PA) chest is approximately 70 mrem, while the effective dose is 10 mrem. The effective (whole-body) dose is much less because much of the body is not included in the primary beam. *(Fosbinder & Kelsey, p. 390)*

80. (D) Proper *alignment* of the x-ray tube, body part, and image recorder is required to avoid image *distortion* in the form of *foreshortening* or *elongation*. *Foreshortening* will usually result when the *part* is out of alignment. *Elongation* is often a result of *angulation of the x-ray tube*. Grid lines or *grid cutoff* will occur when the *grid* itself is off center or not in alignment with the x-ray tube. *(Shephard, p. 232)*

81. (A) Spot-film cameras are rapidly replacing conventional spot film cassettes. A significant advantage of spot film cameras is the big reduction in patient dose that their use permits. However, as the film format increases, so does image quality, patient dose, and heat production. Patient dose, however, is still so much smaller than the dose with conventional spot film cassettes that it is almost insignificant when considering the small improvement in image quality afforded by cassette spot films. *(Bushong, p. 413)*

82. (D); 83. (A); 84. (C) The *stomach* is the dilated, sac-like portion of the gastrointestinal (GI) tract. When the stomach (or a portion of it) is empty, its mucosal lining forms soft folds called *rugae* (L). Exteriorly, the stomach presents a *greater curvature* (K) on its lateral surface and a *lesser curvature* (J) on its medial surface. The proximal opening of the stomach is the cardiac sphincter; the pyloric sphincter is located at its distal end. The portion of the stomach around the distal esophagus is called the cardia; that portion superior to the esophageal juncture is the *fundus* (A). The major portion of the stomach is the *body* (B); the distal portion is the *pylorus* (C). The *incisura angularis* (I) is located on the lesser curvature and marks the beginning of the pylorus (C). The distal opening of the pylorus is the pyloric sphincter. The small intestine is composed of the duodenum, jejunum, and ileum. The duodenum is the shortest portion (approximately 12 inches). It begins just beyond the pyloric sphincter and is divided into four portions: the *duodenal cap or bulb* (D), *descending duodenum* (E), transverse duodenum, and *ascending duodenum* (F). These portions form the C-shaped *duodenal loop* that is occupied by the *head of the pancreas* (G). The ascending duodenum terminates at the duodenojejunal flexure which marks the beginning of the nine foot *jejunum* (H). *(Ballinger & Frank, vol 2, p. 86)*

85. (C) Because the fundus is the most *posterior* portion of stomach, it readily fills with barium when the patient is in the *anteroposterior (AP)* or *left posterior oblique (LPO)* position. With the patient *posteroanterior (PA)* or *right anterior oblique (RAO)*, the barium moves to the more distal portions of the stomach. Figure 17–7 illustrates the RAO position. It is in this position that peristalsis is most active and the stomach's emptying mechanism can be evaluated. In order to evaluate the stomach adequately, preliminary patient preparation is required. The upper gastrointestinal (GI) tract must be empty; patients should be questioned about their preparation, and a preliminary "scout film" taken to check abdominal contents. *(Ballinger & Frank, vol 2, pp. 110, 111)*

86. (C) Major branches of the common carotid arteries (internal carotids) function to supply the anterior brain, while the posterior brain is supplied by the vertebral arteries (branches of the subclavian). The brachiocephalic (innominate) artery is unpaired and is one of the three branches of the aortic arch, from which the right common carotid artery is derived. The left common carotid artery comes directly off the aortic arch. *(Tortora & Grabowski, p. 724)*

87. (B) Most laser film is sensitive to both the Wratten 6B and the GBX safelight filters. Laser film will fog if handled under these safelight conditions. Most laser film is loaded into a film magazine in total darkness. Processing temperatures are the same for laser film as for regular x-ray film. *(Shephard, pp. 92, 94)*

88. (B) Radiographic contrast is described as the difference between densities, or scale of grays, in the radiographic image. Because the function of *grids* is to collect scattered radiation, they serve to shorten the scale of contrast. *Beam restrictors* function to limit the x-ray field size, thereby reducing the production of scattered radiation and shorten the scale of contrast. *Focal spot size* is one of the geometric factors affecting recorded detail, and has no effect on the scale of contrast. It is the function of radiographic contrast to make details visible. The sum of subject contrast and film contrast equals radiographic contrast. *(Carlton & Adler, p. 397)*

89. (C) Some chemical agents used in health care facilities function to kill pathogenic microorganisms, while others function to inhibit the growth/spread of pathogenic microorganisms. *Germicides* and *disinfectants* are used to kill pathogenic microorganisms and *antiseptics* (like alcohol) are used to stop their growth/spread. *Sterilization* is another associated term and refers to killing of all microorganisms and their spores. *(Ballinger & Frank, vol 1, p. 15)*

90. (C) The development of male and female reproductive stem cells has important radiation protection implications. Male stem cells reproduce continuously. However, the female stem cells develop only during fetal life; females are born with all the reproductive cells they will ever have. It is exceedingly important to shield children whenever possible, as they have their reproductive futures ahead of them. *(Bushong, pp. 468–469)*

91. (C) The full length of the nasal septum is best demonstrated in the parietoacanthial (Water's method) projection. This is also the single best view for facial bones. The posteroanterior (PA) axial (Caldwell method) projection superimposes petrous structures over the nasal septum, while the lateral projection superimposes and obscures good visualization of the septum. *(Bontrager, p. 395)*

92. (B) The *quantity* of x-ray photons produced at the target is the function of mAs. The *quality* (wavelength, penetration, energy) of x-ray photons produced at the target is the function of kVp. The kVp also has an effect on exposure rate, because an increase in kVp will increase the number of high energy x-ray photons produced at the target. Exposure rate *decreases* with an increase in source-to-image-receptor distance (SID). *(Selman, pp. 332–333)*

93. (B) Anemia is a blood condition characterized by a decreased number of circulating red blood cells and decreased hemoglobin, and has many causes. Adequate hemoglobin is required to provide oxygen to the body. Anemia is treated according to its cause. Hematuria is the term used to describe blood in the urine and is unrelated to anemia. *(Taber's, p. 96)*

94. (B) In manual processing there is a *stop bath* between the developer and fixer solutions that serves to remove developer solution from the film surface and stop the development process. Automatic processing has no stop bath; film travels directly from the developer into the fixer solution. However, the processor's transport *rollers* serve to squeeze the solution from the film surface, and the acid fixer stops the (alkaline) development process. *Guide shoes* are found in turnaround assemblies and help direct the film as it bends from one direction to another. *(Bushong, p. 197)*

95. (D) Before the radiologic examination begins, patients often need to change their clothing and/or remove radiopaque objects (eg, jewelry, dentures, braided hair) from superimposition on structures of interest. *Figure 17–8* illustrates multiple *braids* of hair superimposed on skull structures. While loose hair is radiolucent, hair that is braided becomes more dense and is often imaged radiographically. The ensuing artifacts can interfere with accurate diagnosis. *(Saia, p. 80)*

96. (C) The greatest effect of and response to irradiation is brought about by a *large dose of radiation, to the whole body, delivered all at one time.* Whole-body radiation can depress many body functions. With a fractionated dose, the effects would be less severe because the body would have an opportunity to repair between doses. *(Bushong, p. 442)*

97. (C) In the *anteroposterior (AP)* projection the proximal fibula is at least partially superimposed on the lateral tibial condyle. *Medial rotation* of 45 degrees will "open" the proximal tibiofibular articulation. *Lateral rotation* will obscure the articulation even more. *(Ballinger & Frank, vol 1, p. 297)*

98. (A) The knee (tibiofemoral joint) is the largest joint of the body, formed by the articulation of the femur and tibia. However, it actually consists of three articulations: the patellofemoral joint, the lateral tibiofemoral joint (lateral femoral condyle with tibial plateau), and the medial tibiofemoral joint (medial femoral condyle with tibial plateau). Although the knee is classified as a synovial (diarthrotic) hinge-type joint, the patellofemoral joint is actually a gliding joint, and the medial and lateral tibiofemoral joints are hinge type. *(Tortora & Grabowski, pp. 264–265)*

99. (B) *Epinephrine* (Adrenalin) is the vasopressor used to treat an anaphylactic reaction or cardiac arrest. *Nitroglycerin* is a vasodilator. *Hydrocortisone* is a steroid that may be used to treat bronchial asthma, allergic reactions, and inflammatory reactions. *Digitoxin* is used to treat cardiac fibrillation. *(Ehrlich et al, p. 135)*

100. (C) Grids are used in radiography to *absorb scatter radiation* before it reaches the image receptor, thus improving radiographic contrast. Contrast obtained with a grid compared to contrast without a grid is termed *contrast improvement factor.* The greater the percentage of scatter radiation absorbed compared to absorbed non-scattered radiation, the greater the "selectivity" of the grid. If a grid absorbs an abnormally large amount of primary radiation due to improper centering, tube angle, or tube distance, *grid cutoff* occurs. *(Selman, p. 370)*

101. (C) Changes in *hormone* levels affect changes in the glandular tissue of the breast. For example, breast tissue changes are seen during breast development, during pregnancy and lactation, and during menopause. Women at higher risk of developing breast cancer include those having had early menses (before age 12 years), late menopause (after age 52 years), and nulliparity (no full- or late-term pregnancies). Risks *other* than hormonal include family history and age. *(Ballinger & Frank, vol 2, p. 428)*

102. (B) Syncope, or fainting, is a result of a drop in blood pressure caused by insufficient blood (oxygen) to the brain. The patient should be helped into a dorsal recumbent position with feet elevated in order to facilitate blood flow to the brain. *(Ehrlich et al, pp. 184, 185)*

103. (D) The advantages of automatic processors are quick, efficient operation and consistent results. Quick operation is attained with increased solution temperatures. The usual temperature of a 90-second processor is 90° to 95°F. Excessively high developer temperature can cause chemical fog. *(Bushong, p. 178)*

104. (A) To test a film's response to processing, the film must first be given a predetermined exposure with a *sensitometer.* The film is then processed and the densities are read using a *densitometer.* Any significant variation from the expected densities is further investigated. A step-wedge is used to evaluate the effect of kVp on contrast, and a spinning top test is used to check timer accuracy. *(Cullinan, p. 91)*

105. (B) Late, long-term, effects of radiation can occur in tissues that have survived a previous irradiation months or years earlier. These late effects, such as carcinogenesis and genetic effects, are "all-or-nothing" effects—either the organism develops cancer or it does not. Most late effects *do not have a threshold dose;* that is, *any* dose, however small, theoretically can induce an effect. Increasing that dose will increase the likelihood of the occurrence, but will not affect its severity; these effects are termed *stochastic. Non-stochastic effects* are those that will not occur below a particular threshold dose, and that increase in severity as the dose increases. *(Sherer et al, p. 136)*

106. (D) The "scapular Y" refers to the characteristic Y formed by the body of scapula, acromion, and coracoid processes. The patient is positioned in a posteroanterior (PA) oblique position—an right anterior oblique (RAO) or left anterior oblique (LAO), depending on which is the affected side. The midcoronal plane is adjusted approximately 60 degrees to the image receptor, and the affected arm is left relaxed at the patient's side. The scapular Y position is employed *to demonstrate anterior (subcoracoid) or posterior (subacromial) humeral dislocation.* The humerus is normally superimposed on the scapula in this position; any deviation from this may indicate dislocation. *(Ballinger & Frank, vol 1, p. 180)*

107. (B) Computed tomography (CT) and magnetic resonance imaging (MRI) are two common examples of *digital imaging.* Special equipment is also available for digital radiography (DR), or computed radiography (CR): images produced by either a fan-shaped x-ray beam received by linearly arrayed radiation detectors or a traditional fan shaped x-ray beam received by a light stimulated phosphor plate. Digital images can also be obtained in digital subtraction angiography (DSA), nuclear medicine, and diagnostic sonography. *Analog* images are conventional images that can be converted to digital images with a device called a digitizer. Pluridirectional tomography refers to conventional tomographic equipment that is capable of several x-ray tube movements. *(Bushong, p. 358)*

108. (C) The *latent image* is the invisible image produced within the film emulsion as a result of exposure to radiation. The developer solution converts this to a visible, manifest image. The exposed silver halide grains in the emulsion undergo chemical change in the developer solution and the *un*exposed crystals are removed from the film during the fixing process. *(Shephard, p. 135)*

109. (D) The ability of x-ray photons to penetrate a body part has a great deal to do with the composition of that part (eg: bone versus soft tissue versus air) and the presence of any pathologic condition. Pathologic conditions can alter the normal nature of the anatomic part. Some conditions such as *osteomalacia, fibrosarcoma,* and *paralytic ileus* (obstruction) result in a *decrease* in body tissue density. When body tissue density *decreases,* x-rays will *penetrate the tissues more readily,* that is, more x-ray penetrability. In conditions such as *ascites,* where body tissue density *increases* as a result of accumulation of fluid, x-rays *will not readily penetrate the body tissues,* that is, *less x-ray penetrability. (Carlton & Adler, p. 258)*

110. (B) In the parieto-orbital projection (Rhese method), the patient is prone with the acanthiomeatal line perpendicular to the image receptor. The head rests on the forehead, nose, and chin, and the MSP should form 53 degrees with the image receptor (37 degrees with the central ray). Radiographically, the optic canal should appear in the *lower outer quadrant* of the orbit. Incorrect *rotation* of the MSP results in *lateral or medial displacement,* and incorrect positioning of the *baseline* results in *longitudinal displacement of the optic canal. (Ballinger & Frank, vol 2, p. 290)*

111. (B) Radiographic contrast is described as the difference between densities in the radiographic image. It is the function of radiographic contrast to make details visible. Radiographs exhibiting many shades of gray are said to possess *long-scale,* or *low,* radiographic contrast; that is, there are *many grays,* and there is only a *little difference between the various shades of gray.* Conversely, radiographs exhibiting *few shades of gray* are said to possess *short scale,* or *high,* radiographic contrast. These images have a very *noticeable difference between radiographic densities. (Shephard, p. 194)*

112. (A) Injectable medications are available in two different kinds of containers. An *ampule* usually holds a single dose of medication. A *vial* is a small bottle which holds several doses of the medication. The term *bolus* is used to describe an amount of fluid to be injected. A *carafe* is a narrow-mouthed container not likely to be used for medical purposes. *(Adler & Carlton, p. 279)*

113. (D) *Orthopnea* is a respiratory condition in which the patient has difficulty breathing *(dyspnea)* in any position other than erect. The patient is usually comfortable in the erect, standing, or seated position. The *Trendelenburg* position places the patient's head lower than the rest of the body. *Fowler's position* is a semi-erect position, and the *recumbent* position is lying down. *(Taber's, p. 1179)*

114. (D) The distal humerus articulates with the proximal radius and ulna to form the elbow joint. At its proximal end the ulna presents the *olecranon process,* found at the proximal and posterior end of the *semilunar (trochlear) notch.* The *coronoid process* is seen at the distal and anterior end of the semilunar notch. Specifically, the semilunar notch of the ulna articulates with the trochlea of the distal medial humerus. The *capitulum* is lateral to the trochlea and articulates with the radial head. *(Saia, p. 90)*

115. (B); 116. (C) Figure 17–9 shows an anteroposterior (AP) projection of the elbow joint. The distal humerus articulates with the radius and ulna to form the elbow joint. The lateral aspect of the distal humerus presents a raised, smooth, rounded surface, the *capitulum* (E), that articulates with the superior surface of the *radial head* (A). The *trochlea* (F) is on the medial aspect of the distal humerus and articulates with the semilunar notch of the ulna. Just proximal to the capitulum and trochlea are the *lateral* (D) and *medial* (C) *epicondyles;* the medial is more prominent and palpable. The coronoid fossa is found on the anterior distal humerus and functions to accommodate the *coronoid process* (B) with the elbow in flexion. *(Saia, pp. 92, 97)*

117. (B) The patient is the most important radiation scatterer during both radiography and fluoroscopy. In general, at 1 m from the patient, *the intensity is reduced by a factor of 1000,* to about 0.1 percent of the original intensity. Successive scatterings can render the intensity to unimportant levels. *(Bushong, p. 513)*

118. (A) Protective aprons and gloves are made of lead-impregnated vinyl or leather. They should be checked annually for cracks via radiographic or fluoroscopic means. Otherwise, minimal care is required. Lead aprons and gloves should always be hung on appropriate hangers. Glove supports permit air to circulate within the glove. Apron hangers provide convenient storage without folding. If lead aprons are folded, or left in a careless heap, cracks are more likely to form. If lead aprons or gloves become soiled, cleaning with a damp cloth and appropriate solution is all that is required. Excessive moisture should be avoided. *(Bushong, p. 560)*

119. (B) Magnification is part of every radiographic image. Anatomic parts within the body are at various distances from the image recorder and therefore have various degrees of magnification. The formula used to determine amount of image magnification is:

$$\frac{\text{image size}}{\text{object size}} = \frac{\text{SID}}{\text{SOD}}$$

Substituting known values:

$$\frac{x}{3''} = \frac{36'' \text{ SID}}{32'' \text{ SOD}} \text{ (SOD = SID minus OID)}$$

$$32\,x = 108$$

$$x = 3.37'' \text{ image width}$$

(Bushong, p. 265)

120. (A) Sternoclavicular joints should be performed posteroanterior (PA) whenever possible to keep OID to a minimum. The *oblique* position (approximately 15 degrees) opens the joint *closest* to the image recorder. The erect position may be used, but is not required. Weight-bearing images are not recommended. *(Ballinger & Frank, vol 1, p. 485)*

121. (D) The greater and lesser tubercles are prominences on the proximal humerus separated by the intertubercular (bicipital) groove. The anteroposterior (AP) projection of the humerus/shoulder places the *epicondyles parallel to the image receptor* and the shoulder in *external rotation*, and demonstrates the *greater tubercle in profile*. The lateral projection of the humerus places the shoulder in extreme internal rotation with the epicondyles perpendicular to the image receptor and demonstrates the lesser tubercle in profile. *(Ballinger & Frank, vol 1, p. 160)*

122. (C) Radiographic examinations of the large bowel generally include the anteroposterior (AP) or posteroanterior (PA) axial position to "open" the S-shaped sigmoid colon, the lateral position especially for the rectum, and the left anterior oblique (LAO) and right anterior oblique (RAO) (or left posterior oblique [LPO] and right posterior oblique [RPO]) to "open" the colic flexures. Left and right decubitus positions are usually employed only in double-contrast barium enemas to better demonstrate double contrast of the medial and lateral walls of the ascending and descending colon. *(Ballinger & Frank, vol 2, pp. 133, 138)*

123. (C) Protective or "reverse" isolation is used to keep the susceptible patient from becoming infected. Patients who have suffered burns have lost a very important means of protection, their skin, and therefore have increased susceptibility to bacterial invasion. Patients whose immune systems are depressed have lost the ability to combat infection, and hence are more susceptible to infection. Active tuberculosis requires airborne precautions. *(Gurley & Callaway, p. 153)*

124. (A) Soft-tissue radiography requires the use of long wavelength, low energy x-ray photons. Therefore, very little filtration is used in mammography. Anything more than 1.0 mm Al would remove the useful soft photons and the desired high contrast could not be achieved. Many dedicated mammographic units have molybdenum targets (for the production of soft, low energy radiation) and a small amount of added molybdenum filtration. *(Selman, p. 345)*

125. (D) The lead strips in a parallel grid are *parallel to each other*, and therefore *not to the x-ray beam*. The more divergent the x-ray beam, the more likely there to be cutoff/decreased density at the lateral edges of the radiograph. This problem becomes more pronounced at short source-to-image-receptor distances (SIDs). If there was a centering or tube angle problem, there would more likely be a noticeable density loss on one side *or* the other. *(Shephard, p. 260)*

126. (A) *Creatinine* is a normal alkaline constituent of urine and blood, but increased quantities of creatinine are present in advanced stages of renal disease. Creatinine and *BUN (blood urea nitrogen)* blood chemistry levels should be checked prior to beginning an intravenous pyelogram (IVP). Increased levels may forecast increased possibility of contrast media induced renal effects and poor visualization of the renal collecting systems. Normal creatinine range is 0.6 to 1.5 mg/100 mL. Normal BUN range is 8 to 25 mg/100 mL. *(Ballinger & Frank, vol 2, p. 168)*

127. (C) The *manubrial or jugular notch* is the depression on the superior border of the manubrium and is located at the level of the *third thoracic* vertebra. The *vertebra prominens* is at the level of the *seventh cervical* vertebra. *(Ballinger & Frank, vol 1, p. 56)*

128. (B) An AEC (automatic exposure control) is calibrated to produce radiographic densities as required by the radiologist for interpretation purposes. Once the part being radiographed has been exposed to produce the required optical density, the AEC automatically terminates the exposure. The manual timer should be used as a *backup timer* should the AEC fail to terminate the exposure, thus protecting the patient from overexposure and the x-ray tube from excessive head load. *Circuit breakers* and *fuses* are circuit devices used to protect circuit elements from overload. In case of current surge the circuit will be broken (opened), thus preventing equipment damage. A *rheostat* is a type of variable resistor. *(Shephard, pp. 286–287)*

129. (C) The cassette is used to support the intensifying screens and x-ray film. It should be strong and provide good screen/film contact. The cassette front should be made of a sturdy material with a low atomic number, because attenuation of the remnant beam is undesirable. Bakelite (the forerunner of today's plastics) and magnesium (the lightest structural metal) are the most commonly used materials for cassette fronts. The high atomic number of tungsten makes it inappropriate as a cassette front material. *(Selman, p. 274)*

130. (C) Category-specific isolations have been replaced by *transmission-based precautions: airborne, droplet,* and *contact.* Under these guidelines, some conditions or diseases can fall into more than one category. *Airborne precaution* is employed with patients suspected or known to be infected with the *tubercle bacillus* (TB), *chickenpox* (varicella), and *measles* (rubeola). Airborne precaution *requires that the patient wear a mask* to avoid the spread of bronchial secretions or other pathogens during coughing. If the patient is unable or unwilling to wear a mask, the radiographer must wear one. The radiographer should wear gloves, but a gown is required only if flagrant contamination is likely. Patients under *airborne precaution* require a *private, specially ventilated (negative pressure) room.*

A private room is also indicated for all patients on *droplet precaution,* that is, diseases transmitted via *large droplets* expelled from the patient while speaking, sneezing, or coughing. The pathogenic droplets can infect others when they come in contact with mouth or nasal mucosa or conjunctiva. *Rubella* ("German measles"), *mumps,* and *influenza* are among the diseases spread by droplet contact; *a private room is required* for the patient, and health care practitioners should use *gown and gloves.* Any diseases spread by direct or close *contact,* such as *MRSA* (methicillin-resistant *Staphylococcus aureus*), *conjunctivitis,* and *hepatitis A,* require *contact precaution. Contact precaution* procedures require a *private patient room,* and the use of *gloves, mask, and gown* for anyone coming in direct contact with the infected individual or his environment. *(Adler & Carlton, p. 215)*

131. (B) When the foot is positioned for a lateral projection, the plantar surface should be perpendicular to the image receptor, so as to superimpose the metatarsals. This may be accomplished with the patient lying on either the affected or unaffected side (usually affected), that is, mediolateral or lateromedial. The talofibular articulation is best demonstrated in the medial oblique projection of the ankle. *(Ballinger & Frank, vol 1, p. 251)*

132. (B) Exposure-type artifacts are those that appear on the radiograph as a result of image formation processes. A *foreign body* in the cassette or within the body part will cast its image on the radiographic film. As the exposed film is removed from the cassette, *static electrical discharge* will expose the film in a characteristic manner. These are *exposure-type artifacts.* In *Figure 17–10,* a right lateral decubitus of the gallbladder, the foam pad and sheet has been imaged to produce the exposure artifact. *Processor artifacts* are not placed on the film during image formation, but rather during chemical processing. They can result from mechanical and/or chemical problems. Several kinds of artifacts can be produced by careless *handling* during production of the radiographic image. X-ray film is sensitive and requires proper handling and storage. Tree-like, branching black marks on a radiograph are usually due to static electrical discharge, especially prevalent during cold dry weather. *(Saia, p. 74)*

133. (D) Factors that regulate the number of x-ray photons produced at the target are be used to control radiographic density, namely milliamperage and exposure time (mAs). Radiographic density is directly proportional to mAs (milliampere-seconds); if the mAs is cut in half, the radiographic density will decrease by one half. Although kilovoltage is used primarily to regulate radiographic contrast, it may also be used to regulate radiographic density in variable kVp (kilovoltage peak) techniques, according to the 15% rule. *(Selman, p. 332)*

134. (B) Perfect film/screen contact is essential to sharply recorded detail. Screen contact can be evaluated with a *wire-mesh test.* A *spinning top test* is used to evaluate timer accuracy and rectifier operation. A *penetrometer* (aluminum step-wedge) is used to illustrate the effect of kVp on contrast. A *star pattern* is used to measure resolving power of the imaging system. *(Selman, pp. 234–235)*

135. (A) The mechanical device used to correct an ineffectual cardiac rhythm is a *defibrillator.* The two paddles attached to the unit are placed on a patient's chest and used to introduce an electric current in an effort to correct the dysrhythmia. A *cardiac monitor* is used to display, and sometime record, electrocardiogram (ECG) readings and some pressure readings. The *crash cart* is a supply cart with various medications and equipment necessary for treating a patient who is suffering from a myocardial infarction or other serious medical emergencies. It is periodically checked and restocked, usually by nursing, although radiographers may be responsible for a daily check of the plastic throwaway locks. These locks are used to ensure that the cart has not been tampered with or supplies inadvertently used in nonemergency situations. A resuscitation bag is used for ventilation, as during cardiopulmonary resuscitation. *(Ehrlich et al, p. 173)*

136. (C) There are many terms (with which the radiographer must be familiar) that are used to describe radiographic positioning techniques. *Cephalad* refers to that which is toward the head, and *caudad* to that which is toward the feet. Structures close to the source or beginning are said to be *proximal,* while those lying close to the midline are said to be *medial. (Ballinger & Frank, vol 1, p. 69)*

137. (A) In the *photoelectric effect,* a relatively low-energy incident photon uses all of its energy to eject an inner-shell electron, leaving a vacancy. An electron from the next shell will drop to fill the vacancy, and *a characteristic ray is given up* in the transition.

This type of interaction is more harmful to the patient, as all the photon energy is transferred to tissue. *(Bushong, pp. 151–154)*

138. (C) Because the anode's focal track is beveled (angled, facing the cathode), x-ray photons can freely diverge toward the cathode end of the x-ray tube. However, the "heel" of the focal track prevents x-ray photons from diverging toward the anode end of the tube. This results in varying intensity from anode to cathode, fewer photons at the anode end, and more photons at the cathode end. *The anode heel effect is most noticeable using large image receptor sizes, short SIDs (source-to-image-receptor distances), and steep target angles. (Saia, p. 336)*

139. (C) The brightness gain of image intensifiers is 5000 to 20,000. This increase is accomplished in two ways. First, as the electron image is focused to the output phosphor, it is accelerated by high voltage (this is *flux gain*). Second, the output phosphor is only a fraction of the size of the input phosphor and this image size decrease represents another brightness gain, termed *minification gain. Total brightness gain is equal to the product of minification gain and flux gain. (Saia, pp. 440–441)*

140. (A) The type of shock associated with pooling of blood in the peripheral vessels is classified as *neurogenic shock.* This occurs in cases of trauma to the central nervous system resulting in decreased arterial resistance and pooling of blood in peripheral vessels. *Cardiogenic shock* is related to cardiac failure, as a result of interference with heart function. It can occur in cases of cardiac tamponade, pulmonary embolus, or myocardial infarction. *Hypovolemic shock* is related to loss of large amounts of blood, either from internal bleeding or hemorrhage associated with trauma. *Septic shock*, as well as *anaphylactic shock,* is generally classified as *vasogenic shock. (Torres, p. 93)*

141. (B) An axial *dorsoplantar* projection is described; the central ray enters the dorsal surface of the foot and exits the plantar surface. The *plantodorsal* projection is done *supine* and requires cephalad angulation. The central ray enters the plantar surface and exits the dorsal surface. *(Ballinger & Frank, vol 1, p. 264)*

142. (D) Surface landmarks, prominences, and depressions are very useful to the radiographer in locating anatomic structures not visible externally. The *costal margin* is at about the same level as L3. The *umbilicus* is approximately at the same level as the L3–L4 interspace. The *xiphoid* tip is at about the same level as T10. The fourth lumbar vertebra is approximately at the same level as the *iliac crest. (Saia, pp. 79–80)*

143. (D) Radiation quality determines degree of penetration and the amount of energy transferred to the irradiated tissue (linear energy transfer [LET]). Certainly, the larger the absorbed radiation dose, the greater the effect. Biologic effect is increased as the size of the irradiated area is increased. The nature of the effect is influenced by the location of irradiated tissue (bone marrow versus gonads and so on). *(Selman, p. 190)*

144. (A) Only two pieces of apparatus are needed to construct a characteristic curve (see Fig. 12–59). First, a *penetrometer* (aluminum step-wedge) is used to expose a film. Once the film is processed, a *densitometer* is needed to read the resulting densities. Log relative exposure is charted along the *x* (horizontal) axis; an increase in log relative exposure of 0.3 results from doubling the exposure. Optical density is plotted on the *y* (vertical) axis and represents the amount of light transmitted through a film compared to the amount of light striking the film (expressed as a logarithm). *(Bushong, pp. 230–238)*

145. (C) X-ray photons are produced in two ways as high speed electrons interact with target atoms. First, if the high speed electron is attracted by the nucleus of a tungsten atom and changes its course, the energy given up as the electron is "braked" in the form of an x-ray photon. This is called *Bremsstrahlung* ("braking") radiation and is responsible for the majority of x-ray photons produced at the conventional tungsten target. Second, a high-speed electron may eject a tungsten K-shell electron, leaving a vacancy in the shell. An electron from a higher energy level, eg: the L shell, drops down to fill the vacancy, emitting the difference in energy as a K characteristic ray. *Characteristic radiation* comprises only approximately 15% of the primary beam. *(Saia, p. 424)*

146. (A) If a radiograph lacks sufficient blackening, an increase in mAs is required. The mAs regulates the *number* of x-ray photons produced at the target. An increase or decrease of *at least 30%* in mAs is necessary to produce a perceptible effect. Increasing the kVp 15% will have about the same effect as *doubling* the mAs. *(Carlton & Adler, p. 370)*

147. (D) Anode target material of *high atomic number* produces higher energy x-rays more efficiently. Because a great deal of heat is produced at the target, the material should have a *high melting point* so as to avoid damage to the target surface. Most of the x-rays generated at the focal spot are directed downward and pass through the x-ray tube's *port window*. The cathode filament receives *low-voltage* current to heat it to the point of thermionic emission. Then *high voltage* is applied to drive the electrons across to the focal track. *(Selman, pp. 204–211)*

148. (C) With inspiration, the diaphragm is depressed, that is, moved into a lower position. The ribs and sternum are elevated. As the ribs are elevated, their angle is decreased. Radiographic density can vary considerably in appearance depending on which phase of respiration the exposure is made. *(Ballinger & Frank, vol 1, p. 516)*

149. (D) The four body types (from largest to smallest) are hypersthenic, sthenic, hyposthenic, and asthenic. The abdominal viscera of the *asthenic* person are generally located quite low, vertical, and toward the midline. The opposite is true of the *hypersthenic* individual: organs are located high, transverse, and laterally. *(Saia, p. 62)*

150. (C) The *wider* dimension of the x-ray film is usually placed on the feed tray and fed into the processor in that direction. The *entrance roller* is the first roller of the transport system located at the end of the feed tray; this is where the microswitch that determines amount of replenishment is located. The *length* of the film (the shorter dimension) activates the microswitch and replenisher is added according to the length of the film; a 10 × 12-inch film will receive less replenisher than will a 14 × 17-inch film. Crossover rollers are located between the different tanks. The receiving bin is where the films exit the processor. The replenishment pump is activated by the microswitch. *(McKinney, p. 106)*

151. (B) An increase in kilovoltage (photon energy) will result in a *greater number* (ie: exposure rate) of scattered photons (Compton interaction). These scattered photons carry no useful information and contribute to radiation *fog*, thus decreasing radiographic contrast. *(Selman, p. 364)*

152. (B) The radiograph in *Figure 17–11* shows the odontoid process superimposed on the base of the skull. The maxillary teeth can be seen very superior to the base of the skull. *Bringing the chin down* will move the base of the skull up and permit visualization of the C1/C2 structures. A diagnostic image of C1–C2 depends on adjusting the flexion of the neck *so that the maxillary occlusal plane and base of the skull are superimposed*. Accurate adjustment of these structures will usually allow good visualization of the odontoid process and the atlantoaxial articulation. Too much flexion superimposes teeth on the odontoid process; too much extension superimposes the base of the skull on the odontoid process. *(Bontrager, p. 292)*

153. (C) The medical word for nosebleed is *epistaxis*. *Vertigo* refers to the feeling of "whirling" or the sensation that the room is spinning. Some possible causes of vertigo include inner ear infection or an acoustic neuroma. *Urticaria* is a vascular reaction resulting in dilated capillaries and edema that cause the patient to break out in hives. An *aura* may be classified as either a feeling or a motor response (such as flashing lights, tasting metal, smelling coffee) that precedes an episode such as a seizure or a migraine headache. *(Ehrlich et al, p. 186)*

154. (B) Changes in hormone levels affect changes in the glandular tissue of the breast. These breast tissue changes are seen during breast development, during pregnancy and lactation, and during menopause. Women at higher risk of developing breast cancer include those having experienced *early menses* (before age 12 years), *late menopause* (after age 52 years), and *nulliparity* (no full- or late-term pregnancies). Risks other than hormonal include *family and personal history* and *age*. The *greatest single risk factor for breast cancer is gender*—being female. Although occurrence of breast cancer in males is not unknown, it is fairly rare. *(Peart, p. 1)*

155. (C) As the colon begins to fill with barium, filling often slows down in the rectosigmoid region. Unless preventative measures are taken, severe abdominal cramping and urge to defecate can occur. *Stopping* the flow of barium momentarily will usually be sufficient to relieve the patient's discomfort. Some patients have repeated cramping throughout the examination. These patients should be instructed to *breathe deeply* through their mouth, and the enema bag should be lowered a few inches to reduce the pressure of barium flow. Many patients benefit from the administration of *glucagon* to relax the intestine. The *Trendelenburg* position is frequently used to separate redundant loops of bowel. *(Ballinger & Frank, vol 2, pp. 130–131)*

156. (D) The *developing fetus* is particularly sensitive to radiation exposure. The Law of Bergonié and Tribondeau states that *stem cells* (which give rise to a specific type of cell, as in hematopoiesis) are particularly radiosensitive, as are *young cells* and tissues. It also states that *cells with a high rate of proliferation* (mitosis) are more sensitive to radiation. Radiation exposure, especially between the second and sixth week following conception (the period of major organogenesis) can cause *organ damage, mental and growth retardation, microcephaly*, and *genital deformities*. *(Sherer et al, p. 129)*

157. (B) *Oral* administration of barium sulfate is used to demonstrate the upper digestive system, esophagus, fundus, body and pylorus of the stomach, and barium progression through the small bowel. The large bowel, including sigmoid colon, is usually demonstrated via *rectal* administration of barium. *(Gurley & Callaway, p. 113)*

158. (B) As the distance from the object to the image receptor (OID) increases, so does magnification distortion. Some magnification is inevitable in radiography, as it is not possible to place anatomic structures directly on the image recorder. However, our understanding of how to minimize magnification distortion is an important part of our everyday work. *(Saia, pp. 290–291)*

159. (A) A *compensating filter* is used when the part to be radiographed is of uneven thickness or density (in the chest, mediastinum versus lungs). The filter (made of aluminum or lead acrylic) is constructed so as to absorb much of the primary radiation that would expose the low-tissue-density area, while allowing the primary radiation to pass unaffected to the high tissue-density area. A *collimator* is used to decrease the production of scattered radiation by limiting the volume of tissue irradiated. The *grid* functions to trap scatter radiation before it reaches the image receptor, thus reducing scatter radiation fog. *(Shephard, p. 193)*

160. (A) An increase in photon *energy* accompanies an increase in *kilovoltage*. Kilovoltage regulates the penetrability of x-ray photons; it regulates their *wavelength*, the amount of *energy* with which they are associated. The higher the related energy of an x-ray beam, the greater its *penetrability* (kilovoltage and photon energy are directly related; kilovoltage and wavelength are inversely related). Adjusting kilovoltage is the preferred method of adjusting radiographic contrast: as kilovoltage (photon energy) is increased, the number of grays increases, thereby producing a longer scale of contrast. In general, as *screen speed* increases, so does contrast (resulting in a shorter scale of contrast). An increase in *mAs* is frequently accompanied by an appropriate decrease in kilovoltage, which would also shorten the contrast scale. SID and radiographic contrast are unrelated. *(Bushong, p. 266)*

161. (C) Inflammation of the *tongue* is termed *glossitis*. Inflammation of the *epiglottis* is epiglottitis. Inflammation of the auditory *ossicles* is termed ossiculitis. Inflammation of the *salivary glands* is usually referred to according to the affected gland, as in parotiditis. *(Taber's, p. 809)*

162. (B) If A and B are reduced to 5 mAs (milliampere-seconds) for mAs consistency, the kVp (kilovoltage peak) would increase in both cases to 85 kVp, thereby balancing radiographic densities. Thus, the greatest density is determined by the shortest source-to-image-receptor distance (SID) (greatest exposure rate). *(Shephard, p. 307)*

163. (C) There are two types of distortion: size and shape. *Shape distortion* relates to the alignment of the x-ray tube, the part to be radiographed, and the image recorder. There are two kinds of shape distortion: *elongation* and *foreshortening*. *Size distortion* is *magnification*, and is related to the object-to-image-receptor distance (OID) and source-to-image-receptor distance (SID). Magnification can be reduced by either increasing the SID or decreasing the OID. However, an increase in SID must be accompanied by an increase in mAs (milliampere-seconds), in order to maintain density. It is therefore preferable, in the interest of exposure, to reduce OID whenever possible. *(Selman, pp. 348, 356)*

164. (B) *Somatic effects* of radiation refer to those effects experienced directly by the exposed individual such as erythema, epilation, and cataracts. *Genetic effects* of radiation exposure are caused by irradiation of the reproductive cells of the exposed individual and transmitted from one generation to the next. *(Sherer et al, pp. 115, 131)*

165. (C) The components of the electromagnetic spectrum are identified in different ways. *Wavelength* is used to identify visible light. *Frequency* is used to identify radio waves. Units of *energy* are used to identify ionizing electromagnetic radiations. The unit *keV (kiloelectron volt)* is used to identify the x-ray photon energies produced by diagnostic x-ray equipment. The unit *kVp (kilovoltage peak)* describes the voltage required to produce the x-rays within the x-ray tube. The units mA and mAs are quantitative units identifying the number or quantity of x-rays available. *(Bushong, p. 62)*

166. (D) The greater the *number of electrons* comprising the electron stream and bombarding the target, the greater the number of x-ray photons produced. Although kV (kilovoltage) is usually associated with the energy of the x-ray photons, because *a greater number of more energetic electrons* will produce more x-ray photons, an increase in kV will also increase the *number* of photons produced. Specifically, the quantity of radiation produced increases as the *square* of the kilovoltage. The material composition of the tube target also plays an important role in the number of x-ray photons produced. The higher the *atomic number*, the denser and more closely packed the atoms comprising the material; therefore, the greater the chance of an interaction between a high speed electron and target material. *(Bushong, pp. 155–157)*

167. (D) This is a modification of the parietoacanthial projection (Water's method) in which the patient is requested to first open the mouth, and then the skull is positioned so that the *orbitomeatal line (OML) forms a 37-degree angle* with the image recorder. The central ray is directed through the *sphenoid sinuses* and *exits the open mouth*. The routine parietoacanthial projection (with mouth closed) is used to demonstrate the maxillary sinuses projected above the petrous pyramids. The frontal and ethmoidal sinuses are best visualized in the posteroanterior (PA) axial position (modified Caldwell method). *(Ballinger & Frank, vol 2, p. 370)*

168. (D) The radiographer must be aware that patient condition has a significant impact on motion control. The patient may wish to be very cooperative, but conditions beyond his or her control may exist. Patients often exhibit uncontrolled motion following a *traumatic injury*. *Medication* can worsen the condition. Traumatized patients are often more sensitive and likely to feel *chilled*. *Peristalsis* is another type of involuntary motion. *(Adler & Carlton, p. 163)*

169. (B) The pregnant radiographer poses a special radiation protection consideration, as the safety of the unborn individual must be considered. It must be remembered that the developing fetus is particularly sensitive to radiation exposure. Established guidelines state that the occupational radiation exposure to the fetus must not exceed 0.5 rem (500 mrem, or 5 mSv) during the entire gestation period. *(Bushong, p. 503)*

170. (B) The female pelvis differs from the male pelvis in that it is more shallow and its bones are generally lighter and more delicate (see Fig. 7–26). The pelvic outlet is wider and more circular in the female, the ischial tuberosities and acetabula are farther apart, the angle formed by the pubic arch is also greater in the female. All these bony characteristics facilitate childbearing and birth. *(Saia, p. 11)*

171. (C) Blood pressure in pulmonary circulation is relatively low, and therefore pulmonary vessels can easily become blocked by blood clots, air bubbles, or fatty masses, resulting in a *pulmonary embolism.* If the blockage stays in place, it results in an extra strain on the right ventricle, which is now unable to pump blood. This occurrence can result in congestive heart failure. *Pneumothorax* is air in the pleural cavity. *Atelectasis* is a collapsed lung or part of a lung. *Hypoxia* is a condition of low tissue oxygen. *(Tortora & Grabowski, p. 651)*

172. (A) The 45-degree oblique position of the lumbar spine is generally performed for demonstration of the *apophyseal joints.* In a correctly positioned oblique lumbar spine, "*Scotty dog*" images are demonstrated. The Scotty's *ear* corresponds to the superior articular process, his *nose* to the transverse process, his *eye* is the pedicle, his *neck* is the pars interarticularis, his *body* is the lamina, and his *front foot* is the inferior articular process. *(Saia, p. 137)*

173. (D) Voltage ripple refers to the percentage drop from maximum voltage each pulse of current experiences. In single phase rectified equipment, the entire pulse (half-cycle) is used; therefore, there is first an increase to maximum (peak) voltage value and a subsequent decrease to zero potential (90 degrees past peak potential). The entire waveform is used; if 100 kV (kilovolts) were selected, the actual average kilovoltage output would be approximately 70. Three phase rectification produces almost constant potential with just small ripples (drops) in maximum potential between pulses. Approximately a 13.5% voltage ripple (drop from maximum value) characterizes the operation of three-phase, six-pulse generators. Three-phase, 12-pulse generators have approximately a 3.5% voltage ripple. *(Selman, p. 254)*

174. (A) The x-ray tube's glass envelope and oil coolant are considered inherent ("built-in") filtration. Thin sheets of aluminum are added to make *a total of at least 2.5 mm Al equivalent filtration in equipment operated above 70 kVp (kilovoltage peak).* This is done in order to remove the low-energy photons that only serve to contribute to patient skin dose. *(Sherer et al, p. 155)*

175. (A) AEC (automatic exposure control) devices are used in today's equipment and serve to produce consistent and comparable radiographic results. In one type of AEC, there is an *ionization chamber* just beneath the tabletop above the image receptor. The part to be examined is centered to it (the sensor) and radiographed. When a predetermined quantity of ionization has occurred (equal to the correct density), the exposure terminates automatically. In the other type of AEC, the *phototimer/photomultiplier,* a small fluorescent screen is positioned beneath the image receptor. When remnant radiation emerging from the patient exposes the film and exits the cassette, the fluorescent screen emits light. Once a predetermined amount of fluorescent light is "seen" by the photocell sensor, the exposure is terminated. A scintillation camera is used in nuclear medicine. A photocathode is an integral part of the image intensification system. *(Saia, p. 433)*

176. (B) The sacroiliac joints angle posteriorly and medially 25 degrees to the median sagittal plane (MSP). Therefore, in order to demonstrate the sacroiliac joints with the patient in the *anteroposterior (AP)* position, the *affected* side must be elevated 25 degrees. This places the joint space perpendicular to the image receptor and parallel to the central ray. Therefore, the *left posterior oblique (LPO)* position will demonstrate the *right* *sacroiliac joint* and the right posterior oblique (RPO) position will demonstrate the left. When performed with the patient *posteroanterior (PA)*, the *unaffected* side will be elevated 25 degrees. *(Bontrager, p. 271)*

177. (A) The spinning top test is used to evaluate *timer accuracy* or *rectifier failure*. With *single-phase*, full-wave rectified equipment (120 pulses/second), individual dots are seen that represent x-ray impulses. *Figure 17–12* was made by using single-phase, full-wave rectified equipment. Because three-phase and high-frequency equipment is almost constant potential, a special synchronous spinning top (or an oscilloscope) is used and a solid black arc is obtained rather than dots. The number of degrees formed by the arc is measured and equated to a particular exposure time. *(Fosbinder & Kelsey, p. 339)*

178. (B) When a spinning top is used to test the timer efficiency of full-wave rectified single-phase equipment, the result is a *series of dots* or dashes, with each dot representing a pulse of radiation. With full-wave rectified current, and a possible 120 pulses (dots) available per second, one should visualize 12 dots at 1/10 second, 6 dots at 0.05 second, etc.

If 4 dots of a possible 120 are seen, then the exposure time was:

$$\frac{4}{120} = \frac{1}{30} \text{ second}$$

The spinning top test may be used to test timer accuracy in single phase equipment. A spinning top is a metal disc with a small hole placed in its outer edge, and placed on a pedestal about 6 inches high. The exposure is made while the top spins. Because three-phase equipment produces almost constant potential—rather than pulsed radiation—the standard spinning top cannot be used. An oscilloscope or synchronous spinning top must be employed to test timers of three phase equipment. *(Selman, p. 233)*

179. (D) A controlled area is one that is occupied by radiation workers trained in radiation safety and who wear radiation monitors. The exposure rate in a *controlled area* must not exceed 100 mR/wk; its occupancy factor is considered to be one, indicating that the area may always be occupied, and therefore requiring maximum shielding. An *uncontrolled area* is one occupied by the general population; the exposure rate there must not exceed 10 mR/wk. Shielding requirements vary according to several factors, one being *occupancy factor*. *(Sherer et al, p. 204)*

180. (B) Because lead content increases as grid ratio increases, more scattered radiation (*and* non-scattered remnant radiation) is absorbed before reaching the image recorder. There are, therefore, fewer x-ray photons interacting with the image recorder, with a resulting *decrease* in optical/radiographic density as grid ratio increases. Scale of contrast would *decrease* with an increase in grid ratio.

181. (A) The trachea (windpipe) bifurcates into left and right *mainstem bronchi,* each entering its respective lung hilum. The *left* bronchus divides into *two* portions, one for each lobe of the left lung. The *right* bronchus divides into *three* portions, one for each lobe of the right lung (Fig. 7–76). The lungs are conical in shape, consisting of upper pointed portions, termed the *apices* (pleural for apex), and the broad lower portions (or *bases*). The lungs are enclosed in a double-walled serous membrane called the *pleura. (Saia, p. 164)*

182. (A) When the shoulders are relaxed, the clavicles are usually carried below the pulmonary apices. To examine the portions of the lungs lying behind the clavicles, the central ray is directed cephalad 15 to 20 degrees to project the clavicles above the apices when the patient is examined in the anteroposterior (AP) position. *(Ballinger & Frank, vol 1, p. 472)*

183. (C) If a radiograph was placed on an illuminator and *100%* of the illuminator's light was transmitted through it, that radiograph must have a density of *0*. According to the equation

$$\text{density} = \log_{10} \frac{\text{incident light intensity}}{\text{transmitted light intensity}}$$

if *10%* of the illuminator's light passes through the film, that film has a density of *1*. If *1%* of the light passes through the film, that film has a density of *2*. *(Bushong, pp. 232, 233)*

184. (A) The approximately 5-foot-long large intestine (colon) functions in the formation, transport, and evacuation of feces. The colon commences at the terminus of the small intestine; its first portion is the sac-like *cecum* in the right lower quadrant (RLQ), located inferior to the ileocecal valve. The *ascending colon* is continuous with the cecum and is located along the right side of the abdominal cavity. It bends medially and anteriorly forming the right colic *(hepatic)* flexure. The colon traverses the abdomen as the *transverse colon* and bends posteriorly and inferiorly to form the left colic *(splenic)* flexure. The *descending colon* continues down the left side of the abdominal cavity and at about the level of the pelvic brim, in the *left lower quadrant (LLQ)*, the colon moves medially to form the S-shaped *sigmoid* colon. The rectum, approximately 5 inches in length, lies between the sigmoid and anal canal. *(Ballinger & Frank, vol 2, p. 89)*

185. (B) A 15% increase kVp (kilovoltage peak) with a 50% decrease in mAs (milliampereseconds) serves to produce a radiograph *similar* to the original, but with some obvious differences. The overall blackness *(radiographic/optical density) is cut in half* because of the decrease in mAs. But the loss of blackness is compensated for by the *addition of grays* (therefore, *longer* scale contrast) from the increased kVp. The increase in kVp also *increases exposure latitude*; a greater margin for error in higher kVp ranges. Recorded detail is unaffected by changes in kVp. *(Shephard, pp. 178, 181)*

186. (B) Single-screen cassettes are made to be used with single emulsion film, such as in mammography. The single fluorescing screen is adjacent to, and exposes, the single emulsion. If double emulsion (duplitized) film is placed in a single screen cassette, it will receive only *one-half the intended exposure* and the resulting image will exhibit decreased density. *(Fauber, p. 146)*

187. (D) With the patient in the anteroposterior (AP) position, the scapula and upper thorax are normally superimposed. With the arm abducted, the elbow flexed, and hand supinated, much of the scapula is drawn away from the ribs. The patient should not be rotated toward the affected side, as this causes superimposition of ribs on the scapula. The exposure is made during quiet breathing to obliterate pulmonary vascular markings. *(Ballinger & Frank, vol 1, p. 202)*

188. (B) The effects of a quantity of radiation delivered to a body are dependent on the amount of radiation received, the size of the irradiated area, and how the radiation is delivered in time. If the radiation is delivered in portions over a period of time, it is said to be fractionated and has a less harmful effect than if the radiation was delivered all at once. Therefore, cells have an opportunity to repair and some recovery occurs between doses. *(Bushong, p. 478)*

189. (B) Because *muscle* and *nerve* tissues perform specific functions and do not divide, they are relatively *insensitive* to radiation exposure. *Epithelial* cells cover the outer surface of the body, and line body cavities as well as tubes and passageways leading to the exterior. They contain very little intercellular substance and are devoid of blood vessels. Because *epithelial* cells constantly regenerate through mitosis, they are very *radiosensitive*. *(Sherer et al, p. 111)*

190. (A) The knee is formed by the proximal tibia, the patella, and the distal femur, which articulate to form the femorotibial and patellofemoral joints. The distal posterior femur presents two large medial and lateral condyles separated by the deep intercondyloid fossa. Two small prominences, the medial and lateral epicondyles, are just superior to the condyles. The femoral and tibial condyles articulate to form the femorotibial joint. In the lateral position, the *medial femoral condyle, being farther from the image receptor, is magnified.* Its magnified image obscures the knee joint space unless correction is made. Computed radiography angulation of 5 degrees cephalad will *superimpose the magnified medial femoral condyle on the lateral condyle* and permit a *better view of the joint space.* *(Ballinger & Frank, vol 1, p. 293)*

191. (D) Insufficient milliamperage and/or exposure time will result in lack of radiographic density. Insufficient kVp (kilovoltage peak) results in underpenetration and excessive contrast. Insufficient source-to-image-receptor distance (SID), however, will result in increased exposure rate and radiographic *overexposure.* *(Selman, pp. 331–333)*

192. (C) When caring for a patient with an indwelling Foley catheter, place the drainage bag and tubing *below the level of the bladder* to maintain the gravity flow of urine. Placement of the tubing or bag above or level with the bladder will allow backflow of urine into the bladder. This reflux of urine can increase the chance of urinary tract infection (UTI) *(Torres, pp. 160–161)*

193. (A) A quality control program requires the use of a number of devices to test the efficiency of various parts of the imaging system. A *slit camera*, as well as a star-pattern or pinhole camera, is used to test focal spot size. A parallel line type resolution test pattern is used to test the resolution capability of intensifying screens. *(Selman, p. 326)*

194. (B) The most effective method of sterilization is moist heat, using steam under pressure. This is known as autoclaving. Sterilization by dry heat requires higher temperatures for longer periods of time than moist heat. Pasteurization is moderate heating with rapid cooling, and is frequently used in commercial preparation of milk and alcoholic beverages such as wine and beer. It is not a form of sterilization. Freezing can also kill some microbes, but is not a form of sterilization. *(Adler & Carlton, p. 208)*

195. (B) Even the smallest exposure to radiation can be harmful. It must, therefore, be every radiographer's objective to keep his or her occupational exposure as far below the dose limit as possible. Radiology personnel should never hold patients during an x-ray examination. *(Bushong, p. 8)*

196. (D) The closer the x-ray source is to the barrier (wall), the greater the thickness necessary. Occupancy factor refers to the degree of occupancy of the room adjacent to the barrier; a stairway would require less shielding than a busy work area. Workload is important in determining barrier thickness, and refers to the number of exams performed in the x-ray room measured in mA-min/wk: the greater the number of exams per week, the greater the barrier thickness required. Use factor is also important in determining barrier thickness, and refers to the amount of time x-rays are directed to a particular wall: the greater the amount of time, the greater the thickness required. *(Sherer et al, pp. 203, 204)*

197. (D) The archival quality of a film refers to its ability to retain its image for a long period of time. Many states have laws governing how long a patient's medical records, including films, must be retained. Very importantly, they must be retained in their original condition. *Archival quality is poor if radiographic films begin to show evidence of stain after being stored for only a short time.* Probably the most common cause of stain, and hence poor archival quality, is *retained fixer* within the emulsion. Fixer may be retained due to poor washing, or because there was insufficient hardener (*underreplenishment*) in the developer, thus permitting fixer to be retained by the swollen emulsion. A test for quantity of retained fixer in film emulsion is often included as part of a quality control program. Stain may also be caused by poor *storage conditions*. Storage in a hot, humid place will cause even the smallest amount of retained fixer to react with silver, causing stain. *(McKinney, p. 79)*

198. (B) A review of the problem reveals that *three changes* are being made: an increase in *SID (source-to-image-receptor distance)*, a change from a 400-*speed system* to a 200-speed system, and a change in *exposure time* (to be considered last). Because the original mAs (milliampere-seconds) was 9, reducing the speed of the system by half (from 400 to 200) will require a doubling of the mAs, to 18, in order to maintain density. Now we must deal with the distance change. Using the density maintenance formula (and remembering that 18 is now the *old* mAs), we find that the required new mAs at 42 inches is 22:

$$\frac{18 \text{ mAs}}{x} = \frac{1444 \ (38''^2)}{1764 \ (42''^2)}$$

$$1444 \ x = 31752$$

$$x = 21.98 \ (22) \text{ mAs}$$

Because we are not changing mA we must determine the *exposure time* that, used with 300 mA, will yield 22 mAs:

$$300 \ x = 22$$

$$x = 0.07 \text{ second exposure}$$

(Selman, pp. 332, 335–336)

199. (C) *Erythema* is the reddening of skin as a result of exposure to large quantities of ionizing radiation. It was one of the first somatic responses to irradiation demonstrated to the early radiology pioneers. The effects of radiation exposure to the skin follow a *non-linear, threshold dose–response relationship.* An individual's response to skin irradiation depends on the dose received, the period of time over which it was received, the size of the area irradiated, and the individual's sensitivity. The dose that it takes to bring about a noticeable erythema is referred to as the *skin erythema dose (SED). (Bushong, p. 468)*

200. (A) The *airway* of the victim is first opened by tilting back the head and lifting the chin. However, if the victim might have suffered a spinal cord injury, the spine should not be moved and the airway should be opened using the jaw-thrust method.

The rescuer next *listens for breathing* sounds and watches for rise and fall of the chest to indicate breathing. If there is no breathing, the rescuer pinches the victim's nose and delivers *two full breaths via mouth-to-mouth rescue* breathing. If rise and fall of the chest is still not present, the Heimlich maneuver is instituted. If ventilation does not take place during the two full breaths, the victims circulation is checked next (using the carotid artery). If there is no pulse, external chest compressions are begun at a rate of 80 to 100/minute for the adult and at least 100/minute for infants. *(Taber's, p. 315)*

Index

Note: Page numbers followed by *f* indicate figures; those followed by *t* indicate tables; those followed by *b* indicate boxed material.